The McGraw-Hill Companies

NOSIS: PRETEST™ SELF-ASSESSMENT AND REVIEW
N
2011

McGraw-Hill Education (Asia), for manufacture and export. This book
ed from the country to which it is sold by McGraw-Hill. This
is not to be sold or purchased in North America and contains content
its North American version.

s Cataloging-in-Publication Data

is : pretest self assessment and review. — 7th ed. /Lisa B. Bernstein.

ical diagnosis / edited by Tyson K. Cobb, Thomas J.
995.
aphical references and index.
07-163301-7
63301-4
osis—Examinations, questions, etc. I. Reteguiz, Jo-Ann. Physical

ical Examination—Examination Questions. 2. Diagnosis—
ns. WB 18.2 B531p 2010]

2010021001

05 04 03 02 01
11 10

title, use ISBN 978-007-108824-4 or MHID 007-108824-5

PreTest™

Physical Diagnosis

PreTest™ Self-Assessment and Review

Notice

Medicine is an ever-changing science. As new research and clinical experience broaden our knowledge, changes in treatment and drug therapy are required. The authors and the publisher of this work have checked with sources believed to be reliable in their efforts to provide information that is complete and generally in accord with the standards accepted at the time of publication. However, in view of the possibility of human error or changes in medical sciences, neither the authors nor the publisher nor any other party who has been involved in the preparation or publication of this work warrants that the information contained herein is in every respect accurate or complete, and they disclaim all responsibility for any errors or omissions or for the results obtained from use of the information contained in this work. Readers are encouraged to confirm the information contained herein with other sources. For example and in particular, readers are advised to check the product information sheet included in the package of each drug they plan to administer to be certain that the information contained in this work is accurate and that changes have not been made in the recommended dose or in the contraindications for administration. This recommendation is of particular importance in connection with new or infrequently used drugs.

Physica

PreTest™ Self-

Seve

Lisa B.
Associate
Co-Director, Be
Emory Univ
A

New York Chicago San Fran
Milan New Delhi San Ju

PHYSICAL DIAG
SEVENTH EDIT
International Editio

Library of Congre

Bernstein, Lisa
Physical diagno
p. ; cm.
Rev. ed. of: Phy
Motycka. 2nd ed. c
Includes bibliog
ISBN-13: 978-0
ISBN-10: 0-07-
1. Physical diag
diagnosis. II. Title.
[DNLM: 1. Phy
Examination Questi
RC76.P5 2010
616.07'54076—dc2

10 09 08 07 06
20 15 14 13 12
CTP ANL

When ordering th

Printed in Singapore

Dedicated to my father, Arnold Bernstein, M.D.,
who instilled in me his passion for teaching
and the importance of truly caring for patients.

Student Reviewers

Amanda Cooper
New York College of Osteopathic Medicine
Class of 2012

David Scoville
Medical Scientist Training Program
University of Kansas School of Medicine
Class of 2012

Contents

Endocrinology

Hematology and Oncology

Rheumatology

Musculoskeletal System

Neurology

Geriatrics

Infectious Diseases

Obstetrics and Gynecology

Pediatrics and Neonatology

Bonus Chapter: The Ten Toughest Physical Diagnosis Questions Ever Written

High-Yield Facts

Introduction

An astute clinician must be able to perform a careful history and physical examination and apply knowledge of pathophysiology to the clinical manifestations of common and not-so-common diseases. These skills are ideally learned and honed at the bedside. If you understand the normal and recognize the abnormal characteristics of each organ system, you can unlock many diagnostic dilemmas. Expertise results from time, practice, and experience.

The purpose of this book is to provide medical students and physicians with a comprehensive and convenient method for review and self-assessment of their physical diagnosis skills. Over 500 revised and updated questions cover the most relevant and pertinent topics in medicine.

The questions have been designed to parallel the format and degree of difficulty of the questions contained in the United States Licensing Examination (USMLE) Step 1 and Step 2 CK examinations. Students in medical school physical diagnosis courses, those preparing for an OSCE or for the USMLE Step 2 CS, and practicing physicians will find this book to be an excellent resource. This will be a true test of your mastery of physical diagnosis from beginning to end. Each chapter of the book is based on a specific organ system, so learners can assess and target their specific weaknesses and strengths. There is also a section on important miscellaneous subjects, such as geriatrics, infectious diseases, obstetrics and gynecology, and pediatrics. A bonus chapter of 10 master-level physical diagnosis questions will challenge and strengthen your knowledge in the Oslerian method of bedside diagnosis.

Each question in this book is accompanied by a thorough explanation of the answers and a specific page reference to a current textbook for further study if desired. A special "High-Yield Facts" section filled with helpful mnemonics is included at the back of the book for quick review before examinations.

When answering the questions in a chapter, try to approximate the time limits imposed by board examinations by taking no more than 1 minute to answer each question. You should then spend as much time as you need verifying your answers by carefully reading the explanations. Although you should pay special attention to the explanations for the questions you answered incorrectly, you should ideally read every single explanation. Even a question you answer effortlessly is accompanied by a unique collection of physical diagnosis pearls. If, after reading the explanations for a given chapter, you feel you need more information about the material covered, you should consult and study the reference indicated. For your convenience, I have limited the number of references to seven:

Fauci AF, Braunwald E, Kasper DL, et al. *Harrison's Principals of Internal Medicine.* 17th ed. New York, NY: McGraw-Hill; 2008.

Kliegman RM, Behrman RE, Jenson HB, et al. *Nelson's Book of Pediatrics.* 18th ed. Philadelphia, PA: Saunders; 2007.

LeBlond RF, Brown DD, DeGowin RL. *DeGowin's Diagnostic Examination.* 9th ed. New York, NY: McGraw-Hill; 2009.

McPhee SJ, Papadakis MA. *Current Medical Diagnosis & Treatment 2010.* 49th ed. New York, NY: McGraw-Hill; 2010.

Seidel HM, Ball JW, Dains JE, et al. *Mosby's Guide to Physical Examination.* 6th ed. St. Louis, MO: Mosby; 2006.

Simel DL, Rennie D. *The Rational Clinical Examination: Evidence-Based Clinical Diagnosis.* New York, NY: McGraw-Hill; 2009.

Wolff K, Johnson RA. *Fitzpatrick's Color Atlas & Synopsis of Clinical Dermatology.* 6th ed. New York, NY: McGraw-Hill; 2009.

It is my hope that after completion of this book you will be better able to recognize and understand the clinical characteristics of many important medical diagnoses. With the aid of this book, as well as in taking a thorough history and skillfully performing the proper physical examination, you will move further down the road to becoming a master diagnostician. Good luck with physical diagnosis at the bedside!

Acknowledgments

I wish to acknowledge the administration and faculty of the Emory University School of Medicine for their exceptional commitment to patient care and medical education. I am also tremendously grateful to my students and patients who continually inspire me to learn; to my parents and in-laws for their boundless love, support, and encouragement; and to my sister, Debra, for being my best friend and for allowing me to practice my physical examination skills on her as a medical student.... Finally, I want to thank the three great loves of my life—my husband, Jay, and my sons, Aaron and Daniel—who make every moment of life sweeter and more exciting.

General Inspection and Vital Signs

Questions

1. A 47-year-old woman is referred to your office for two consecutive blood pressure readings of 139/89 mm Hg and 124/86 mm Hg. She has no complaints, and physical examination is normal. Which of the following best describes her stage of hypertension?

a. Stage 1 hypertension
b. Stage 2 hypertension
c. Stage 3 hypertension
d. Prehypertension
e. Normal blood pressure

2. A patient with chronic kidney disease (his most recent glomerular filtration rate, GFR, was 15 mL/min/1.73 m^2) comes in for follow-up. He complains of fatigue, anorexia, and difficulty concentrating. On physical examination he is hypertensive, with yellowish skin and mild lower extremity edema. Which of the following is the most appropriate diet to recommend for this patient?

a. Regular diet
b. Low-calorie diet
c. Low-salt diet
d. Low-fat, low-carbohydrate diet
e. Low-potassium, low sodium, low-protein diet

3. A 46-year-old man presents to your office because of the recent onset of blackouts. He has no past medical history and admits to smoking cigarettes and drinking beer socially more recently since his divorce. His blackouts usually occur on weekends, when he is out with his friends relaxing at the neighborhood bar. His physical examination is normal. Which of the following is the next best diagnostic step for this patient?

a. CAGE questionnaire
b. Liver function tests
c. Percussion of the liver for hepatomegaly
d. Mini-mental status examination (MMSE)
e. Check for macrocytic anemia

4. A 36-year-old woman, accompanied by her attentive husband throughout the visit, presents to the emergency room complaining of right wrist pain. She states that she fell down a flight of stairs and is concerned that the wrist may be fractured. On physical examination, the wrist has minimal swelling and is nontender, with a full range of motion. There is a bruise over the right forearm above the wrist, which appears to be several days old. She was also seen in the ER last month for chest pain. Which of the following must you consider first as her diagnosis?

a. Recurrent falls
b. Alcohol intoxication
c. Opiate use
d. Benzodiazepam abuse
e. Domestic violence victim

5. A 47-year-old man with mild shortness of breath and increased expiratory phase of respiration on examination admits that he has a problem with cigarettes. He is committed to stopping smoking and has come to your office to seek help on how to do it. Which of the following best describes the stage of behavior change in this addicted patient?

a. Precontemplation
b. Contemplation
c. Preparation
d. Action
e. Maintenance
f. Termination

6. A 17-year-old high-school student presents to your office with a 6-month history of menstrual irregularities. She has no past medical history and does not smoke cigarettes, drink alcohol, or use illicit drugs. She is not sexually active. Her menarche was at the age of 12 years. The patient is 66 in tall and has weighed 115 lb for nearly 3 years. Mouth examination reveals dental enamel erosion. She has enlarged parotid glands bilaterally. Examination of the extremities reveals scars on the dorsal surfaces of the hands. Which of the following is the most likely diagnosis?

a. Bulimia
b. Premature menopause
c. Substance dependence
d. Anorexia nervosa
e. Personality disorder

7. A 34-year-old woman presents with left-sided chest pain for 8 months. She describes the pain as sharp, intermittent, and associated with palpitations, dizziness, trembling, nausea, paresthesias, and diaphoresis. She experiences three episodes per week. The episodes last 15 minutes each and may occur at rest or with exertion. The episodes are unpredictable, and the patient often feels as if she is going to die because of the chest pain. The patient does not smoke cigarettes, drink alcohol, or use drugs. She has no family history of heart disease. Her blood pressure and pulse are normal. Physical examination is normal. Electrocardiogram (ECG) is normal. Which of the following is the most likely diagnosis?

a. Acute myocardial infarction (AMI)
b. Unstable angina
c. Mitral valve prolapse (MVP)
d. Panic disorder
e. Malingering
f. Hyperthyroidism
g. Post-traumatic stress disorder (PTSD)

8. A 48-year-old woman with poorly controlled non-insulin-dependent diabetes and hypertension comes in for follow-up. She has struggled with weight issues since adolescence and has "tried every diet there is." Because of peripheral neuropathy and degenerative joint disease of her knees, she has not been able to tolerate much exercise. Upon evaluating her today, her BMI is 38 and her blood sugar is 256 mg/dL. She has been researching her options and is interested in gastric bypass surgery. What should you advise her?

a. Her body mass index (BMI) is not high enough to qualify for gastric bypass surgery.
b. You can refer her to a bariatrician who will educate her and prepare her for surgery.
c. Bariatric surgery will not help her obesity.
d. Bariatric surgery will not improve her weight-related conditions.
e. She needs to enroll in a formal exercise program first.

Questions 9 and 10

For each patient, select the most likely type of allergic reaction. Each lettered option may be used once, multiple times, or not at all.

a. Type I allergic reaction
b. Type II allergic reaction
c. Type III allergic reaction
d. Type IV allergic reaction

9. A 26-year-old graduate student presents with a photosensitive cutaneous facial rash after starting a 2-week course of tetracycline.

10. A 61-year-old woman develops hemolysis and thrombocytopenia after receiving a blood transfusion prior to elective surgery.

General Inspection and Vital Signs

Answers

1. The answer is d. *(Fauci, p 1553.)* The classification of blood pressure according to the most recent Joint National Committee on Prevention, Detection, Evaluation, and Treatment of High Blood Pressure (JNC 7) is based on the average of readings on at least two separate visits. In contrast to the recommendations of JNC 6, the category of prehypertension has been added and stages 2 and 3 have been combined. If a systolic measurement is in one category and the corresponding diastolic blood pressure is in another, the highest classification should be used.

Category of Blood Pressure	Systolic Blood Pressure (mm Hg)	Diastolic Blood Pressure (mm Hg)
Normal	<120	and <80
Prehypertension	120-139	or 80-89
Stage 1 hypertension	140-159	or 90-99
Stage 2 hypertension	≥160	or ≥100

2. The answer is e. *(McPhee, p 830.)* An important part of managing chronic illnesses is dietary counseling. Patients with **chronic kidney disease** should have **protein intake restricted** to not more than 1 g/kg/d in order to slow progression to end-stage renal disease. In addition, **sodium, water, potassium, and phosphorus should be limited** in the diet and, because magnesium is almost exclusively excreted renally, magnesium-containing over-the-counter medications should be avoided. Patients with hypertension should be on a sodium-restricted diet and patients with diabetes should have limited fat and carbohydrates. Patients needing to lose weight should restrict calories.

3. The answer is a. *(Fauci, p 1920.)* Although liver function tests (LFTs), macrocytic red blood cell changes, and hepatomegaly are good tests for establishing whether the patient has complications of alcoholism, the

CAGE questionnaire is the best screening tool for alcohol dependence. If patients respond "yes" to more than one question, alcoholism is likely. There are four CAGE questions:

1. Have you felt the need to **C**ut down on your drinking?
2. Have you ever felt **A**nnoyed by criticisms of your drinking?
3. Have you ever felt **G**uilty about your drinking?
4. Have you ever needed an **E**ye-opener in the morning?

4. The answer is e. *(Fauci, p 2723.)* The patient most likely is a victim of **domestic violence**. Patients may present to a physician with a poorly explained injury, an obvious injury, or a subtle, pain-related complaint (headache, chest pain, or abdominal pain). One in five patients presenting to a primary care practice is involved in a relationship where abuse exists, and all physicians should screen for this problem. The **SAFE questionnaire** may be used to screen for domestic violence:

S = Do you feel **S**afe or **S**tressed in a relationship?
A = Have you ever been **A**bused or **A**fraid in a relationship?
F = Are your **F**riends and **F**amily aware of your relationship problem?
E = Do you have an **E**mergency plan if needed?

5. The answer is c. *(Fauci, pp 2738-2739.)* There are **six stages of behavior change in addicted personalities:**

1. Precontemplation = denies problem; no intention of changing
2. Contemplation = acknowledges problem; seriously thinks about solving it
3. Preparation = committed to action; needs to plan
4. Action = modifies behavior and surroundings
5. Maintenance = at risk for relapse if not committed to following through with changes
6. Termination = no continuing effort needed; addiction no longer a threat

This patient is in the **preparation stage** because he is committed to quitting but has come to the physician for a plan.

6. The answer is a. *(Fauci, pp 476-477.)* The patient most likely has **bulimia** which is more common than **anorexia nervosa**. Patients typically maintain their body weight by induced vomiting or the use of laxatives or diuretics. Patients present with dental enamel erosion, excessive dental caries, parotid enlargement, and scars on the dorsal surfaces of the hands from inducing vomiting. Electrolytes may reveal abnormalities from chronic use of laxatives, diuretics, and enemas. Patients with **anorexia nervosa** present below their ideal body weight. Characteristics of anorexia nervosa include cold intolerance, emaciated appearance, hypothermia, hypotension, and bradycardia. Irregularities in the menstrual cycle may be a presenting sign in both bulimia and anorexia nervosa.

7. The answer is d. *(Fauci, p 2710.)* The patient has no risk factors for coronary artery disease, such as family history or tobacco or cocaine use, and her ECG is normal. **Hyperthyroidism** is unlikely without tachycardia and other physical examination findings. A click and murmur are often found on heart auscultation in patients with **MVP**. The patient has no known previous traumatic event in her life to have caused **PTSD**. The patient has symptomatology consistent with **panic disorder**. Four of five criteria are needed for the diagnosis of panic disorder: **PANIC** = **P**alpitations; **A**bdominal pain; **N**ausea; **I**ncreased perspiration; and **C**hest pain, **C**hills, or **C**hoking.

8. The answer is b. *(Fauci, pp 472-473.)* Assessment of **body mass index (BMI)** (weight in kg divided by height in m^2 or weight in pounds divided by [height in inches]$^2 \times 703.1$) is useful in assessing both over- and undernutrition. It is a useful measure to predict the risk of certain diseases associated with obesity. For example, non-insulin-dependent diabetes mellitus (NIDDM) is rare in persons with a BMI below 22 kg/m^2.

Normal BMI is defined as 18.5 to 24.9 kg/m^2.
Overweight is a BMI of 25 to 29.9 kg/m^2.
Obesity is a BMI of 30 to 39.9 kg/m^2.
Morbid obesity is a BMI of more than 40 kg/m^2.
Mild malnutrition is defined as a BMI of 17 to 18.4 kg/m^2.
Moderate malnutrition is a BMI of 16 to 16.9 kg/m^2.
Severe malnutrition is a BMI of less than 16.0 kg/m^2.

Roux-en-Y gastric bypass may be considered for patients with a BMI of 40 or greater who have been obese for more than 5 years and have failed diet and exercise, are well-informed, and are good surgical candidates, as well as those with a BMI greater than 35 who have concomitant weight-related medical issues (diabetes, sleep apnea, severe osteoarthritis).

Bariatric surgery not only improves weight loss, but also markedly improves or resolves weight-related medical conditions, though there are risks.

9 and 10. The answers are 9-d, 10-b. *(McPhee, p 784.)* **Type I** allergic reactions are IgE-mediated and cause urticaria and anaphylaxis. They are often caused by penicillin, insulin, sulfonamides, morphine, and contrast media. **Type II** antibody-mediated reactions are due to transfusions (ABO mismatch), newborn Rh hemolytic disease, or use of medications (quinidine, heparin, phenacetin, sulfonamides) and typically cause hemolysis, thrombocytopenia, and nephritis. **Type III** allergic reactions are immune complex mediated and seen with chronic infections, penicillin, propylthiouracil, hydralazine, and procainamide, leading to serum sickness. **Type IV** delayed hypersensitivity reactions are mediated by T cells and result from tetracyclines, nitrofurantoin, neomycin, parabens, and sulfonamides. These medications and contact with topical agents like poison ivy or nickel can cause a contact dermatitis, pulmonary fibrosis, photosensitivity, and toxic epidermal necrolysis.

The Systems

Dermatology

Questions

11. A 10-year-old girl presents with multiple pigmented macules on the vermilion border of her lower lip and the mucus membranes of her mouth. The dark brown lesions are 2 to 5 mm in size and are arranged in a cluster. The patient's older brother has similar lesions. The patient complains of recurrent bouts of abdominal pain. Which of the following is the patient also at risk for?

a. Acanthosis nigricans
b. Cutaneous lymphoma
c. Disseminated intravascular coagulation
d. Hamartomatous polyps in the small bowel
e. Ulcerations of the extremities

12. A 16-year-old student with a recent history of herpetic gingivostomatitis develops a generalized and symmetric rash primarily on her face and extremities, including her palms and soles. The rash consists of 1- to 2-cm target-like lesions which are burning and pruritic. A few erosive lesions are visible in the oral mucosa. Which of the following is the most likely diagnosis?

a. Erythema multiforme
b. Secondary syphilis
c. Systemic lupus erythematosus
d. Pemphigus vulgaris
e. Urticaria

13. A 17-year-old patient presents with severe pruritus that is worse at night. On examination of the skin, areas of excoriated papules are observed in the interdigital area of the hands. Family members report similar symptoms. Which of the following is the most likely diagnosis?

a. Scabies
b. Cutaneous larva migrans
c. Contact dermatitis
d. Dermatitis herpetiformis
e. Enterobius vermicularis

14. A 35-year-old woman, who had been camping in Wisconsin 2 weeks ago, develops an erythematous rash on her inner thigh. The macular lesion is 10 cm in diameter and has a distinct red border with central clearing. The patient reports no fever, chills, or other symptoms. She has no medical problems or allergies and takes no medications. She does not recall any spider or tick bites. The rest of the physical examination is normal. Which of the following is the most likely etiology of the lesion?

a. Brown recluse spider bite
b. *Borrelia burgdorferi* infection
c. *Bartonella henselae* infection
d. *Mycobacterium marinum* infection
e. *Rickettsia rickettsii* infection

15. A 27-year-old man presents to the emergency room 3 days after undergoing a hernia repair operation. He is febrile and hypotensive. The symptoms began with the sudden onset of a diffuse maculopapular rash that was pruritic and erythematous. Cutaneous examination reveals that the erythroderma involves the palms and soles and is beginning to desquamate. The patient has no other illnesses and takes no medications. Which of the following is the most likely diagnosis?

a. Toxic epidermal necrolysis
b. Toxic shock syndrome
c. Necrotizing fasciitis
d. Scarlet fever
e. Cellulitis

16. A 6-year-old child presents with patchy hair loss on the back of the scalp. Examination reveals well-demarcated areas of erythema and scaling, and although there are still some hairs in the area, they are extremely short and broken in appearance. Which of the following is the most likely diagnosis?

a. Androgenic hair loss
b. Psoriasis of the scalp
c. Seborrheic dermatitis
d. Tinea capitis
e. Carbuncle

17. A 27-year-old woman with a history of Crohn disease complains of painful, red tender bumps on both of her legs, accompanied by a low-grade fever and joint aches, primarily in her ankles. On examination you see the red lesions (see following figure) and on palpation appreciate a nodular, indurated quality to them. Which of the following is the most likely diagnosis?

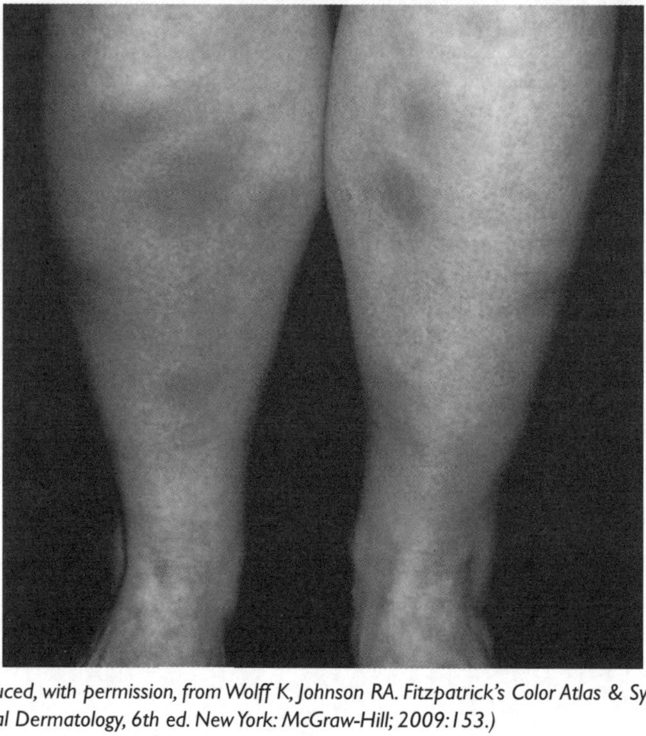

(Reproduced, with permission, from Wolff K, Johnson RA. Fitzpatrick's Color Atlas & Synopsis of Clinical Dermatology, 6th ed. New York: McGraw-Hill; 2009:153.)

a. Bacillary angiomatosis
b. Erythema nodosum
c. Sweet syndrome
d. Ecthyma gangrenosum
e. Disseminated fungal infection

18. A 51-year-old homeless man presents to the emergency room in winter complaining of numbness of his feet. Physical examination of the feet reveals erythema, edema, and the presence of several clear blisters. Peripheral pulses are palpable. You suspect frostbite. Which of the following is the best way to initially manage the patient's injuries and prevent further cold injury?

a. Rewarm his feet by rubbing them.
b. Rewarm his feet using dry heat.
c. Rewarm his feet by immersing in a warm bath.
d. Start him on empiric antibiotics.
e. Unroof the blisters to allow them to heal.

19. Five days after going on a nature walk, a 13-year-old adolescent develops well-demarcated erythematous plaques and vesicles over his arms and face. The plaques are arranged in a linear fashion and are crusting. The boy has some facial edema. He has no history of fever or chills but complains of pruritus. Which of the following is the most likely diagnosis?

a. Rubeola
b. Atopic dermatitis
c. Allergic contact dermatitis
d. Impetigo
e. Erythema infectiosum

20. A 6-year-old child presents with flesh-colored papules on the hand that are not pruritic. Examination reveals lesions that are approximately 4 mm in diameter with central umbilication. A halo is seen around those lesions undergoing regression. Which of the following is the most likely diagnosis?

a. Verruca vulgaris
b. Molluscum contagiosum
c. Keratoacanthoma
d. Herpetic whitlow
e. Hemangioma

21. A 42-year-old man presents with blisters and erosions of his hands for 6 months. He has noticed excessive hair growth on his temples lateral to his eyebrows. Physical examination reveals tense, fragile bullae and erosions on otherwise normal skin of the dorsa of the hands. The patient complains of generalized malaise but has no other symptoms. Which of the following will definitively confirm your suspected diagnosis?

a. Elevated liver enzymes
b. Elevated blood glucose
c. Anemia
d. Green fluorescence of skin examined under a Wood lamp
e. Orange-red fluorescence of urine examined under a Wood lamp

22. A 19-year-old man comes in with a mildly pruritic rash that began over a week ago on his upper abdomen and has now spread to the rest of his trunk and proximal extremities. After examining him and seeing the rash in the following figure, what can you tell him?

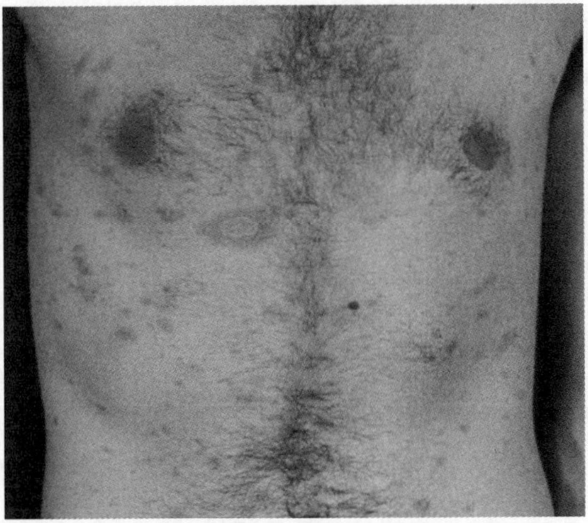

(Reproduced, with permission, from Wolff K, Johnson RA. Fitzpatrick's Color Atlas & Synopsis of Clinical Dermatology, 6th ed. New York: McGraw-Hill; 2009:123.)

a. Ultraviolet B (UVB) phototherapy is the best treatment at this point.
b. The rash will remit spontaneously.
c. The rash will soon spread to her face.
d. The rash will likely scar without steroid treatment.
e. The rash will probably come back in the future.

23. A 41-year-old woman is brought to the emergency room after sustaining a burn in a house fire. She shows some evidence of smoke inhalation but is improving with oxygen. Her heart and lung examinations are normal. Her left arm has a 12-cm burn that extends to the papillary layer of the dermis. Which of the following best describes the severity of the burn?

a. First-degree burn
b. Second-degree burn
c. Third-degree burn
d. Fourth-degree burn
e. Fifth-degree burn

24. A 23-year-old Japanese man attends a party where he drinks three glasses of wine. In a short period of time, he develops facial erythema and experiences severe facial flushing. Which of the following is the most likely diagnosis?

a. Alcohol dehydrogenase deficiency
b. Glucuronyl transferase deficiency
c. Aldehyde dehydrogenase deficiency
d. Angioedema
e. Photosensitivity reaction

Questions 25 to 27

For each patient with skin abnormalities, select the most likely diagnosis. Each lettered option may be used once, multiple times, or not at all.

a. Discoid lupus
b. Melasma
c. Acne vulgaris
d. Spider angioma
e. Atopic dermatitis
f. Rosacea
g. Lichen simplex chronicus

25. A 15-year-old adolescent presents with inflammatory papules, pustules, and crusting on the forehead and cheeks.

26. A 51-year-old woman presents with pustules and papules with sebaceous hyperplasia around the central parts of her face. She complains of facial flushing after drinking alcohol or hot fluids.

27. A 22-year-old woman in her fifth month of pregnancy presents with well-demarcated, hyperpigmented macules on her cheek, nose, and forehead.

Questions 28 to 30

For each patient with ulcer formation, select the most likely diagnosis. Each lettered option may be used once, multiple times, or not at all.

a. Venous ulcer
b. Arterial ulcer
c. Neuropathic ulcer
d. Aphthous ulcer
e. Pressure ulcer

28. A 64-year-old patient with a history of previous strokes is chronically bedridden. Her nutritional intake is poor, and she has fecal and urinary incontinence. She complains of pain in her lower back and has a low-grade fever.

29. A 67-year-old woman presents with a long history of aching and swelling of her legs, relieved by elevation. Over the last several weeks, she has developed two blue-red, irregular, punched-out patches over the medial malleolus of her left leg.

30. A 55-year-old diabetic patient presents with complaints of a painful right leg when walking and at rest. The pain is worse at night and improves with dependency. His distal leg is porcelain white and cool to the touch. No dorsalis pedis pulse is palpable. A sharply demarcated, punched-out ulcer is visible over the supramalleolar area.

Questions 31 to 35

For each patient with abnormal nail findings, select the most likely nail finding. Each lettered option may be used once, multiple times, or not at all.

a. Leukonychia
b. Koilonychia
c. Muehrcke nails
d. Terry nails
e. Blue nails
f. Beau lines
g. Pitting nails
h. Brown nails
i. Mees lines
j. Splinter hemorrhages
k. Yellow-nail syndrome
l. Brittle nails

31. A 34-year-old woman presents with concavity of the outer surfaces of her fingernails. When a drop of water is placed on the nail bed surface, it does not roll off. Her past medical history is significant for menorrhagia.

32. A 61-year-old man has early nephrotic syndrome secondary to diabetes mellitus; he presents with fingernails containing two white lines parallel to the lunula. The lines do not appear to progress with the growth of the nail.

33. A 55-year-old woman with a history of alcohol abuse and evidence of ascites has fingernails that are white proximally with a distal pink rim.

34. A 62-year-old man is recovering from a myocardial infarction. Transverse white grooves are visible on each fingernail.

35. A 41-year-old woman presents with fingernails that are half white (proximally) and half brown (distally). She has a history of hypotension, hyponatremia, hyperkalemia, and eosinophilia.

Questions 36 and 37

For each patient with skin abnormalities, select the most likely vitamin deficiency. Each lettered option may be used once, multiple times, or not at all.

a. Vitamin D deficiency
b. Zinc deficiency
c. Niacin deficiency
d. Vitamin C deficiency
e. Thiamine deficiency

36. A 71-year-old woman presents with ecchymoses and perifollicular hemorrhage on her legs in a saddle distribution (how a rider would touch the saddle). She is edentulous with bleeding gums and is anemic. She lives alone and eats a diet with no added fruits or vegetables.

37. A bottle-fed infant presents with the triad of acral dermatitis, alopecia, and diarrhea.

Questions 38 and 39

For each patient with skin abnormalities, select the most likely HIV-associated skin disorder. Each lettered option may be used once, multiple times, or not at all.

a. Kaposi sarcoma
b. Seborrheic dermatitis
c. Molluscum contagiosum
d. Eosinophilic folliculitis
e. Herpes zoster

38. A 47-year-old man with AIDS presents with the lesions on his face, shown in the following figure.

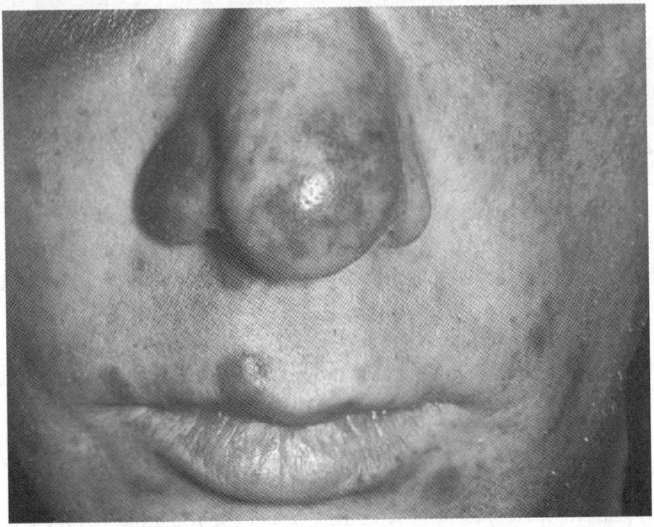

(Reproduced, with permission, from Wolff K, Johnson RA. Fitzpatrick's Color Atlas & Synopsis of Clinical Dermatology, 6th ed. New York: McGraw-Hill; 2009:541.)

39. A 28-year-old HIV-positive woman presents with the rash on her face, shown in the following figure.

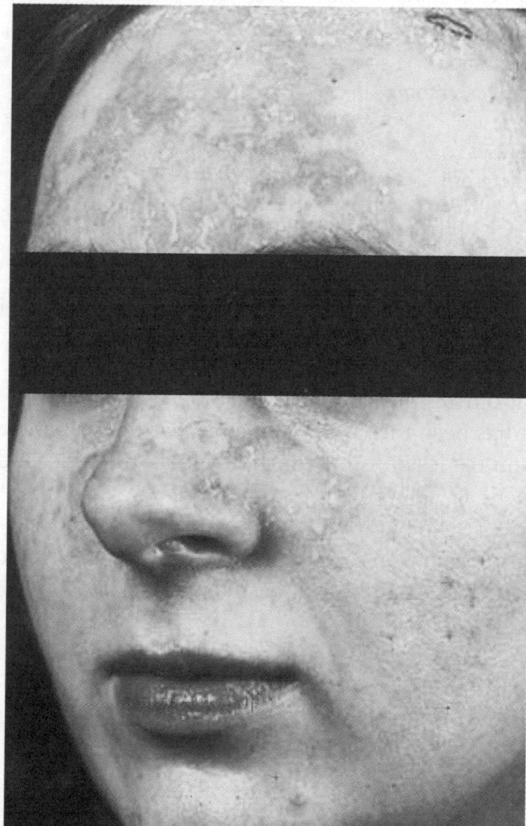

(Reproduced, with permission, from Wolff K, Johnson RA. Fitzpatrick's Color Atlas & Synopsis of Clinical Dermatology, 6th ed. New York: McGraw-Hill; 2009:50.)

Questions 40 to 42

For each patient with skin abnormalities, select the most likely disorder. Each lettered option may be used once, multiple times, or not at all.

a. Superficial spreading melanoma
b. Basal cell carcinoma
c. Squamous cell carcinoma
d. Bowen disease
e. Actinic keratoses
f. Seborrheic keratoses
g. Leukoplakia

40. A 50-year-old construction worker who smokes presents with a slow-growing nonhealing ulcer on his lower lip. He has a small, palpable supraclavicular node.

41. A 57-year-old red-headed female is concerned about a spot on her lower leg that has been there for a while but has grown and gotten darker. On examination the lesion is brownish-black, asymmetric, and raised with irregular borders.

42. A 42-year-old man presents with a single firm, pearly nodule on his nose that, upon close examination, has telangiectasias.

Dermatology

Answers

11. The answer is d. *(Wolff, p 498.)* The most likely diagnosis in this patient is **Peutz-Jeghers syndrome (PJS).** This is an autosomal dominant polyposis characterized by multiple small macules (lentigines) on the lips and oral membranes. Abdominal pain and GI bleeding may occur in late childhood because of **multiple benign hamartomatous polyps** in the small and large bowel as well as in the stomach. These polyps have the potential to develop into adenocarcinoma. PJS is not associated with any of the other answer choices.

12. The answer is a. *(Wolff, pp 148-151.)* This patient has most likely developed **erythema multiforme (EM)** minor following a herpes infection. EM classically consists of **generalized target lesions that may be burning and pruritic.** They often involve the oral mucosa, face, and extremities, **including the palms and soles.** EM major is often a reaction to drugs such as phenytoin, sulfonamides, barbiturates, and allopurinol. Finger pressure in the vicinity of a lesion in EM major leads to a sheetlike removal of the epidermis or extension of a blister **(Nikolsky sign)**. **Pemphigus vulgaris** is a chronic bullous autoimmune disease usually seen in middle-aged adults. The Nikolsky sign is also positive in pemphigus vulgaris. **Secondary syphilis** appears up to 6 months after a primary infection and consists of round to oval maculopapular lesions 0.5 to 1.0 cm in diameter. The eruptions typically involve the palms and soles. Secondary syphilis lesions that are flat and soft with a predilection for the mouth, perineum, and perianal areas are called **condylomata lata**. The skin lesions of systemic **lupus erythematosus (SLE)** range from the classic butterfly malar rash to the discoid plaques of **chronic cutaneous lupus erythematosus (CCLE). Urticaria** is an allergic reaction characterized by pruritic wheals typically lasting several hours.

13. The answer is a. *(Wolff, pp 868-876.)* The history is classic for **scabies**, an infestation by the mite *Sarcoptes scabiei* that is spread by skin-to-skin contact. Patients usually complain of intense pruritus and may have burrows most visible in the intertriginous areas, such as the webs of the hands. **Contact dermatitis** is unlikely only in this location on the hands, and **cutaneous larva migrans** (most commonly from *Ancylostoma brasiliense* due to the dog and cat hookworm) typically has large, erythematous, serpiginous tracks. **Dermatitis herpetiformis** is associated with a gluten-sensitive enteropathy and is characterized by tiny papules, vesicles, and urticarial wheals. ***Enterobius vermicularis*** is the pinworm, the most common intestinal parasite in the United States, and usually results in anal pruritus.

14. The answer is b. *(Wolff, pp 684-691.)* The rash described is **erythema migrans (EM)**, the early pathognomonic eruption of Lyme disease, caused by the spirochete, ***B. burgdorferi,*** transmitted to humans by the bite of an infected deer tick. Most cases in the United States involve the northeastern or northcentral areas of the country. The rash typically occurs 1 to 2 weeks after the bite, but less than 20% of patients recall being bitten. The bite of the **brown recluse spider** (*Loxosceles*) begins as an area of erythema and in some cases progresses to become a painful bulla and deep necrotic ulcer. ***Rickettsia rickettsii***, transmitted by dog or wood ticks, is the etiologic agent of **Rocky Mountain spotted fever**. This infection has a characteristic maculopapular rash that begins peripherally and often involves the palms and soles. ***Bartonella henselae*** (formerly *Rochalimaea henselae*) is the etiologic agent responsible for **cat-scratch disease (CSD)**. ***Mycobacterium marinum*** infections follow a traumatic inoculation in aquariums and swimming pools.

15. The answer is b. *(Wolff, pp 629-631.)* **Toxic shock syndrome (TSS)** is the most likely diagnosis in this patient. This disease is a toxin-mediated multisystem infection caused by *Staphylococcus aureus*. Risk factors for TSS include surgical wounds, nasal packs, burns, skin ulcers, postpartum infections, eye injuries, and use of vaginal tampons. The rash is generalized and erythematous and involves the mucous membranes of the mouth and eyes. Desquamation of the epithelium of the palms and soles and subsequent multisystem failure often occur in TSS. **Toxic epidermal necrolysis (TEN)** is a mucocutaneous, primarily drug-induced eruption characterized by a generalized erythema and exfoliation that may lead to multisystem failure. TEN is a more severe variant of **Stevens-Johnson syndrome (SJS)** and begins 1 to 3 weeks after drug exposure. Drugs that have been implicated include sulfa derivatives, allopurinol, and hydantoins. **Necrotizing fasciitis** begins as a painful induration of the underlying soft tissues with rapid development of an eschar and necrotic mass. **Scarlet fever** is seen in children and is due to an exotoxin-producing strain of group A *Streptococcus*. It has a characteristic confluent (scarlatiniform) erythema, which begins centrally, spreads to the extremities, and then desquamates. **Cellulitis** is an acute infection of the dermal and subcutaneous tissues characterized by erythema, warmth, and tenderness of the skin at the site of the entry of the bacteria.

16. The answer is d. *(Wolff, pp 709-714.)* The history is most consistent with **tinea capitis** due primarily to *Trichophyton tonsurans* or *Microsporum canis*. It is usually seen in school-age children and may be transmitted from person to person, causing broken hair and scaling or inflammation of the scalp. **Androgenic hair loss** is progressive and hereditary bitemporal, frontal, or vertex balding that may begin any time after puberty and is more common in males. **Psoriasis** is a hereditary disorder characterized by scaling patches and plaques appearing in specific areas of the body, such as the scalp, elbows, lumbosacral region, and knees. The lesions are salmon pink with a silver-colored scale that, on removal, produces blood **(Auspitz sign)**. The **Koebner phenomenon** (with trauma, the lesion jumps to a new location) is also elicited in patients with psoriasis. **Seborrheic dermatitis** is a common chronic dermatosis occurring in areas with active sebaceous glands (face, scalp, and body folds) and may be seen either in infancy or in people over the age of 20. The eczematous plaques of seborrheic dermatitis are yellowish red and are often greasy with a sticky crust. A **carbuncle** is a deep infectious collection of interconnecting abscesses **(furuncles)** arising from several hair follicles.

17. The answer is b. *(Wolff, pp 152-153.)* This patient is presenting with **erythema nodosum (EN)**, which tends to affect women more than men, usually peaking in the third decade of life. Lesions are **erythematous, indurated, tender nodules** (hence the name!) located **bilaterally in the subcutaneous fat usually of the anterior lower legs**. EN is a cutaneous reaction to a variety of etiologies ranging from inflammatory bowel disease and sarcoidosis to bacterial, viral, and fungal infectious etiologies and drugs such as sulfonamides and oral contraceptives. The lesions respond to anti-inflammatory agents and resolve spontaneously, **never ulcerating** or scarring. **Bacillary angiomatosis** is caused by *Bartonella* species and causes erythematous, nonblanching nodules and friable lesions in AIDS patients. **Sweet syndrome** is more common in women and is caused by an infection with *Yersinia*, resulting in tender red or blue edematous nodules on the face, neck, and extremities, mimicking erythema nodosum. **Disseminated fungal infections** cause fluctuant subcutaneous nodules in immunocompromised individuals. **Ecthyma gangrenosum** is caused by gram-negative rods (usually *Pseudomonas*) and is an ulcerated plaque that evolves into a hemorrhagic bulla which sloughs to form an eschar.

18. The answer is c. *(McPhee, pp 1405-1406.)* The patient has **second-degree frostbite**. **Frostnip** is a superficial cold injury that causes paresthesias but no tissue loss. **First-degree frostbite** is characterized by partial skin freezing, erythema, edema, no blisters, and desquamation several days later. **Second-degree frostbite** involves full-thickness skin freezing, erythema, edema, and the presence of clear blisters. Patients complain of throbbing and numbness. **Third-degree frostbite** injuries are characterized by damage that extends into the subdermal plexus. The skin is blue or gray, and there are hemorrhagic blisters. Patients complain of burning, shooting pains, and the feeling that the involved area feels like a block of wood. Prognosis is poor. **Fourth-degree frostbite** injuries extend into the subcutaneous tissue, muscle, and bone. There is typically no edema, and the skin is mottled and cyanotic; eventually these injuries form a mummified eschar. The best way to prevent further tissue necrosis in frostbite is through **rapid rewarming, best accomplished by immersing the affected area in a warm bath.** Use of dry heat increases the risk of accidental burns and warming through exercise or friction is contraindicated early on. Blisters should be left intact and antibiotics should be reserved for infections that do not respond to local wound care.

19. The answer is c. *(Wolff, pp 26-29.)* This patient presents with typical symptoms of **allergic contact dermatitis** due to poison ivy resin. This is a type IV cell-mediated delayed hypersensitivity reaction which results in an eruption within a week of exposure. Contact dermatitis due to poison ivy is usually pruritic, localized to the region of exposure, and often consists of linear vesicles or crusts. **Atopic dermatitis**, or **eczema**, is an autosomal dominant pruritic inflammation with a predilection for the neck, face, flexor areas, feet, wrists, and hands. Usually there is a personal or family history of asthma, allergic rhinitis, or hay fever. **Rubeola (measles)** is a viral infection characterized by **conjunctivitis, coryza, and cough (the**

three C's) and a confluent erythematous maculopapular rash that spreads centrifugally. **Koplik spots** (bright red spots with blue-white specks in the center), which appear on the buccal mucosa opposite the premolar teeth, are pathognomonic for rubeola. **Impetigo** is an epidermal bacterial infection seen on the face and characterized by vesicles that rupture and crust. **Erythema infectiosum**, or **fifth disease**, is a childhood disease due to parvovirus B19 and is characterized by edematous, erythematous plaques on the cheeks **("slapped cheek" disease)**.

20. The answer is b. *(Wolff, pp 771-775.)* The description of the skin lesions is most consistent with **molluscum contagiosum**. This is a self-limited viral infection due to a poxvirus (molluscum contagiosum virus) seen in children, sexually active adults, and HIV-infected patients. These lesions characteristically have a central keratotic plug that gives them the appearance of being dimpled (umbilication). The lesions in children occur on exposed skin and resolve spontaneously. Common warts, or **verrucae vulgaris**, are due to human papillomavirus (HPV). Warts are firm, hyperkeratotic, round papules 1 to 10 mm in diameter. They have no umbilication but have a predilection for sites of trauma including hands, fingers, and knees. A **keratoacanthoma** is a single dome-shaped nodule with a central hyperkeratotic core usually found on the face and considered a variant of squamous cell cancer. **Herpetic whitlow**, due to herpes simplex virus, consists of a painful group of vesicles on the volar surface of the finger. Capillary **hemangiomas** are bright red or purple nodules or plaques that develop at birth and spontaneously disappear by the fifth year.

21. The answer is e. *(Wolff, pp 252-256.)* This patient presents with **porphyria cutanea tarda (PCT)**, a disease of adults that affects males and females equally. Although the disease is often hereditary, drugs (estrogens including oral contraceptives, chloroquine, and alcohol), chemicals, and illnesses (hepatitis C virus, diabetes, and hemachromatosis) may induce PCT. The disease occurs gradually, with formation of fragile, tense bullae and hypermelanosis on sun-exposed areas such as the dorsa of the hands and is also associated with hypertrichosis of the face. Though patients may have elevated liver enzymes from associated hepatitis C or alcohol abuse, as well as elevated blood glucose in concomitant diabetes, eliciting an **orange-red fluorescence of the urine with a Wood lamp confirms the diagnosis**. Funguses fluoresce green under a Wood lamp.

22. The answer is b. *(Wolff, pp 122-123.)* This patient has a rash characteristic of **pityriasis rosea (PR)**, which usually presents in younger patients in the spring and fall and is associated with a reactivation of herpesviruses. In the majority of affected people, the rash begins on the trunk as an oval, slightly raised, light red **herald patch** with scale attached at the edges. Over the next week or two, scattered oval lesions appear on the trunk and proximal extremities in a characteristic **"Christmas tree" pattern, sparing the face** and often accompanied by pruritus. **Phototherapy is only helpful if begun in the first week** of the rash, though antihistamines or topical steroids may be used to treat the pruritus. You can reassure your patient that the rash will **resolve spontaneously, without long-term sequelae, over 6 to 12 weeks and rarely recurs**.

23. The answer is b. *(McPhee, pp 1408-1409.)* A **first-degree burn** involves the epidermis and retains normal capillary refill. Burns that blister are **second-degree burns**, resulting from partial thickness dermal injury. **Third-degree burns** involve the entire thickness of the skin and **fourth-degree burns** extend through the skin to subcutaneous fat, muscle, and bone. The **rule of 9's** is often used to calculate burn surface area in adults: 9% for each arm and the head and 18% for each leg and each side of the torso. There is no fifth-degree burn.

24. The answer is c. *(McPhee, p 978.)* The first step in elimination of alcohol is mediated by **alcohol dehydrogenase** which metabolizes ethanol to acetaldehyde. However, it is the lack of the enzyme involved in the next step, **aldehyde dehydrogenase (ALDH),** that results in **accumulation of acetaldehyde after ingestion of alcohol. Up to 50% of Chinese and Japanese people lack ALDH and develop facial flushing and erythema after ingestion of alcohol.**

Crigler-Najjar syndrome, a familial nonhemolytic jaundice due to high levels of unconjugated bilirubin, results from **glucuronyl transferase deficiency**.

Angioedema is an IgE-mediated allergic response that involves swelling of the lips, eyelids, hands, and feet and may progress to laryngeal edema and hypotension.

Photosensitivity is a tendency to sunburn more readily when exposed to ultraviolet radiation and can be caused by medications and lupus erythematosus, among other conditions.

25 to 27. The answers are 25-c, 26-f, 27-b. *(Wolff, pp 2-13; 34-43.)* **Acne vulgaris (common acne)** is an inflammation of the pilosebaceous units of the face and trunk occurring usually in adolescence. It manifests itself as comedones, papulopustules, or nodules and cysts. **Rosacea** is a chronic acneform disorder of the facial pilosebaceous units coupled with an increased reactivity of capillaries to heat, leading to flushing and the formation of telangiectasia. **Melasma** is an acquired hyperpigmentation that occurs in sun-exposed areas, especially the face. It is common in women with brown or black skin color and may occur in pregnancy or with oral contraceptive use. **Discoid lupus** presents with facial plaques that may result in dyspigmentation and scarring. A **spider angioma** is a pulsatile arteriolar lesion that blanches with pressure and is seen in patients with cirrhosis (hyperestrogenism). **Atopic dermatitis** usually begins in childhood, is familial, and is characterized by dry skin and pruritus, resulting in an "itch-scratch cycle." In **lichen simplex chronicus**, repetitive scratching results in plaques of thickened skin and accentuated skin markings.

28 to 30. The answers are 28-e, 29-a, 30-b. *(Wolff, pp 471-479.)* **Pressure, or decubitus, ulcers** are common in patients who are chronically ill and bedridden. Risk factors for development of pressure ulcers include immobility, incontinence, poor nutritional status, and hypoalbuminemia. Sixty percent of pressure ulcers occur over the sacrum. Prevention is possible by turning immobile patients (every 1-2 hours) to prevent skin compression and subsequent ischemic necrosis. **Venous ulcers** usually develop in the medial calf or over the malleolus (both lateral and medial). Chronic venous insufficiency precipitates the formation of these shallow, painful ulcers. Peripheral arterial disease leads to **arterial ulcers**, which are typically in the lower leg over pressure sites and are painful at night, improving with dependency. Patients present with complaints of claudication. Arterial insufficiency may lead to atrophic skin changes (shiny and white) and loss of hair on the feet and legs. **Neuropathic ulcers** occur in diabetics; early symptoms may include paresthesias of the leg and foot. Trauma usually precedes the formation of the neuropathic ulcers of the toe, heel, or metatarsal areas **(Charcot joint). Aphthous ulcers** are painful, gray-based ulcers with erythematous rims occurring in the oropharynx.

31 to 35. The answers are 31-b, 32-c, 33-d, 34-f, 35-h. *(Wolff, pp 1021-1027.)* **Koilonychia**, also called **spoon nails** (due to a thin and soft nail plate), is seen in iron-deficiency anemia and may be demonstrated when a drop of water on the nail does not roll off. White lines parallel to the lunula, separated by normal nail, that remain immobile as the nail grows (they are located in the nail bed, not the nail plate) are called **Muehrcke nails**. They are seen in patients with severe hypoalbuminemia, such as those with nephrotic syndrome. **Terry nails** is a nail abnormality seen in patients with cirrhosis whereby the proximal four-fifths of the nail is white and the distal rim is pink. Times of severe stress (ie, myocardial infarction) may cause a temporary growth arrest and horizontal depressions across the nail plate, called **Beau lines**. Multiple **brown nails** occur with Addison disease, hemochromatosis, gold therapy, and arsenic intoxication. **Leukonychia** occurs when there are white patches (subungual air bubbles) between the nail and its bed; it may be congenital or a result of trauma. **Blue nails** (azure half-moons) may be due to Wilson disease, hemochromatosis, use of antimalarial drugs, or exposure to silver nitrate. **Pitting** of the nails is seen in psoriasis. In contrast to the immobile lines of Muehrcke nails, **Mees lines** are transverse white lines that move with the growth of the nail plate and are caused by arsenic poisoning, chemotherapy, Hodgkin lymphoma, and severe cardiac and renal disease. **Splinter hemorrhages** are brown or red streaks in the midportion of the nail and may be seen in patients with endocarditis or trichinosis, or as the result of trauma. **Yellow nails** are characterized by a yellowish color of the nail plates due to poor lymphatic circulation. **Brittle nails** (frayed and irregular) may be seen with hyperthyroidism, malnutrition, or calcium or iron deficiency.

36 and 37. The answers are 36-d, 37-b. *(Wolff, pp 440-446.)* **Scurvy, or vitamin C deficiency**, is seen in infants under 1 year of age or in older adults who lack fruits and vegetables in their diet. Perifollicular hemorrhage and areas of ecchymosis are common, especially on the back of the lower legs, arms, and inner thighs **(saddle distribution)**. Loose teeth and bleeding gums are also seen with scurvy. Genetic **zinc deficiency** causes **acrodermatitis enteropathica** in infancy, characterized by the **classic triad of acral dermatitis, alopecia, and diarrhea.** Adults may also develop zinc deficiency. **Vitamin D deficiency leads to rickets**, defective mineralization of the growing skeleton. **Niacin (vitamin B_3) deficiency** is seen in alcoholic patients and causes **pellagra**, which is characterized by a triad of the three Ds—dementia, diarrhea, and dermatitis. **Thiamine (vitamin B_1)** deficiency causes **beriberi** (which affects the cardiovascular and neurologic systems) and **Wernicke-Korsakoff syndrome**, characterized by inability to form new memories, ataxia, hallucinations, and abnormal eye movements.

38 and 39. The answers are 38-a, 39-b. *(Wolff, pp 48-49; 538-543; 771-775; 942-960.)* **Kaposi sarcoma** is a multisystem vascular neoplasm associated with human herpesvirus type 8 that may be seen in elderly males of eastern European heritage on the feet and legs and in immunocompromised patients also on the face and trunk. Macules develop into patches, papules, plaques, nodules, and tumors, which are initially pinkish red and later purple brown. The disease can be localized or widespread. **Seborrheic dermatitis** is more common in males and is characterized by redness and scaling on the face, scalp, and in body folds. It is the cause of "cradle cap" in infants and the mild form of this on the scalp is commonly called "dandruff." **Molluscum contagiosum** is caused by a poxvirus and skin-colored papules have a characteristic central umbilication. In immunocompromised patients the lesions most often occur on the face and do not spontaneously regress as they do in children and immunocompetent adults. **Eosinophilic folliculitis** presents as erythematous follicular papules and pustules, usually on the face, upper trunk, and proximal extremities that may be intensely pruritic. **Herpes zoster** is a reactivation of latent varicella zoster virus. It is preceded by paresthesias and a prodromal phase and then presents as vesicular eruptions in dermatomal distributions, though it may be disseminated and more severe in immunocompromised hosts such as HIV patients. Vesicles progress to crusts and often are followed by postherpetic neuralgia.

40 to 42. The answers are 40-c, 41-a, 42-b. *(Wolff, pp 274-293; 315-319.)* **Oral leukoplakia** is a white macular lesion found in the buccal mucosa. Predisposing factors include tobacco use, alcohol use, human papillomavirus, and syphilis. It may lead to squamous cell carcinoma. **Actinic (solar) keratoses** are dry, rough, adherent, scaly lesions occurring in sun-exposed areas of adults. These lesions are premalignant and may develop into squamous cell carcinoma. **Bowen disease** is otherwise known as **squamous cell carcinoma in situ** and refers to well-demarcated pink or red macules, papules, or plaques with scaling or a crusted surface that results from sun exposure. **Squamous cell carcinoma** may result from Bowen disease or actinic keratoses. It often manifests in patients with a long history of sun exposure as a nonhealing ulcer or nodule which **may metastasize**, especially in lesions involving the lip, tongue, oral cavity, or genitalia. **Seborrheic keratosis** is the most common benign epithelial tumor and range from barely elevated papules to plaques with a characteristic "stuck on" appearance. **Basal cell carcinoma (BCC)** is the most common type of skin cancer. It is invasive and aggressive but rarely metastasizes. These lesions are usually **round, firm, glistening (pearly), and shiny with telangiectasias**. Histologically, basal cell carcinomas have **palisading nuclei**. Superficial **spreading melanomas (SSMs)** have five cardinal features **(ABCDE rule):** **A**symmetry, **B**order that is irregular, **C**olor that is a haphazard range of colors, **D**iameter that is larger than a pencil eraser, and **E**nlargement over time/**E**levation that is irregular.

Head, Ears, Eyes, Nose, and Throat

Questions

43. A 71-year-old woman presents to your office complaining of unilateral hearing loss. She denies vertigo and tinnitus. A Weber test lateralizes to the deaf ear, and bone conduction is greater than air conduction on the Rinne test. The tympanic membranes are bilaterally normal. Which of the following best explains her hearing loss?

a. Conductive hearing loss
b. Sensorineural hearing loss
c. Electrical hearing loss
d. Hysterical hearing loss
e. Mixed hearing loss

44. A 31-year-old man comes to your office complaining of fullness and decreased hearing in his left ear for nearly a week following a viral upper respiratory tract infection. He tells you that he hears a popping sound in that ear with yawning but has no fever or discharge from the ear. Physical examination reveals a normal right ear canal and tympanic membrane but the left tympanic membrane is noninflamed, retracted, and immobile. Which of the following should you tell him?

a. He should be placed on systemic antibiotics.
b. Systemic and intranasal decongestants may help this condition.
c. This condition does not increase his risk of serous otitis media.
d. This condition does not increase his risk of acute otitis media.
e. There is no contraindication to flying on an airplane with this condition.

45. A 48-year-old man presents complaining that his vision has been deteriorating over the last several months. His pupils are equal and reactive to light and accommodation. Extraocular muscle movements and visual field examinations are intact. He has decreased visual acuity as determined by a Snellen chart. Funduscopic examination is normal. Which of the following is the most appropriate next step in diagnosis?

a. Slit-lamp examination
b. Pinhole test
c. Pseudochromatic plate test
d. Schiötz tonometry
e. Amsler grid test
f. Fluorescein stain

46. A 52-year-old man comes to your office complaining of an itchy feeling in his right ear. He has been trying to scratch the itchiness using a cotton swab applicator. He denies tinnitus or hearing loss. On physical examination, the patient is afebrile and complains of pain when the pinna is pulled for the examination. The ear canal is red and swollen with some areas of white debris. Because of the debris, you cannot visualize the tympanic membrane. There is no adenopathy. Which of the following is the most likely diagnosis?

a. Otitis media
b. Serous otitis
c. Otitis externa
d. Cerumen blockage
e. Malignant otitis

47. A 74-year-old man with a history of previous myocardial infarction and stroke presents with the sudden onset of left-sided vision loss. Blood pressure is 135/85 mm Hg. Heart rate is 80 beats per minute and regular. Heart and lungs are normal. Funduscopic examination of the left eye reveals a bright yellow refractile deposit wedged at the bifurcation of a peripheral arteriole. The deposit appears to be migrating down the vessel. Which of the following is the most appropriate next step in diagnosis?

a. Holter monitor
b. Cardiac isoenzymes
c. Carotid dopplers
d. Echocardiogram
e. Electrocardiogram
f. Computed tomographic (CT) scan of the head

48. A 14-year-old adolescent presents to your office after being hit in the face by a soccer ball. He complains of left eye pain, and on physical examination you see blood in the anterior chamber. Pupils are equal and reactive to light, and extraocular muscles are intact. Which of the following is the most likely diagnosis?

a. Hyphema
b. Esotropia
c. Amblyopia
d. Subconjunctival hemorrhage
e. Hypopyon

49. A 31-year-old man is brought into the emergency room after blunt trauma to the right eye. He complains of diplopia on upward gaze. A step-off is felt at the inferior rim of the orbit. Palpation of the surrounding tissue reveals subcutaneous crepitus. Subconjunctival air bubbles are obvious with a penlight. Extraocular muscle movement examination reveals that the patient is unable to gaze upward. Which of the following is the most likely diagnosis?

a. Blowout fracture
b. Preseptal cellulitis
c. Dyschromatopsia
d. Subconjunctival hemorrhage
e. Pterygium

50. A 70-year-old man with hypertension and diabetes complains of seeing flashing lights and then a curtain spreading upward across his field of vision, but thus far he has retained his central vision. He does not have ocular pain or headache. Which of the following is the most likely diagnosis?

a. Diabetic retinopathy
b. Retinal vein occlusion
c. Retinal artery occlusion
d. Ischemic optic neuropathy
e. Retinal detachment
f. Hypertensive retinopathy

51. A 43-year-old woman who is HIV positive presents with painful vesicles of the right ear canal and eardrum. Physical examination reveals right facial paralysis, hyperacusia, and unilateral loss of taste. Which of the following is the most likely diagnosis?

a. Sweet syndrome
b. Bullous myringitis
c. Sturge-Weber disease
d. Ramsay Hunt syndrome
e. Behçet syndrome

52. A 41-year-old man with a 10-year history of sarcoidosis presents with the chief complaint of nose disfiguration. His nose is not enlarged, but he has a nonblanching purple discoloration of the skin of the external nose. There is no history of trauma, and he denies epistaxis. He has no other skin lesions. Which of the following best describes the nose abnormality?

a. Rhinophyma
b. Nasal fracture
c. Septal hematoma
d. Lupus pernio
e. Saddle nose deformity
f. Polychondritis

53. A 32-year-old woman presents to your office complaining of "a sinus infection." She states that she had a cold, with a runny nose and cough, and now has sinus congestion with pain under her eyes and a headache. She has had this before and is requesting antibiotics. Which of the following signs and symptoms increase the likelihood of her self-diagnosis of sinusitis being correct?

a. History of clear nasal drainage
b. History of maxillary toothache
c. Facial pain does not change with movement
d. Recent good response to nasal decongestants
e. Good transmission of light to the hard palate using a transilluminator on the maxillary sinuses

54. A 57-year-old man presents with hoarseness for 3 months, which has kept him from singing with his church choir. He has no other symptoms or complaints. He had a cold at the beginning of the symptoms but this seemed to resolve. He has no past medical history and takes no medications, but he has smoked a pack of cigarettes per day for 40 years and drinks one beer per day. He uses no illicit drugs. Which of the following is at the top of your differential?

a. Acute laryngitis
b. Cancer of the larynx
c. Reflux esophagitis
d. Voice strain
e. Postnasal drip syndrome

55. A 66-year-old woman with a history of hypertension and asthma presents for her annual eye examination. She has been seeing floaters recently but has no other complaints. Intraocular pressure measurement by Schiötz tonometry is 15 mm Hg. Red reflex is normal, pupils are equal and reactive to light, and extraocular muscles are intact. Examination of the fundi reveals narrow, tortuous arterioles, with arteriovenous nicking. There are no hard exudates, hemorrhages, cotton-wool spots, or microaneurysms. The optic cup constitutes 25% of the optic disc, and there is no papilledema. Which of the following is the most likely diagnosis?

a. Glaucoma
b. Early cataract
c. Macular degeneration
d. Hypertensive retinopathy
e. Retinitis pigmentosa
f. Early retinal detachment

56. A 32-year-old woman presents with a 2-day history of "the room spinning." She states that this occurs when she suddenly moves her head, like when she rolls over in bed, and lasts for a minute or so. She complains of nausea accompanying the spinning sensation but has no upper respiratory symptoms, tinnitus, hearing loss, or facial numbness. On physical examination, she is afebrile and her tympanic membranes are bilaterally normal. Which of the following tests would confirm her likely diagnosis?

a. MRI of the brain with thin cuts through the internal auditory meatus
b. MRA of the brain
c. Dix-Hallpike maneuver
d. Audiometry
e. CT scan of the brain

57. A 48-year-old man presents with inability to move the right side of his mouth. On physical examination, the patient has difficulty raising his right eyebrow, puffing out his right cheek, and smiling using the left side of his mouth. His nasolabial fold on the right is absent. Blinking is difficult on the right compared to the left, but extraocular muscles are intact and pupils are equal and reactive. The patient's tongue is midline but he complains of food tasting funny. Which of the following is the most likely diagnosis?

a. Paralysis of cranial nerve V
b. Lower motor neuron paralysis of cranial nerve VII
c. Paralysis of cranial nerve XII
d. Horner syndrome
e. Central paralysis of cranial nerve VII

58. A 71-year-old man complains of increasing difficulty in seeing street signs when driving and some difficulty with vision when reading. The patient's vision is 20/100 in his right eye and 20/80 in his left eye. The pinhole test does not improve vision in either eye. There is dullness of the red reflex bilaterally and fundi are difficult to visualize with the ophthalmoscope. Intraocular pressure is measured to be 15 mm Hg in both eyes. Which of the following is the most likely diagnosis?

a. Glaucoma
b. Macular degeneration
c. Presbyopia
d. Cataract
e. Arcus senilis

59. A 15-year-old adolescent presents with a sore throat. Which presentation accompanying the sore throat would lead him to most likely test positive for streptococcal pharyngitis?

a. Runny nose, headache, and cough but no fever, lymphadenopathy or tonsillar exudates
b. Fever, runny nose, sinus pain, and cervical lymphadenopathy
c. Fever, cervical lymphadenopathy, tonsillar exudates, and no cough
d. Cough, tonsillar exudates, and cervical lymphadenopathy, but no fever
e. Cough, fever, nasal drainage, and cervical lymphadenopathy

60. A 22-year-old woman presents with complaints of runny nose, itchy throat, and sneezing that seem to occur every year in the springtime. She has no history of known allergies, but her mother and sister have similar symptoms. What findings on physical examination would support a diagnosis of seasonal allergic rhinitis?

a. Erythematous nasal turbinates
b. Dullness on transillumination of the maxillary sinuses
c. Expiratory wheezing
d. Strawberry tongue
e. Nasal salute

61. A 21-year-old man presents with a sore throat. He also complains of dysphagia, odynophagia, and otalgia. His temperature is 39.2°C (102.5°F). The patient speaks with a hot potato voice and is drooling. Examination of the throat reveals a hypertrophied right tonsil that appears to be displaced inferiorly and medially. There is contralateral deflection of the uvula. The patient has trismus and cervical lymphadenopathy. Which of the following is the most likely diagnosis?

a. Retropharyngeal abscess
b. Peritonsillar abscess
c. Exudative pharyngitis
d. Cancer of the right tonsil
e. Mononucleosis

Questions 62 to 64

For each patient with ear complaints, select the most likely diagnosis. Each lettered option may be used once, multiple times, or not at all.

a. Bullous myringitis
b. Nasopharyngeal carcinoma
c. Acoustic neuroma
d. Cholesteatoma
e. Ramsay Hunt syndrome

62. A 30-year-old woman complains of severe left ear pain. On physical examination, there is hemorrhagic blistering of the left eardrum.

63. A 47-year-old man complains of hearing loss and otorrhea. On physical examination, there is a perforation of the tympanic membrane.

64. A 51-year-old man complains of vertigo, hearing loss, and tinnitus of the left ear.

Questions 65 and 66

For each patient with eye complaints, select the most likely diagnosis. Each lettered option may be used once, multiple times, or not at all.

a. Adenoviral conjunctivitis
b. Bacterial conjunctivitis
c. Blepharitis
d. Hordeolum
e. Keratitis
f. Iritis
g. Allergic conjunctivitis

65. A 17-year-old student complains of bilateral red eyes with a watery discharge. Physical examination reveals some preauricular lymphadenopathy.

66. A 22-year-old man with a history of hilar adenopathy and lung disease presents with eye pain and photophobia. Eye examination reveals an irregular pupil and ciliary flush.

Questions 67 and 68

For each patient with pupil abnormalities, select the most appropriate diagnosis. Each lettered option may be used once, multiple times, or not at all.

a. Argyll Robertson pupil
b. Adie tonic pupil
c. Marcus Gunn pupil
d. Anisocoria
e. Oculomotor nerve palsy

67. A 59-year-old woman presents with a history of multiple sexual partners and has been treated for *Chlamydia* in the past. Pupils are small and irregular and do not respond to light but respond to accommodation.

68. A 25-year-old woman presents with a hyperemic and swollen left optic disc. The swinging flashlight test is positive.

Questions 69 to 71

For each of the following patient presentations, select the appropriate cranial nerve involved. Each lettered option may be used once, multiple times, or not at all.

a. Cranial nerve I
b. Cranial nerve III
c. Cranial nerve IV
d. Cranial nerve V
e. Cranial nerve VI
f. Cranial nerve VII

69. A 57-year-old man with diabetes presents with ptosis and an eye that is slightly depressed and laterally deviated, but with a normal pupillary response.

70. A 62-year-old woman complains that her favorite ice cream "tastes funny" but its smell is intact.

71. A 50-year-old woman complains of a 1-week history of recurrent, excruciating pain in her lips and left cheek that lasts for seconds and is exacerbated by washing her face or brushing her teeth. On physical examination there is no sensory deficit of her face.

Head, Ears, Eyes, Nose, and Throat

Answers

43. The answer is a. *(Seidel, pp 333-334.)* The **Weber test** is performed by placing a tuning fork on the midline vertex of the head. In **conductive hearing loss** the Weber lateralizes to the deaf ear, while in sensorineural hearing loss the Weber lateralizes to the better ear. The **Rinne test** is performed by placing a 512-Hz tuning fork over the mastoid process. When the vibration is no longer heard via bone conduction, the tuning fork is placed near the ear to determine whether the vibration is heard. If the vibration is heard, then **air conduction is greater than bone conduction and the test is considered positive or normal**. If the vibration is not heard, then bone conduction is greater than air conduction and this **negative Rinne test denotes conductive hearing loss**. **Sensorineural hearing loss** occurs when a positive or normal Rinne test in the involved ear is complemented by a Weber test that lateralizes to the unaffected ear. **Mixed hearing loss** is a combination of sensorineural and conductive etiologies. Hearing loss may be addressed through **electrical stimulation** for high-frequency sound by a hearing aid or cochlear implant. **Hysterical hearing** loss is nonorganic and often psychiatric in origin.

44. The answer is b. *(McPhee, pp 182-183.)* This patient with decreased hearing and fullness in his ear following an upper respiratory infection suffers from **eustachian tube dysfunction.** His physical examination corroborates this diagnosis, and while the condition is usually self-limited over a few weeks, **systemic and intranasal decongestants may speed symptom relief**. As there is no evidence of acute infection, antibiotics would not be the appropriate treatment at this time; however, eustachian tube dysfunction does predispose patients to both acute otitis media and serous otitis media. In addition, air travel and underwater diving should be avoided as patients with this condition are unable to equalize the barometric pressure in the middle ear.

45. The answer is b. *(Seidel, p 287.)* For patients whose visual acuity is less than 20/20, first use the **pinhole test** to diagnose refractive errors as the cause of the decreased acuity. Pinholes allow only paraxial parallel light rays through to the center of the lens and improve visual acuity if refractory errors are present (most commonly myopia). The **slit-lamp examination** is a direct visualization of the eye and its components. The **pseudochromatic plate test** detects color blindness, and **Schiötz tonometry** measures intraocular pressure. **Visual field testing** determines whether the patient has any blind spots. The **Amsler grid test** screens for macular degeneration. **Fluorescein staining** is used to detect abrasions of the cornea. A **cobalt blue light** is used to detect foreign bodies after the fluorescein is instilled into the affected eye.

46. The answer is c. *(McPhee, p 179.)* This patient has **otitis externa**, an infection of the external ear canal that may be due to trauma or water in the ear canal **(swimmer's ear).** Either of these may lead to maceration of the epithelium and subsequent colonization by bacteria or fungi. Diabetic patients are especially at risk for this ear infection. Physical examination often reveals a tender, erythematous ear occluded with debris. Patients complain of pain when the examiner pulls on the pinna or tragus. The treatment is removal of debris with antibiotic otic drops or the placement of a wick to facilitate drainage. **Acute otitis media** is a bacterial infection of the middle ear, causing otalgia and often erythema, dullness, and bulging of the tympanic membrane, but patients rarely complain of pain with moving the pinna. **Serous otitis media** is more common in children and involves a dull tympanic membrane with bubbles in the middle ear as well as a conductive hearing loss. **Malignant otitis** (often seen in diabetic patients and usually due to *Pseudomonas*) causes severe, unrelenting otorrhea and otalgia and a foul-smelling discharge. Malignant otitis requires the use of systemic antibiotics for nearly 2 months. **Cerumen blockage** is the leading cause of conduction hearing loss.

47. The answer is c. *(McPhee, p 164.)* The patient described has experienced **amaurosis fugax**, or transient monocular blindness. On examination, he has a **Hollenhorst plaque**, or cholesterol embolus, at the bifurcation of a retinal arteriole that usually originates from an ulcerated atheromatous plaque in the ipsilateral internal carotid. Thus, a **carotid doppler ultrasound** would be helpful in discerning the source of the embolus. These plaques are bright, refractile, and yellow. They appear to migrate down the vessel; carefully massaging the eyeball can actually facilitate migration. A **Holter monitor** would be used to discern an arrhythmia, which you do not suspect in this case. An **electrocardiogram** and **cardiac isoenzymes** are used to rule out myocardial ischemia and infarction. An **echocardiogram** helps diagnose problems with cardiac contractility and valvular abnormalities while a **CT scan of the head** would be helpful in diagnosing strokes or other brain pathology.

48. The answer is a. *(McPhee, p 171.)* A common sequela of blunt trauma to the eye is a **hyphema** (blood in the anterior chamber). This is caused by rupture of the small blood vessels lying close to the cornea. **Esotropia** is a kind of strabismus, or misalignment of the eyes, in which one eye is deviated inward. **Amblyopia** (lazy eye) is loss of visual acuity in an otherwise healthy deviated eye to avoid the discomfort of diplopia. This is treatable if discovered early. A **subconjunctival hemorrhage** (between the conjunctiva and sclera) causes the sudden appearance of a bright red spot. A **hypopyon**, which often accompanies uveitis or bacterial keratitis, is a collection of white cells in the anterior chamber.

49. The answer is a. *(McPhee, p 171.)* The signs in this patient are consistent with **blowout fracture** of the floor of the orbit. Crepitus and air bubbles are due to air escaping from the fractured sinus. The inability to gaze upward and diplopia are due to entrapment of the inferior rectus muscle. **Preseptal cellulitis** involves only the eyelids; ocular motility remains normal. **Dyschromatopsia** is acquired color blindness (instead of congenital color blindness) due to optic nerve disease or degenerative disease of the macula. Bleeding under the conjunctiva, or **subconjunctival hemorrhage**, is harmless and often induced by sneezing or violent coughing, as well as trauma. A **pterygium** is a raised extension of conjunctiva onto the nasal side of the cornea due to exposure to wind or dust.

50. The answer is e. *(McPhee, pp 161-168.)* Visual acuity is recorded as a fraction in which the numerator is the distance of the patient from the chart (usually 20 ft) and the denominator is the distance at which the average person can read the same line (20 ft). This patient has **retinal detachment**. Patients complain of acute vision loss after noticing flashing lights, floaters, and then a shade over the eye. An eye examination showing the retina appears elevated and often has folds. **Ischemic optic neuropathy** usually occurs in patients with giant cell arteritis or a history of diabetes or hypertension (underlying vascular disease). The disc is pale and swollen, with splinter hemorrhages. This disorder is due to occlusion of the posterior ciliary arteries, with subsequent production of edema. **Retinal artery occlusion** is sudden and painless. It is usually due to infarction from a thrombus or embolus and causes the retina to become pale. The thin tissue of the macula area appears like a **cherry-red spot. Occlusion of the retinal vein** occurs from slow venous blood flow and thrombosis, which results in a slowly progressive loss of vision. The funduscopic image of retinal vein occlusion is so dramatic that it is often described as "**blood and thunder.**" **Diabetic retinopathy** may be proliferative or nonproliferative. In nonproliferative (background) disease, retinal findings include microaneurysms, dot-and-blot hemorrhages, hard exudates, and macular edema. **Proliferative diabetic retinopathy** (neovascularization with the formation of fragile vessels) is a response to continuous retinal ischemia and is responsible for most of the blindness seen in diabetes mellitus. **Hypertensive retinopathy** is classified by the **Keith-Wagener-Barker classification:**

Grade 1: arteriolar narrowing and copper wiring
Grade 2: grade 1 changes and arteriovenous nicking
Grade 3: grade 2 changes with the addition of hemorrhages and exudates
Grade 4: grade 3 changes with the addition of papilledema

51. The answer is d. *(McPhee, p 192.)* **Ramsay Hunt syndrome** is involvement of the geniculate ganglion by herpes zoster. Patients may present with facial paresis, hyperacusia, unilateral loss of taste, reduced tear formation, reduced salivation, pain in the ear, and vesicles in the ear canal and eardrum. **Bullous myringitis** is an inflammation of the tympanic membrane due to the presence of vesicles; patients complain of earache, hearing loss, and bloody discharge. It occurs in several viral and bacterial infections (ie, *Mycoplasma pneumoniae*). **Sturge-Weber disease** is characterized by a port-wine nevus on the scalp and vascular abnormalities that may lead to seizures and cerebellar calcifications; examination of the ear may reveal auricle ecchymoses. **Sweet syndrome** is characterized by dark red nodules that are often ulcerated, located over the hands, face, arms, and legs; it is seen in patients with leukemias or other proliferative disorders.

Behçet syndrome is characterized by the presence of aphthous ulcers of the mouth and genitalia; the ulcers are associated with arthritis, uveitis, and neurological disorders.

52. The answer is d. *(Wolff, p 417-419.)* **Lupus pernio** is a doughy, purple discoloration and enlargement of the nose, cheeks, or earlobes seen in active **sarcoidosis**. **Rhinophyma** is rubbery thickening of the nasal skin due to longstanding rosacea, especially in those with excessive alcohol use; the nose may appear enlarged and is covered with multiple telangiectasias. The best example of rhinophyma is the nose of comedian W. C. Fields. **Septal hematoma** is a result of trauma; a red, painful nodule is visible in the nasal septum. **Saddle nose deformity** (destruction of the bony nose) may be acquired or congenital; it may be a complication of Wegener granulomatosis or congenital syphilis. **Polychondritis** can cause **pseudosaddle nose deformity**, but cartilage is destroyed rather than bone. **Nasal fractures** follow trauma; patients present with severe pain and significant anterior bilateral epistaxis. Periorbital ecchymoses, septal hematoma, and septal deviation are complications of septal fractures. All nasal fractures require antibiotics to prevent osteomyelitis.

53. The answer is b. *(Simel, pp 593-598.)* In patients presenting with nasal congestion, headache, and cough, the astute clinician must differentiate causes of rhinitis (viral infection, allergies, or vasomotor instability) from **infectious sinusitis**. On history, symptoms that increase the likelihood of sinusitis include **fever, maxillary toothache, colored nasal discharge, headache, facial pain worsened with bending forward and little improvement with nasal decongestants**. On examination, these patients will have tenderness to palpation of the sinuses and the two best predictors: **abnormal transillumination** (poor light reflex transmitted to the hard palate) and **purulent secretions on otoscopic examination of the nasal mucosa.** Clear nasal drainage is found in vasomotor and allergic rhinitis.

54. The answer is b. *(McPhee, p 207-211.)* **Hoarseness** may be due to edema or swelling of the larynx or vocal cords or to external compression of the larynx or the recurrent laryngeal nerve. **Laryngeal carcinoma** must be ruled out first in patients with a history of heavy tobacco use who complain of a hoarse voice for more than 2 weeks. **Acute laryngitis** is the most common cause of hoarseness and may remain for a week or more after a viral upper respiratory infection has resolved. Certain occupations, such as being a singer or a telephone operator, place people at risk for **voice strain** due to overuse. **Gastroesophageal reflux** disease may cause hoarseness, but the patient would also complain of heartburn, nocturnal cough, chronic sore throat, and excess phlegm production. **Postnasal drip** syndrome leads to chronic throat clearing, and physical examination reveals **cobblestoning** of the posterior pharynx. A helpful mnemonic for hoarseness is **VINDICATE: V**ascular (thoracic aneurysm), **I**nflammation, **N**eoplasm, **D**egenerative (ie, amyotrophic lateral sclerosis), **I**ntoxication (smoking, alcohol), **C**ongenital (laryngeal web), **A**llergies, **T**rauma, and **E**ndocrine (thyroiditis).

55. The answer is d. *(McPhee, pp 167.)* This patient presents with eye findings consistent with **hypertensive retinopathy: copper-wiring of the retinal arterioles, with venous compression at the place where arteries and veins cross in the retina (arteriovenous nicking)**, though she lacks the **flame hemorrhages** that may occur as well. Acute blood pressure elevations may result in cotton-wool spots (white, indistinct, opaque areas of the inner or superficial retina), retinal hemorrhages and yellowish deep retinal hard exudates, as well as papilledema. **Retinal hemorrhages** are due to leaky and damaged retinal capillaries. Depending on their retinal layer location, they may be **dot-and-blot** (due to diabetes and hypertension), **flame-and-splinter** (due to intracranial hemorrhage, papilledema, and glaucoma), or white-centered (**Roth spots** seen in endocarditis, leukemia, and diabetes). **Normal intraocular pressure (IOP)**, measured with a **Schiötz tonometer**, is in the range of 10 to 21.5 mm Hg. IOP is determined by the outflow of aqueous humor from the eye; the greater the resistance to outflow, the higher the IOP. This patient lacks the increased IOP and enlarged cup-to-disc ratio (30%) usually seen with **glaucoma**. The **red reflex** is present, meaning that all of the light-transmitting media of the eye will be transparent and visible. **Cataracts and retinal detachment obscure the presence of a red reflex. Drusen bodies**, which are absent in this patient, are yellow, deep epithelial pigment deposits located in the macula; they are the earliest sign of **macular degeneration. Microaneurysms** are outpouchings of the retinal capillaries and are almost always associated with diabetes mellitus. In **retinitis pigmentosa**, the fundi are covered with a bony spicule formation.

56. The answer is c. *(Simel, pp 709-713.)* **Vertigo** is an illusion of movement that gives the sensation of spinning. This patient, with attacks lasting several seconds that are provoked by head movements, likely has **benign paroxysmal positional vertigo (BPPV)** caused by the detachment of calcium carbonate crystals from the affected side into the semicircular canal. The **Dix-Hallpike maneuver** (having the patient go from a sitting to supine position while quickly turning the head to the side) will reproduce the vertigo of BPPV and cause rotary nystagmus with the fast component to the dependent side. The history does not suggest **Ménière disease** (hydrops), a disorder of endolymph control in which patients often complain of disabling imbalance, vomiting, tinnitus, and sensorineural hearing loss confirmed on **audiometry**. **Magnetic resonance angiography (MRA)** would confirm arterial occlusions in the posterior circulation which could also cause vertigo in someone with risk factors for atherosclerosis. Patients with cerebellopontine angle tumors, such as **schwannomas (acoustic neuromas)**, complain of vertigo, tinnitus, hearing loss, and facial numbness and weakness as the tumor compresses on the adjacent cranial nerves (VII and VIII) and brainstem. The best initial screening test for acoustic neuromas is **audiometry**, followed by **magnetic resonance imaging (MRI)** with thin cuts thorough the internal auditory meatus.

57. The answer is b. *(McPhee, p 928.)* **Bell palsy**, or **lower motor neuron paralysis of cranial nerve VII,** causes ipsilateral drooping of the mouth and facial muscles, inability to close the ipsilateral eye, and difficulty eating and speaking (due to the mouth droop or weakness), with occasional altered taste and hyperacusis. Bell palsy may be idiopathic or due to trauma, multiple sclerosis, or infections such as reactivation of herpes simplex virus infection. A **central cranial nerve VII palsy** would spare the forehead due to dual innervation in this area. **Horner syndrome** is caused by a lack of sympathetic innervation to one side of the face and neck. With loss of this innervation, the pupil becomes constricted, the eyelid droops, and there is loss of sweating on the ipsilateral side of sympathetic loss. Horner syndrome is often secondary to a Pancoast tumor. **Cranial nerve V** controls the muscles of mastication, and **cranial nerve XII** innervates the muscles of the tongue.

58. The answer is d. *(McPhee, p 161.)* This patient presents with gradually increasing blurry vision without pain, most likely because of a **cataract**, an opacity of the lens. In the presence of cataracts, which affect older patients or may be congenital, the red reflex is diminished and it becomes difficult to see the fundus through the opacity. Patients with **macular degeneration** present with central vision loss, and **drusen bodies** (yellow-white lesions), retinal atrophy, and neovascularization are often found on funduscopic examination. **Presbyopia** is a decreased ability to focus on near objects (because of loss of accommodation) that occurs with aging. **Glaucoma** is an insidious disease in which patients complain of peripheral vision loss (central vision is spared until late in the disease) and scotomas. Whereas intraocular pressure in this patient is normal, in glaucoma it is usually elevated. **Arcus senilis** is a gray or white arc or ring caused by lipid deposits along the outer rim of the cornea.

59. The answer is c. *(Simel, pp 615-625.)* Sore throat is one of the most common presenting complaints to outpatient practices and may result from a multitude of illnesses ranging from gastroesophageal reflux disease and allergic rhinitis to viral illnesses and strep throat. It is important to correctly diagnose **strep throat** to prevent antibiotic overuse in negative cases and to appropriately treat patients with the illness to prevent suppurative complications such as peritonsillar abscesses and rheumatic fever. A simple validated four-item prediction rule, **the Centor score, can help identify patients who should be tested for strep throat,** though it has not been validated in younger patients. **The presence of three or four of the following increases the likelihood of strep throat: history of fever, anterior cervical adenopathy, tonsillar exudates, and absence of cough.** The Centor score has been modified for age (< 15 years old gets another point and > 45 years old subtracts a point) which has improved its accuracy. **In this modified Centor model, adults with a score of 4 should be treated with antibiotics and those with 2 and 3 points should receive a rapid strep test; all children with a score of 2 to 5 should get a rapid strep test, followed by a culture if the rapid test is negative.**

60. The answer is e. *(McPhee, p 196-197.)* The patient has symptoms consistent with **seasonal allergic rhinitis (AR).** Fifty percent of patients have a family history of seasonal rhinitis. Symptoms include runny nose, pruritus, sneezing, itchy throat, congestion, stuffiness, conjunctival erythema, tearing, and frequent throat clearing. Physical examination may reveal nasal mucosa that is **boggy (pale and swollen)** or **blue-gray (severe AR)** and often accompanied by polyps, while turbinates are erythematous in viral rhinitis. A **nasal salute** (a transverse crease across the nose resulting from repeated rubbing), **allergic shiners** (dark circles under the eyes), and **Dennie-Morgan lines** (folds below the margin of the inferior eyelids) may be visible. The pharynx may have a **cobblestone** appearance (due to lymphoid tissue hypertrophy), and postnasal drip may be visible. Multiallergen screening tests are the most sensitive and specific of all the screening options to confirm the diagnosis. Patients with sinusitis will often have tenderness on palpation and percussion of the frontal and maxillary sinuses and absent light reflex on transillumination. Expiratory wheezing results from bronchospasm, as in asthma, and strawberry tongue is associated with scarlet fever and Kawasaki disease.

61. The answer is b. *(McPhee, p 205.)* The patient has a **peritonsillar abscess**, which is an accumulation of pus between the tonsillar capsule and the superior constrictor muscle of the pharynx. Patients present with a **hot potato voice**, fever, cervical lymphadenopathy, **trismus** (inability to open the mouth), and a **displaced uvula** due to a unilaterally enlarged tonsil. Patients complain of dysphagia, odynophagia, and otalgia. A **retropharyngeal abscess** is an infection of the deep spaces of the neck (from the base of the skull to the tracheal bifurcation); patients are often young children who present with fever, cervical lymphadenopathy, neck pain, neck swelling, **torticollis** (rotation to the affected side), difficulty breathing, and stridor. Patients with an **exudative pharyngitis** have fever, cervical lymphadenopathy, bilateral tonsillar enlargement, erythema, edema of the midline uvula, and discrete tonsillar exudate. The two most common **neoplasms of the tonsil** are squamous cell carcinoma and lymphoma which often present as a neck mass with cervical lymphadenopathy. **Mononucleosis** is a viral illness presenting as fatigue, headache, a sore throat with exudative tonsillitis, lymphadenophathy, and often splenomegaly.

62 to 64. The answers are 62-a, 63-d, 64-c. *(McPhee, pp 244, 184, 191.)* **Bullous myringitis** is associated with *M. pneumoniae* infection but may be seen with viral infections as well. **Cholesteatomas** (sacs) are a complication of chronic otitis media and consist of keratinized squamous epithelium that has entered the middle ear through a perforation from the external canal. These form in relationship to a perforation and can become infected, leading to bone (ossicular chain) destruction. **Acoustic neuromas** or **schwannomas** arise from cranial nerve VIII (vestibular division), and their growth within the internal auditory canal produces tinnitus and hearing loss. **Nasopharyngeal carcinomas** are rare, usually squamous cell in origin and produce symptoms that mimic rhinitis; thus any adult with unilateral nasal symptoms (pain, bleeding) or new otitis media should be evaluated by a specialist. **Ramsay Hunt syndrome** is due to herpes zoster (shingles) infection of the face that involves the seventh nerve and causes paralysis of the facial muscles.

65 and 66. The answers are 65-a, 66-f. *(McPhee, pp 153-154.)* The most common cause of **red eye** is **viral conjunctivitis** due to **adenovirus**. This is a highly contagious keratoconjunctivitis usually accompanied by preauricular adenopathy. **Bacterial conjunctivitis** is usually associated with a purulent discharge but no adenopathy. **Allergic** insults may cause itching and watery discharge of the eyes, but usually the patient complains of hypersensitivity to a specific agent. **Iritis (acute anterior uveitis or iridocyclitis)** is an inflammation of the iris and ciliary muscle. It may be a systemic marker for ankylosing spondylitis, Reiter syndrome, or sarcoidosis. The patient complains of eye pain and photophobia, and eye examination reveals a **ciliary flush** (engorgement of the deep pericorneal blood vessels, which is never seen in a superficial infection) and an irregular pupil. **Keratitis**, or **corneal inflammation**, may be due to trauma, including overuse of contact lenses. Patients complain of diminished visual acuity, photophobia, and a sensation of a foreign body in the eye. They are at risk for further vision loss. A **hordeolum** is an infection (pustule) of the eyelid gland, usually due to *Staphylococcus aureus*, which causes pain and swelling of the lid margin **(stye). Blepharitis** is a chronic inflammation of the eyelid margins that causes burning, itching, and irritation of the lids. Patients often complain of sticky eyelids on awakening in the morning.

67 and 68. The answers are 67-a, 68-c. *(Seidel, pp 307-308.)* The patient with a history of sexually transmitted infections has **Argyll Robertson pupils**, commonly referred to as "the prostitute pupil(s)," because they do not react (to light) but will accommodate (constrict with convergence). Pupils are miotic bilaterally and this defect is often caused by neurosyphilis infection that affects the light reflex pathway. The description of a hyperemic and swollen disc is consistent with **optic neuritis**, which is an inflammation of the optic nerve sometimes seen in patients with multiple sclerosis. A **Marcus Gunn pupil** (afferent pupillary defect) is diagnosed using the swinging flashlight test, in which bright light is moved from one eye to the other, and pupillary reactions are observed. In unilateral lesions of the retina or optic nerve (optic neuritis), the affected eye will not perceive light as well, so it will constrict appropriately with the consensual reflex but will appear to dilate when the flashlight comes back to directly shine on it. An **Adie tonic pupil** is a dysfunction of the constrictor muscle in which the affected pupil is dilated and does not respond to direct light or accommodation. Often, the patient has **absent deep tendon reflexes. Anisocoria** implies pupils of unequal size and is found in up to 20% of normal subjects. **Oculomotor nerve (cranial nerve III) palsies** due to compression manifest as a dilated and fixed pupil accompanied by ptosis and deviation of the eye laterally and downward ("**down and out**").

69 to 71. The answers are 69-b, 70-f, 71-d. *(LeBlond, pp 685-689.)* Problems with **cranial nerve I** impact the patient's ability to smell. Patients with diabetes, hypertension, and temporal arteritis may present with an **isolated third nerve palsy** in which there is ptosis and extraocular movements are restricted, except laterally and with looking down at the nose. With medical causes, pupillary reaction is preserved, but if pupils do not respond to light, compressive lesions of the third nerve should be considered. **Fourth nerve paralysis** causes double vision (diplopia) and the eye is deviated upward and cannot look at the nose (superior oblique muscle). The patient with fleeting but excruciating pain in the lips and cheek **has tic douloureux, or trigeminal neuralgia**. Patients will have recurrent episodes and report triggers (such as washing the face, brushing the teeth or experiencing cold drafts of air), which set off an attack. On physical examination of patients with this condition, there will be **no objective sensory deficit**. Paralysis of **cranial nerve VI** impacts the lateral rectus muscle, thus patients cannot abduct the affected eye and experience diplopia when trying to look to the side with that eye. In addition to supplying the motor fibers to the face, **cranial nerve VII** is also responsible for supplying taste to the anterior two-thirds of the tongue. Patients with problems with this nerve will not be able to taste sweet items on the tip of the tongue.

Pulmonary/Critical Care

Questions

72. A 59-year-old woman presents complaining of a cough productive of sputum for nearly 10 years. Her cough occurs during the day, and she produces sputum daily. The woman states that as a child, she had several episodes of pneumonia requiring hospital admissions and antibiotics. Several times a year, her sputum becomes purulent and she requires antibiotic therapy. She has never smoked cigarettes and has worked as a seamstress all of her life. On physical examination, the lungs are clear without wheezes, rhonchi, or crackles. A chest radiograph reveals tram-track markings at the bases. Which of the following is the most likely diagnosis?

a. Asthma
b. Cystic fibrosis
c. Chronic bronchitis
d. Emphysema
e. Bronchiectasis

73. A 71-year-old woman has been in the hospital for 4 days after suffering a stroke in the distribution of the middle cerebral artery. She is not ambulating but is able to eat a pureed diet with assistance from hospital personnel. On the fifth hospital day, she develops a fever and a cough productive of purulent sputum. Lung examination reveals increased fremitus and crackles at the right base. Chest radiograph reveals a right lower-lobe patchy infiltrate. Which of the following is the most likely causal organism?

a. *Pseudomonas aeruginosa*
b. *Chlamydia pneumoniae*
c. Atypical *Mycobacterium*
d. Influenza virus
e. Parainfluenza virus
f. *Moraxella catarrhalis*

74. A 33-year-old woman comes to the emergency department complaining of sharp, pleuritic chest pain on the right, 3 days following the onset of an upper respiratory infection which includes nasal drainage and nonproductive cough. She has no significant past medical history and takes no medication except an oral contraceptive. She does smoke occasionally and has not traveled recently. She has no family history of venous thromboembolism. On physical examination she is not in respiratory distress, with no tachypnea or tachycardia, though she is preventing full inspiratory effort due to pain. Her legs are not swollen. A pregnancy test is negative. Which is the appropriate first step in ruling out a pulmonary embolism in this patient?

a. Ventilation-perfusion scan (V/Q scan)
b. Doppler ultrasound of the lower extremities
c. Spiral computed tomography (CT) of the chest
d. D-dimer
e. Chest x-ray

75. A healthy 50-year-old man presents with a 1-month history of low-grade fever, exertional dyspnea, and cough productive of clear phlegm. He denies hemoptysis and hematuria. He has been taking two antibiotics for the symptoms without relief. He does not smoke cigarettes and works as an accountant. On physical examination, his temperature is 38.3°C (101.0°F) and his lung examination reveals inspiratory crackles. A chest radiograph reveals bibasilar fibrosis and air-space densities in the lower lobes. Which of the following is the most likely diagnosis?

a. Cryptogenic organizing pneumonitis
b. Sarcoidosis
c. Allergic bronchopulmonary aspergillosis
d. Wegener granulomatosis
e. Goodpasture syndrome

76. A 39-year-old man has a seizure in your clinic. On physical examination he is unresponsive and cyanotic. Vital signs reveal a temperature of 38°C (100.5°F), heart rate of 110 beats per minute, and blood pressure of 150/85 mm Hg. Lung examination reveals decreased breath sounds bilaterally. Heart examination is normal and he has a gag reflex. Pulse oximetry reveals a hemoglobin saturation of 80% on 100% oxygen. Which of the following is the most appropriate first step in management?

a. Chest tube placement
b. Endotracheal intubation
c. Arterial blood gas analysis
d. Stat portable chest radiograph
e. Head tilt–chin lift maneuver

77. A 65-year-old woman being treated for lung cancer presents with the sudden onset of pleuritic chest pain and shortness of breath. She has been doing well until 3 days ago, when she noticed some swelling of her left lower extremity. She is not a smoker and denies any recent trauma. On physical examination, she is afebrile but has a respiratory rate of 32 breaths per minute. Her heart rate is 120 beats per minute and her blood pressure is normal. An accentuated (loud) S_2 is heard on heart auscultation. The left lower extremity is swollen, tender to palpation, and erythematous. Lung examination and chest radiograph are normal. Arterial blood analysis on room air shows a Pco_2 of 30 mm Hg and a Po_2 of 58 mm Hg. Which of the following is the most appropriate next diagnostic step?

a. Transesophageal echocardiogram
b. Transthoracic echocardiogram
c. Cardiac catheterization
d. Helical CT
e. D-dimer assay

78. A thin 35-year-old woman presents with a 2-day history of cough. She complains of some mild dyspnea and left-sided pleuritic chest pain. On physical examination, her temperature is 38.5°C (101.4°F) and her respiratory rate is 26 breaths per minute. Her blood pressure is 110/65 mm Hg and her heart rate is 125 beats per minute. Which of the following physical examination findings would most likely be found if she has an uncomplicated left-sided pneumonia?

a. Inspiratory stridor
b. Vesicular breath sounds on the left
c. Absence of egophony on the left
d. Decreased tactile fremitus on the left
e. Increased tactile fremitus on the left

79. A 34-year-old nursing student is referred to your office because of the onset of a recent cough productive of dark-colored sputum. She is febrile but does not appear ill. She has been able to continue working with her symptoms. Examination of the posterior thorax is normal, but there is dullness at the anterior right hemithorax below the fifth rib. Crackles, as well as localized pectoriloquy, are audible over the same area. Which of the following is the most likely diagnosis?

a. Right lower-lobe pneumonia
b. Left lower-lobe pneumonia
c. Right lower-lobe atelectasis
d. Right middle-lobe pneumonia
e. Right upper-lobe pneumonia

80. A 14-year-old adolescent presents with a history of chronic sinusitis and frequent pneumonias. He was born at 38 weeks and had an uneventful delivery. On physical examination, the patient has normal vital signs and is afebrile. He has mild frontal and maxillary sinus tenderness with palpation. Transillumination of the sinuses is normal. Heart sounds are best heard on the right side of the chest. The boy is coughing copious amounts of yellowish sputum. Which of the following is the most likely diagnosis?

a. Cystic fibrosis
b. Kartagener syndrome
c. Bronchopulmonary dysplasia
d. Tuberculosis
e. Pulmonary hypertension

81. A 30-year-old woman presents with the chief complaint of shortness of breath with minimal activity. In retrospect, she feels she has been dyspneic for at least 1 year but has now progressed to the point where she has difficulty climbing stairs and walking short distances. She denies fever, cough, or chest pain. On physical examination, the patient has jugular venous distension (JVD) and a palpable right ventricular lift. On heart auscultation, there is a loud S_2 and a systolic murmur that increases with inspiration. Lungs are clear. There is no clubbing. Which of the following is the most likely diagnosis?

a. Sarcoidosis
b. Coronary heart disease
c. Idiopathic pulmonary fibrosis
d. Primary pulmonary hypertension
e. Systemic lupus erythematosus

82. A 44-year-old obese woman presents with the chief complaint of hemoptysis. She states that over the last day she has coughed up approximately 10 mL of blood-streaked sputum. She denies fever, chills, chest pain, or shortness of breath. She had a recent upper respiratory tract infection with cough and a copious amount of sputum production. She has smoked one pack of cigarettes per day since high school. Examinations of the pharynx and lungs are normal. Which of the following is the most likely diagnosis?

a. Acute bronchitis
b. Tuberculosis
c. Adenocarcinoma of the lung
d. Congestive heart failure
e. Pulmonary infarction

83. A 70-year-old man with a history of smoking since age 14 complains of worsening shortness of breath for the last several days. At baseline he has a dry cough and wheezes daily, but now he is coughing large amounts of yellow-colored sputum and is receiving no relief from his β_2-agonist and ipratropium aerosolized pumps. On physical examination, the patient's respiratory rate is 40 breaths per minute and his heart rate is 110 beats per minute. His blood pressure is 150/85 mm Hg. The patient is afebrile. He is using his accessory muscles of respiration (sternocleidomastoids and intercostals) to assist in breathing. Lung examination reveals diffuse inspiratory and expiratory wheezing with a prolonged expiratory phase. Which of the following is the most likely diagnosis?

a. Acute exacerbation of chronic obstructive pulmonary disease (COPD)
b. α_1-Antitrypsin deficiency
c. Chronic bronchitis
d. Exacerbation of asthma
e. Pneumonia

84. A 53-year-old woman presents with a 4-month history of cough productive of bloody sputum. She denies fever, chills, and night sweats but has occasional flushing that she feels is secondary to menopause. She has had two pneumonias over the last 3 years that required short-term hospitalization. Physical examination reveals wheezing localized to the left midlung field. Chest radiograph is normal. Which of the following is the most appropriate next diagnostic step?

a. Pulmonary function tests
b. Pulmonary angiography
c. Fiberoptic bronchoscopy
d. Ventilation-perfusion scan
e. Video-assisted thoracoscopy

85. A man is stabbed and arrives at the emergency room within 30 minutes. You notice that the trachea is deviated away from the side of the chest with the puncture. The most likely lung finding on physical examination of the traumatized side is which of the following?

a. Increased fremitus
b. Increased breath sounds
c. Dullness to percussion
d. Hyperresonant percussion
e. Wheezing
f. Stridor

86. A 65-year-old man with longstanding emphysema presents with the sudden onset of sharp right-sided chest pain associated with shortness of breath. He denies any history of trauma. On physical examination, the patient is afebrile with a respiratory rate of 28 breaths per minute. His blood pressure is 100/70 mm Hg and his heart rate is 120 beats per minute. Neck examination reveals no tracheal deviation. On lung auscultation, the patient has decreased fremitus, hyperresonance, and diminished breath sounds over the right posterior hemithorax. Which of the following is the most likely diagnosis?

a. Tension pneumothorax
b. Secondary pneumothorax
c. Pulmonary embolus
d. Primary pneumothorax
e. Pneumonia

87. A 41-year-old woman with a past medical history significant for rheumatoid arthritis presents with shortness of breath and dyspnea on exertion. She has right-sided chest pain that worsens with cough and deep breath. Her cough is nonproductive; she denies fever, chills, and night sweats. Physical examination reveals diminished breath sounds halfway down the right posterior hemithorax with an audible pleural rub. Chest radiograph reveals a right-sided pleural effusion. Which of the following is most likely to be seen on thoracentesis?

a. High amylase level
b. High glucose level
c. Bloody fluid
d. High complement levels
e. Cholesterol crystals

88. A 66-year-old man presents with a scanty cough and pleuritic chest pain. He also complains of fever and watery diarrhea. He smokes one pack of cigarettes per day and lives in an apartment building that is undergoing plumbing renovation. He has no past medical history and takes no medications. Physical examination reveals a toxic-appearing man with a temperature of 40°C (104°F). His heart rate is 60 beats per minute. Chest auscultation reveals bilateral scattered crackles. Abdominal examination reveals diffuse tenderness. Laboratory results reveal hyponatremia, hypophosphatemia, elevated liver function tests, and thrombocytopenia. A chest radiograph reveals patchy bilateral infiltrates. Which of the following is the most likely diagnosis in this patient?

a. Pontiac fever
b. Legionnaires disease
c. Influenza
d. Tuberculosis
e. Psittacosis

89. A 37-year-old woman was recently extubated after requiring a ventilator for 10 days for an exacerbation of her asthma. After the uncomplicated extubation, the patient complains of hoarseness and dyspnea. On physical examination, her lungs are clear, with normal fremitus and dullness. There is no tracheal deviation, and heart examination is normal. The patient's chest radiograph is normal. Which of the following is the most likely diagnosis?

a. Oxygen toxicity
b. Premature extubation
c. Hospital-acquired pneumonia
d. Tracheal stenosis
e. Aspiration pneumonia

90. A 41-year-old woman presents to the emergency room after being given naloxone by paramedics for a probable heroin overdose. The paramedics state that the patient began to vomit excessively, and they fear she may have aspirated gastric contents. Physical examination reveals a respiratory rate of 32 breaths per minute, and pulse oximetry reveals a saturation of 82%. The patient appears cyanotic. Lung examination is significant for bilateral crackles. There is no S_3 gallop. Chest radiograph reveals bilateral basilar alveolar infiltrates. The patient is immediately intubated and stabilized. Which of the following is the most appropriate next step in management?

a. High-dose steroids
b. Broad-spectrum antibiotics
c. β-Agonist therapy
d. Intravenous theophylline
e. No other therapy is needed

91. A 23-year-old college student presents to the emergency room unresponsive. He has been depressed at school and may have ingested 20 phenobarbital pills his roommate had for a seizure disorder. Paramedics report that the patient was found in the supine position. Vital signs reveal a blood pressure of 90/50 mm Hg, a heart rate of 54 beats per minute, and a respiratory rate of 10 breaths per minute. Pupils are equally dilated and constrict to light. Lung examination reveals right-sided crackles. Neurologic examination is significant for decreased muscle tone and hyporeflexia. Gag reflex is not tested. You suspect that the patient has aspirated. Which of the following is the most likely lung segment to be affected?

a. Medial segment of the right middle lobe
b. Lateral segment of the right middle lobe
c. Posterior segment of the right upper lobe
d. Apical segment of the right upper lobe
e. Anterior segment of the right upper lobe

92. A 65-year-old man presents with severe right-sided chest pain over several months. He has been a lifelong smoker and worked most of his life as a shipbuilder. On physical examination, the patient appears to be dyspneic at rest. Lung auscultation reveals scattered rhonchi anteriorly and posteriorly. The patient has clubbing. Chest radiograph reveals the lungs to have a ground-glass appearance, and bilateral pleural plaques with some areas of calcification and pleural thickening are evident. Which of the following is the most likely diagnosis?

a. Byssinosis
b. Bagassosis
c. Silicosis
d. Asbestosis
e. Farmer's lung

93. A 45-year-old obese man with a history of hypertension presents with his wife complaining of daytime sleepiness, to the extent that he falls asleep if he sits still for any length of time. His wife reports that he snores very loudly and occasionally even stops breathing for a few seconds, eventually snorting and then resuming his normal breathing pattern. On examination, he has a large neck and centripetal obesity with an elevated blood pressure. He has a pendulous uvula but his heart, lung, and abdominal examinations are normal. What is the most appropriate first step in diagnosing his complaint?

a. Polysomnography
b. Pulmonary function tests
c. Chest radiograph
d. Pulse oximetry
e. Arterial blood gas analysis

94. A 21-year-old college student who lives in an apartment off campus presents with a 2-month history of anterior and posterior cervical lymphadenopathy. He denies recent illness, weight loss, fever, and night sweats. His physical examination reveals scattered nontender 1-cm cervical nodes bilaterally. Lung, heart, and abdominal examinations are normal. His chest radiograph shows bulky hilar lymph nodes with no parenchymal abnormality. Which of the following is the most likely diagnosis?

a. Pneumonia
b. Sarcoidosis
c. Tuberculosis
d. Berylliosis
e. Idiopathic fibrosing interstitial pneumonia

95. A 45-year-old woman with no past medical history presents with a 2-year history of nonproductive cough. The cough is not associated with time of day or year, and the patient denies any occupational or environmental exposures. She has never smoked cigarettes. She finds herself clearing her throat frequently during the day and night. She has no nasal discharge, heartburn, or cardiac symptoms. She denies fever, chest pain, or shortness of breath. She takes no medications. On physical examination, her nasopharynx reveals mucopurulent secretions and a cobblestone-appearing mucosa. Lung examination is normal. Chest radiograph is normal. Which of the following is the most likely diagnosis?

a. Gastroesophageal reflux disease
b. Asthma
c. Bronchitis
d. Postnasal drip
e. Use of angiotensin-converting enzyme (ACE) inhibitors
f. Congestive heart failure

96. A 30-year-old homeless man presents with a 3-month history of left-sided pleuritic chest pain, shortness of breath with exertion, and night sweats. He admits to a 10-lb weight loss over the last several months. He is a nonsmoker and does not use illicit drugs. He reports being heterosexual. He recalls a negative purified protein derivative (PPD) when he was incarcerated 2 years ago. On physical examination, his temperature is 38.3°C (100.9°F) and his respiratory rate is 24 breaths per minute. Lung examination reveals decreased fremitus, dullness to percussion, and diminished breath sounds over the left posterior lung. A pleural friction rub is audible at the left lung base. Which of the following is the most likely diagnosis?

a. Pneumonia
b. Pneumothorax
c. Pleural effusion
d. Lung abscess
e. Pulmonary nodule

97. A 26-year-old woman presents complaining of dyspnea on exertion and bilateral pleuritic chest pain with a recent 30-lb weight loss. On social history she reports occasional intravenous drug use and sex with multiple partners since her teens. On physical examination, heart rate is 124 beats per minute, respiratory rate is 28 breaths per minute, blood pressure is 100/70 mm Hg, and temperature is 39.1°C (102.4°F). Pulse oximetry reveals a saturation of 85% on room air. She has thrush in her mouth and lung auscultation reveals scattered bilateral crackles posteriorly. Chest radiograph reveals bilateral interstitial infiltrates and no cardiomegaly. Which of the following is the most likely diagnosis?

a. Pulmonary edema
b. *Pneumocystis jiroveci* pneumonia
c. Cytomegalovirus pneumonia
d. Kaposi sarcoma
e. Varicella zoster pneumonia

98. An 18-year-old college student presents with a 2-week history of a dry cough. Her symptoms include sore throat at the start of the illness, headache, low-grade fever, and generalized malaise. She is otherwise healthy and does not drink alcohol or smoke cigarettes. Several of her colleagues at school are ill with a similar illness. Physical examination reveals normal vital signs, and lung examination reveals some crackles at the right midaxillary line. Which of the following is the most likely diagnosis?

a. Pneumococcal pneumonia
b. *Mycoplasma* pneumonia
c. Aspiration pneumonia
d. Primary pulmonary hypertension
e. *Legionella* pneumonia

99. A 55-year-old man with emphysema will have which pattern of breathing?

a. Biot respiration
b. Apneustic breathing
c. Cheyne-Stokes respiration
d. Rapid and shallow breathing
e. Kussmaul breathing

100. A 22-year-old man is brought to the emergency room after being found unconscious in a swimming pool. The patient is mildly cyanotic. Blood pressure is 80/50 mm Hg, heart rate is 60 beats per minute, and respiratory rate is 26 breaths per minute. His core body temperature is 31.7°C (89°F). Pupils are 4 mm bilaterally and reactive. The patient is moving all extremities and responds appropriately to questions. Crackles are heard bilaterally on lung auscultation. Pulse oximetry reveals a saturation of 94% on 50% oxygen. Chest radiograph reveals bilateral perihilar infiltrates with a normal-sized heart. Which of the following is the most likely diagnosis?

a. Partial fracture of the C5 vertebral body
b. Subdural frontal hematoma
c. Congestive heart failure
d. Noncardiogenic pulmonary edema
e. Drowning

101. Forty-eight hours after a motor vehicle accident, a 47-year-old man develops restlessness and hypoxemia. He has retinal and conjunctival hemorrhages, and fat is seen in the retinal vessels. A petechial rash is visible in the upper chest and supraclavicular areas. Lung examination reveals bilateral crackles, and chest radiograph shows interstitial bilateral infiltrates. Fat globules are present in the urine. The patient requires immediate endotracheal intubation. Which of the following is the most likely diagnosis?

a. Fat embolism
b. Hospital-acquired pneumonia
c. Mendelson syndrome
d. Cardiac pulmonary edema
e. *Pneumocystis jiroveci* pneumonia

102. A 60-year-old man with an 80-pack-per-year history of cigarette smoking presents to the emergency room complaining of some dyspnea on exertion. He has an asthenic body habitus and pursed-lip breathing. He has an increased anteroposterior thickness of the thorax. Lung examination reveals decreased fremitus, hyperresonance on percussion, and diminished breath sounds. Which of the following signs most indicates respiratory distress signifying possible need for intubation?

a. Pursed-lip breathing
b. Prolonged expiratory phase of breathing
c. Nasal flaring
d. Clubbing
e. Productive cough

103. A 45-year-old alcoholic man with a history of blackouts when intoxicated presents with fever, chills, and cough productive of putrid, foul-smelling sputum. On physical examination the patient appears inebriated. He is febrile with a temperature of 39.5°C (103.2°F). Mouth examination reveals numerous dental caries and poor dental hygiene. Which of the following is the most likely diagnosis?

a. Spontaneous pneumothorax
b. Bronchogenic carcinoma
c. Lung abscess
d. Pleural effusion
e. Community-acquired pneumonia

104. A 53-year-old woman with diabetes and COPD was initially admitted with pyelonephritis and sepsis. On her second day of admission, she complains of significant shortness of breath. The patient is tachypneic with use of accessory muscles and on lung examination has crackles anteriorly and posteriorly. Her cardiac examination is only significant for tachycardia. Arterial blood gas reveals a Po_2 of 50 mm Hg on 100% oxygen. The chest radiograph reveals bilateral whiteout of the lungs, consistent with interstitial and alveolar infiltrates, without cardiomegaly. V/Q scan is read as low probability. Which of the following is the most likely diagnosis?

a. Acute respiratory distress syndrome
b. Hospital-acquired pneumonia
c. Pneumothorax
d. Cardiogenic pulmonary edema
e. Pulmonary embolism

105. A 62-year-old man with a history of cirrhosis presents to the hospital with discomfort due to ascites. While hospitalized he is noted to have an increased alveolar-arterial gradient on room air and upon further discussion admits to baseline shortness of breath over the past few months. What might you expect to find on this patient?

a. Greater dyspnea and deoxygenation when supine
b. Greater dyspnea and deoxygenation when upright
c. Greater dyspnea and deoxygenation when laying on his left side
d. Greater dyspnea and deoxygenation when laying on his right side
e. Complete improvement of his symptoms with paracentesis of his ascitic fluid

106. A 6-year-old boy who had a mild respiratory tract infection for 2 days awakens in the middle of the night with shortness of breath and difficulty breathing, and his parents bring him to the emergency room. His respiratory rate is 36 breaths per minute and his heart rate is 150 beats per minute. He has a prolonged expiratory phase when breathing. He is afebrile. Lung auscultation reveals high-pitched, squeaky, musical breath sounds in all lung fields during inspiration and expiration. Which of the following is the most likely diagnosis?

a. Epiglottitis
b. Asthma
c. Croup
d. Tonsillitis
e. Pneumonia

107. A 26-year-old incoming medical resident develops a positive PPD skin test. The area of induration is 12 cm in diameter at 48 hours. A previous PPD skin test was negative. The patient has no past medical history and does not know of any contact with patients with tuberculosis. She has not received the BCG (extract of *Mycobacterium bovis*) vaccine. She has no fever, chills, night sweats, weight loss, or respiratory symptoms. Her chest x-ray is negative. Which of the following statements is the next best step?

a. She does not have tuberculosis and therefore needs no therapy.
b. She requires a booster purified protein derivative (PPD).
c. She should receive isoniazid chemoprophylaxis.
d. She should have anergy testing.
e. This is likely a false-positive test.

108. A 36-year-old woman complains of frequent headaches accompanied by abdominal pain, nausea, weakness, and palpitations. A mass located in the posterior mediastinum is seen on chest radiograph. Which of the following masses is most likely to be found in this compartment of the mediastinum?

a. Thymoma
b. Teratoma
c. Thyroid adenoma
d. Parathyroid adenoma
e. Bronchogenic cyst
f. Pericardial cyst
g. Pheochromocytoma

109. A 59-year-old patient presents with fever and agitation. On physical examination, his temperature is 39.5°C (103.2°F). His respirations are 26 breaths per minute, pulse is 126 beats per minute, and blood pressure is 100/70 mm Hg. He appears warm and flushed. A Swan-Ganz catheter is inserted that demonstrates increased cardiac output, decreased peripheral vascular resistance, and normal pulmonary capillary wedge pressure (PCWP). The patient's urine Gram stain reveals pyuria and gram-negative rods. Which of the following is the most likely diagnosis?

a. Late septic shock
b. Early septic shock
c. Cardiogenic shock
d. Hypovolemic shock
e. Neurogenic shock

110. A 45-year-old woman presents to the emergency room with altered mental status. On physical examination, her temperature is 38.9°C (102°F), pulse is 120 beats per minute, and respirations are 24 breaths per minute. She has increased fremitus and bronchial breath sounds at the left base. Neurologic examination reveals no focal deficits, but the patient is disoriented to place and time. Chest radiograph confirms the diagnosis of pneumonia. The patient's $PaCO_2$ is 30 mm Hg. Which of the following best categorizes this patient's illness?

a. The patient has bacteremia.
b. The patient has systemic inflammatory response syndrome (SIRS).
c. The patient has multiple-organ dysfunction syndrome (MODS).
d. The patient has severe sepsis.
e. The patient has septic shock.

111. A 28-year-old woman is brought to the emergency room in a coma. Her respiratory rate is 6 breaths per minute and shallow. Blood pressure is 90/60 mm Hg, heart rate is 50 beats per minute, and temperature is 35.5°C (96°F). Her pupils are pinpoint but reactive to light and accommodation. She has no focal neurologic deficits. Which of the following is the most likely diagnosis?

a. Carbon monoxide poisoning
b. Opiate overdose
c. Ethylene glycol poisoning
d. Methanol poisoning
e. Cocaine abuse

112. A 41-year-old man presents to the emergency room complaining of itchiness and difficulty breathing. He states that his symptoms started after attending a party where he ate some fish and peanuts. On physical examination, the patient is anxious, tachypneic, and tachycardic. He has urticaria over his chest, neck, and extremities. Lung examination reveals inspiratory and expiratory wheezes. Heart examination is normal. Which of the following is the most likely diagnosis?

a. Angioedema
b. Exacerbation of asthma
c. Pulmonary embolus
d. Toxic shock syndrome
e. Anaphylaxis

113. A 16-year-old student has recurrent episodes of facial swelling without urticaria. Family history reveals that two siblings and both parents have similar symptoms. Which of the following is the most likely diagnosis?

a. Familial C1 inhibitor deficiency
b. Cystic fibrosis
c. Exacerbation of asthma
d. Acquired C1 inhibitor deficiency
e. Serum sickness

114. A 6-year-old girl with spina bifida is admitted to the intensive care unit because of rapidly progressive swelling of her lips, wheezing, and stridor. She had been playing with balloons at a birthday party. Which of the following is the most likely diagnosis?

a. Food anaphylaxis
b. Latex anaphylaxis
c. Severe drug allergy
d. Exercise-related anaphylaxis
e. Idiopathic anaphylaxis

115. A 22-year-old man develops shortness of breath and difficulty breathing while mountain climbing at an altitude of 12,000 ft. His temperature is 36.1°C (97°F). He has a blood pressure of 120/80 mm Hg, respirations of 24 breaths per minute, and a heart rate of 114 beats per minute. He has retinal hemorrhages on funduscopy examination. He has no heart murmur. Bilateral crackles are audible on lung examination. Which of the following is the most likely diagnosis?

a. Carbon monoxide poisoning
b. Acute mountain sickness
c. Hypothermia
d. Exhaustion
e. Dehydration

116. Paramedics bring a 41-year-old man to the emergency room. He is complaining of headache, dizziness, nausea, and abdominal pain. The paramedics state that the patient's apartment has a coal furnace. His blood pressure is 110/70 mm Hg, respirations are 20 breaths per minute, and pulse is 100 beats per minute. The patient has a cherry-red appearance most noticeable around the lips and nail beds. Neurologic examination reveals a disoriented and confused man without focal deficits. Oxygen saturation by pulse oximetry is normal. Which of the following is the most likely diagnosis?

a. Drug overdose
b. Carbon monoxide poisoning
c. Alcohol intoxication
d. Methemoglobinemia
e. Dysbarism

Questions 117 and 118

For each chest description, select the appropriate skeletal deformity. Each lettered option may be used once, multiple times, or not at all.

a. Pectus excavatum
b. Kyphosis
c. Barrel chest
d. Pectus carinatum
e. Lordosis

117. A 4-year-old boy has a marked depression of the sternum below the clavicular-manubrial junction.

118. A 9-year-old girl has a chest deformity in which the sternum protrudes from the thorax.

Questions 119 and 120

For each patient with a sleep disturbance, select the most appropriate disorder. Each lettered option may be used once, multiple times, or not at all.

a. Narcolepsy
b. Depression
c. Obstructive sleep apnea syndrome
d. Obesity hypoventilation syndrome
e. Cataplexy
f. Somnambulism

119. A 35-year-old man complains of daytime sleepiness and disruptive snoring. He admits to falling asleep several times a day while at work. He does not smoke. He is 72 in tall and weighs approximately 210 lb.

120. A morbidly obese woman is admitted to the intensive care unit after being found in bed with lethargy, cyanosis, and hypoxemia.

Questions 121 to 123

For each patient with a specific breath odor, select the most likely etiology. Each lettered option may be used once, multiple times, or not at all.

a. Diabetic ketoacidosis
b. Cyanide poisoning
c. Marijuana use
d. Mercaptan poisoning
e. Arsenic poisoning
f. Naphthalene ingestion

121. A 30-year-old man presents to the emergency room with headache, dizziness, abdominal pain, nausea, vomiting, and confusion. The odor of bitter almonds is detected on his breath. Venous oxygen saturation is more than 90%.

122. A 19-year-old college student is brought to the emergency room by ambulance. She has no past medical history and takes no medications. She does not smoke cigarettes, drink alcohol, or use illicit drugs. She is unresponsive and hyperpneic. Her breath has a fruity odor.

123. A 44-year-old factory worker presents with a 12-hour history of abdominal pain, vomiting, watery diarrhea, and muscle cramps. An odor of garlic is detected on his breath. He has diminished vibration sensation of the lower extremities.

Pulmonary/Critical Care

Answers

72. The answer is e. *(McPhee, p 240.)* **Bronchiectasis** is an acquired disease that causes abnormal dilatation of the bronchi leading to pooling of secretions in the airways and recurrent infections. Patients typically present with cough productive of purulent sputum, shortness of breath, and pleuritic chest pain. Lung auscultation may be normal or remarkable for wheezes, rhonchi, or crackles at the lung bases. Chest radiograph may be normal, but occasionally the damaged, dilated airways will appear as **tram tracks** or **ring shadows**. Bronchiectasis may be a sequela of foreign body aspiration, cystic fibrosis, rheumatic diseases (rheumatoid arthritis, Sjögren disease), recurrent pulmonary infections (tuberculosis, pertussis, *Mycoplasma*), AIDS, or allergic bronchopulmonary aspergillosis (ABPA). **Chronic bronchitis** and **emphysema** are both forms of **chronic obstructive pulmonary disease (COPD)** resulting from cigarette smoking, which this patient denies. Patients with chronic bronchitis have a daily productive cough for at least 3 months in 2 or more years in a row, while those with emphysema complain of shortness of breath and wheezing due to alveolar destruction. Patients with **asthma** have chronic inflammation of the airways and usually present with expiratory wheezing, shortness of breath and dry cough that are often worse at night or exacerbated by allergens or exercise. **Cystic fibrosis** is a fatal autosomal recessive disorder most often affecting Caucasians and resulting from abnormal membrane chloride transport which leads to impaired mucocilliary function. Patients manifest with recurrent episodes of bronchitis and pneumonia and pancreatic insufficiency with steatorrhea, among other symptoms.

73. The answer is a. *(McPhee, pp 248-249.)* The patient has been in the hospital for more than 48 hours and has developed a **hospital-acquired pneumonia**. Patients develop fever, leukocytosis, cough productive of purulent sputum, and a new or progressive infiltrate on chest radiograph.

The most likely organisms are *P aeruginosa*, *Staphylococcus aureus* (often methicillin resistant), *Enterobacter*, *Klebsiella pneumoniae*, and *Escherichia coli*. The other answer choices are usually etiologies of pulmonary infection on presentation to the hospital, rather than acquired during hospitalization.

74. The answer is d. (*Simel, pp 561-575.*) Pulmonary embolism (PE) occurs in 1 to 2 persons per 1000 annually in the United States. Most patients who have a PE present with risk factors for hypercoagulability (pregnancy, use of oral contraceptives, family or personal history of clotting, prolonged immobility), pleuritic chest pain, dyspnea, and occasionally hemoptysis. On examination patients will be hypoxic, tachypneic, and tachycardic with an accentuated pulmonary component (P_2) of the second heart sound (S_2) due to pulmonary hypertension. A clinician's pretest probability greatly impacts the prevalence of PEs. The simplified Wells scoring system is one model that can be used to assess pretest probability (see scoring system below). This patient does take oral contraceptives and smokes, which puts her at risk for a PE, but she has no other risk factors or clinical signs and more likely has viral pleuritis, giving her a **Wells score of zero. If pretest probability is low, as in this patient, a negative D-dimer assay helps reliably exclude PE, eliminating needless anticoagulation therapy.** If she had unilateral lower extremity edema suggesting a DVT, a **Doppler ultrasound** would be a good choice, and a **spiral CT or V/Q scan** would confirm the presence of a PE in someone with a higher pretest probability. A **chest x-ray** is best used to rule out other causes such as pneumonia or rib fracture, as a wedge-shaped pulmonary infarct accompanying a PE is fairly uncommon.

SIMPLIFIED WELLS SCORING

System	Score
Clinical signs/symptoms of DVT (leg swelling)	3.0
No alternative diagnosis more likely than PE	3.0
Heart rate > 100 bpm	1.5
Immobilization or surgery in last 4 weeks	1.5
History of DVT or PE	1.5
Hemoptysis	1.0
Cancer treated within last 6 months	1.0

Wells score is a sum of the predictor variables. Score < 2 is low; 2 to 6 is moderate; > 6 is high.

75. The answer is a. *(Fauci, p 1648.)* This patient has **cryptogenic organizing pneumonitis, also known as idiopathic bronchiolitis obliterans with organizing pneumonia (BOOP)**. Usually, patients present with an acute flu-like illness followed by exertional dyspnea. On examination there are inspiratory crackles and hypoxemia with a restrictive defect on pulmonary function tests. Chest x-ray reveals alveolar opacities and high-resolution CT shows air-space consolidation, nodular and ground glass opacities, and bronchial wall thickening and dilation, primarily in the lower lung and periphery. Correct diagnosis of patients with **allergic bronchopulmonary aspergillosis (ABPA)** is almost assured if the first six of these seven criteria are present: a history of asthma, peripheral eosinophilia, elevated serum IgE levels, skin reactivity to *Aspergillus* antigen, precipitating antibodies to *Aspergillus* antigen, a chest radiograph showing transient or fixed infiltrates, and central bronchiectasis. Patients with **pulmonary sarcoidosis** present with malaise and dyspnea and chest x-ray reveals hilar adenopathy, parenchymal involvement, or a combination of the two. **Wegener granulomatosis** typically involves the upper airways (ie, nasal ulcers, sinus infections), lungs, joints, and kidneys, with positive antineutrophil cytoplasmic antibodies (c-ANCA). **Goodpasture syndrome** causes glomerulonephritis and pulmonary hemorrhage, and patients have antibodies to renal and lung alveolar basement membranes.

76. The answer is e. *(McPhee, p 1421.)* The tongue may fall posteriorly to obstruct the oropharynx and is the major cause of airway obstruction. This may occur in patients with a decreased level of consciousness and may be corrected by utilizing the **head tilt–chin lift maneuver.** All of the other answer options may be appropriate after first securing the airway.

77. The answer is d. *(McPhee, pp 266-273.)* This patient has several symptoms (shortness of breath and pleuritic chest pain, in the setting of cancer) and signs (tachypnea, tachycardia, lower extremity edema, increased alveolar-arterial gradient, loud S_2) suspicious for **pulmonary embolus (PE)**. A deep venous thrombosis (DVT) in the lower extremities is the most common source of PE. Common settings for PE include malignancy, prolonged immobilization, sedentary lifestyle, use of oral contraceptives, obesity, recent surgery, burns, severe trauma, congestive heart failure, pregnancy, sickle cell anemia, polycythemias, inherited deficiencies of the anticoagulating proteins (protein C, protein S, antithrombin III), and the Factor V Leiden

V mutation. This patient's Wells score is 8.5, representing **high pretest probability**. The best next step in making the diagnosis, of the options given, would be to order a **helical CT, which has become the initial diagnostic test of choice for PE and is comparable to the ventilation-perfusion (V/Q) scan**. A normal helical CT, in the setting of a high pretest probability, should be followed by further studies, such as pulmonary arteriogram or venous ultrasonography of the lower extremity. **Chest radiograph** in PE may be normal but may demonstrate a peripheral wedge-shaped density above the diaphragm **(Hampton hump)**, focal oligemia **(Westermark sign)**, or abrupt occlusion of a vessel **(cutoff sign)**. A **D-dimer assay** is only helpful in ruling out a PE in a low-probability clinical setting, while this patient is at high risk. If the patient was too unstable to be scanned, a bedside **transthoracic echocardiogram** might confirm increased pulmonary pressures, though a **cardiac catheterization and transesophageal echocardiogram** would not be helpful in diagnosing a PE.

78. The answer is e. *(Seidel, p 400.)* The patient described most likely has **community-acquired pneumonia (CAP)** due to *Streptococcus pneumoniae*. Other pathogens responsible for CAP include *M pneumoniae*, viruses, and *C pneumoniae*. In smokers, even without documented chronic lung disease, *Haemophilus influenzae* must be considered. On examination, patients with consolidation from pneumonia have **dullness to percussion and increased tactile fremitus** (vibrations that are perceived on palpation). On auscultation, instead of normal vesicular breath sounds, patients often have **bronchial breath sounds** (like breathing through a straw, normally heard only over the trachea) and **inspiratory crackles**, as well as other findings like **bronchophony** (sounds like "99" are louder and clearer), **egophony** (long "e" perceived as short "a," like a goat bleating), and **whispered pectoriloquy** (whispered sounds are louder and clearer). Areas of atelectasis or pleural effusion have dullness to percussion with decreased tactile fremitus. Patients with an obstructed airway develop stridor, a high-pitched inspiratory sound.

79. The answer is d. *(Seidel, p 372.)* The best areas to listen for **right middle lobe** findings would be (1) the right anterior midclavicular line between the fifth and sixth ribs and (2) the right midaxillary line between the fourth and sixth ribs. The right middle lobe is not heard posteriorly, and the lung examination is incomplete if the physician does not listen anteriorly or medially.

80. The answer is b. *(Fauci, p 1629.)* This patient has **Kartagener's syndrome**, due to a defect that causes the cilia within the respiratory tract epithelium to become immotile, thereby predisposing patients to frequent pneumonias. Patients also have **situs inversus, chronic sinusitis (with the formation of nasal polyps), and bronchiectasis**. Cilia of the sperm are also affected, thereby rendering **most males infertile**. While **cystic fibrosis** can lead to pneumonias and infertility in adolescents as well, sinusitis is less likely and it is not associated with situs inversus. The patient does not have an accentuated P_2 as seen in **pulmonary hypertension** and does not present with fever, night sweats, or other signs or symptoms of **tuberculosis**. **Bronchopulmonary dysplasia** is a chronic lung disease that develops in preterm neonates treated with oxygen and mechanical ventilation; patients have lung scarring and recurrent infections early in life.

81. The answer is d. *(McPhee, pp 273-275.)* **Primary pulmonary hypertension (PPH)** is of unknown etiology and primarily affects women in their thirties or forties. The underlying problem in the disorder is a fixed increased resistance to pulmonary blood flow. Pulmonary function in PPH is usually normal, but the elevation in pulmonary artery pressure causes a decrease in cardiac output and eventually right ventricular failure. Patients become dyspneic and hypoxemic due to the mismatch of pulmonary ventilation and perfusion and the reduced cardiac output. Physical examination, as in this patient, reveals signs of right ventricular hypertrophy, right- and left-sided heart failure, and tricuspid and pulmonic regurgitation. The mean survival for this disease is 2 to 3 years from the time of diagnosis. **Coronary artery disease** may present with dyspnea on exertion, but would be unlikely in a young female and this, as well as **sarcoidosis and systemic lupus erythematosus,** would not cause the described physical findings of pulmonary hypertension and right ventricular failure. Patients with **idiopathic pulmonary fibrosis** have dry crackles on examination and may also have clubbing.

82. The answer is a. *(McPhee, p 27.)* Massive **life-threatening hemoptysis** is more than 200 mL of blood in 24 hours. The most common cause for nonmassive hemoptysis (< 30 mL/d) in smokers and nonsmoking patients with a normal chest radiograph is **acute or chronic bronchitis**. While all of the other diagnoses may cause hemoptysis, it is more likely that this patient has **acute bronchitis** with cough productive of bloody sputum.

She has no associated fever or night sweats usually seen in **TB,** she has never smoked (diminishing her risk for **adenocarcinoma** of the lung at such a young age) and is less likely to have a **pulmonary infarction**. Patients with **CHF** often present with rose-colored frothy sputum rather than gross blood.

83. The answer is a. *(McPhee, p 234-236.)* This patient has an exacerbation of **chronic obstructive pulmonary disease (COPD)**, a condition in which there is chronic obstruction to airflow due to chronic bronchitis or emphysema. This patient appears to have baseline **emphysema**, with chronic cough, dyspnea, and wheezing. An exacerbation of COPD occurs when the patient develops the acute onset of marked dyspnea and tachypnea due to airflow obstruction, requiring the use of accessory muscles. Often patients are unresponsive to their home medication regimen and may require antibiotics for a superimposed infection. **Chronic bronchitis** is characterized by excessive secretions manifested by a productive cough, often purulent or bloody, for 3 months or more for 2 consecutive years in the absence of any other disease to explain the symptoms. Patients are often obese and cyanotic **(blue bloater)**. The mnemonic is **BBB** = **B**ronchitis/**B**lue **B**loater. While this patient could have a **pneumonia** complicating his underlying COPD, he does not have fever or other signs of an infiltrate on exam. **Asthma** manifests much earlier in life and usually results in a dry cough and wheezing, as opposed to this presentation. **α_1-antitrypsin deficiency** should be suspected in nonsmokers who present with **COPD of the lung bases** in their fifties without any predisposing history, such as occupational exposure, to support the diagnosis. α_1-Antitrypsin deficiency is rare in African Americans and Asian–Pacific Islanders.

84. The answer is c. *(McPhee, p 261.)* **Carcinoid and bronchial gland tumors** are called **bronchial adenomas** but are actually low-grade malignant neoplasms. They are resistant to radiation and chemotherapy. Patients present usually before the age of 60 years; common symptoms include hemoptysis, chronic cough, focal wheezing, and recurrent pneumonia (due to obstruction and atelectasis). The chest radiograph may be normal. The classic presentation of flushing, diarrhea, wheezing, and hypotension **(carcinoid syndrome)** is rare. These tumors are **centrally located,** and **fiberoptic bronchoscopy** will offer tissue diagnosis of a tumor in a central airway. CT scanning and octreotide scintigraphy also may help to localize the lesion. **Video-assisted thoracoscopy** is useful for diagnosis of lung cancers and pleural diseases, but bronchoscopy in this case is a better choice for a central lesion. Though she is wheezing, **pulmonary function tests** would likely not help as her symptoms are localized to the left mid-lung. Her presentation is not consistent with a PE, thus **angiography** or a **V/Q scan** is unnecessary.

85. The answer is d. *(McPhee, p 286.)* The patient has a **tension pneumothorax**, as evidenced by the **trachea deviating away from the side of the traumatized lung**. This occurs secondary to trauma or during mechanical ventilation. **Breath sounds will be faint or distant, percussion will be hyperresonant, and fremitus will be decreased**. The increased air on the affected side is in the pleural space, not in the lung. As an attempt is made to inflate the lung, air moves into the pleural space from the puncture site, resulting in a collapsed lung with a large pleural space. The contralateral lung is also at risk for collapse. Anytime the trachea is deviated from the involved side, it is considered a medical emergency and the tension pneumothorax must be relieved or the patient will die from hypoxemia or inadequate cardiac output.

86. The answer is b. *(Tierney, p 299.)* The patient most likely has a **secondary spontaneous pneumothorax, likely due to ruptured blebs resulting from his emphysema**. Patients with COPD, cystic fibrosis, *Pneumocystis jiroveci* pneumonia (PCP), and tuberculosis may have blebs and are at risk for secondary pneumothoraxes. **Primary pneumothorax** affects tall, thin men and may be recurrent. It is thought to be due to the rupture of subpleural blebs in response to high negative intrapleural pressures. In a patient with a pneumothorax, physical examination often reveals unilateral chest expansion, decreased fremitus, hyperresonance, and diminished breath sounds. This patient's presentation is not consistent with **tension pneumothorax**, which often results from trauma and leads to tracheal deviation to the opposite side, **pneumonia** (which would cause fever and increased fremitus on examination) or **pulmonary embolism**.

87. The answer is e. *(McPhee, p 284.)* The pleural effusion of **rheumatoid arthritis** is **exudative** with a high lactate dehydrogenase, low complement level, **low glucose level**, high rheumatoid factor, and characteristic **cholesterol crystals**. The fluid is usually **greenish-yellow** in color, not grossly bloody (as seen with pulmonary infarction and with malignancy). Malignancy and infections may present with low glucose as well. Pancreatitis and esophageal rupture produce pleural effusions that have elevated amylase levels; these effusions are typically left-sided. On physical exam, patients with pleural effusions have dullness to percussion, decreased breath sounds and decreased tactile fremitus over the effusion, with bronchial breath sounds and increased fremitus immediately above the pleural effusion.

88. The answer is b. *(Fauci, pp 929-932.)* The clinical presentation of **pulmonary and gastrointestinal complaints** is most consistent with **legionnaires disease (*Legionella* pneumonia)**. Patients are usually elderly, immunocompromised, or have chronic lung disease. Air conditioners, whirlpools, water-using machinery, and cooling towers have been linked to outbreaks of the disease. Clinical symptoms and signs of the disease include **ubiquitous high fever above 40 degrees celsius, bradycardia relative to the fever, abdominal complaints (diarrhea in up to half of cases and nausea and vomiting as well), scanty cough that is occasionally blood-streaked, and laboratory abnormalities such as hyponatremia, elevated liver function tests and elevated creatine phosphokinase**. **Pontiac fever** is an acute, self-limited, flu-like illness due to *Legionella,* but it does not cause pneumonia. **Psittacosis** *(Chlamydia)* is pneumonia associated with the handling of birds. **Tuberculosis** can present with fever and hemoptysis and **influenza** causes fever and occasional pulmonary and GI symptoms, but neither cause the constellation of findings in this case.

89. The answer is d. *(McPhee, p 215.)* **Tracheal stenosis** may occur days to months after intubation and is a sequela of the balloon cuff of the tracheal tube pressing against the tracheal wall, causing necrosis and scar tissue formation. Patients are typically hoarse and dyspneic, with an inability to effectively clear secretions, increasing risk for pneumonia and respiratory failure. She does not have signs of a **pneumonia,** with clear lungs, and neither **oxygen toxicity** nor **premature extubation** would result in hoarseness.

90. The answer is e. *(McPhee, p 278.)* The patient most likely has **Mendelson syndrome (acute aspiration of gastric contents), which leads to a chemical pneumonitis and potentially acute respiratory distress syndrome (ARDS)** due to extensive desquamation of the bronchial epithelium with subsequent pulmonary edema. Patients cough, wheeze, and have fever and tachypnea, with crackles at the lung bases and possible hypoxemia. There is no evidence to support the use of antibiotics or high-dose steroids. **Treatment consists of supplemental oxygen and other supportive measures.**

91. The answer is c. *(Fauci, p 1002.)* The right main stem bronchus is wider, shorter, and vertically placed, and therefore, if the patient aspirates while supine, the **posterior segment of the right upper lobe as well as** the **superior segments of both lower lobes** are anatomically susceptible to aspiration. These three segments are often referred to as the **aspiration segments of the lung**. The **basilar segments of the lower lobes of both lungs** are susceptible to **aspiration if the patient aspirates while erect or sitting up**.

92. The answer is d. *(McPhee, p 279.)* Persons in certain occupations, such as asbestos mining, shipbuilding, construction, insulation, pipe fitting, plumbing, electrical repair, and railroad engine repair are at risk for **asbestos** exposure. Even persons handling the clothes of the person exposed to asbestos are at risk for asbestosis (bystander exposure). Patients with asbestosis present 15 years or more after exposure with increasing dyspnea, inspiratory crackles, and even cyanosis. On chest radiographs, patients have bilateral nodular interstitial pulmonary fibrosis with **honeycomb changes, as well as characteristic calcified pleural plaques**. Patients with asbestosis are at risk not only for lung cancer and **mesothelioma** but also for pharyngeal, gastric, and colon cancers. This patient has clubbing, and malignancy must be considered. **Farmer's lung** results from exposure to moldy hay containing spores. **Bagassosis** is a hypersensitivity pneumonitis from exposure to moldy sugarcane. Patients who work as miners, sandblasters, stonecutters, or foundry or quarry workers are at risk for exposure to **silica**. The chest x-ray typically reveals eggshell calcification of the hilar nodes. **Byssinosis** occurs with exposure to cotton, flax, or hemp.

93. The answer is a. *(McPhee, pp 288-289.)* This obese patient with daytime somnolence and witnessed snoring and apneic episodes has **obstructive sleep apnea**. Large neck circumference has specifically been linked to this disorder in which the pharynx collapses during inspiration in sleep. The first step to diagnosing this problem is an overnight sleep study or **polysomnography** which will reveal the apneic episodes in which oxygen saturation precipitously falls. Treatment includes significant weight loss and **continuous positive airway pressure (CPAP)**, but compliance is poor. None of the other tests listed would help diagnose sleep apnea. **Pulmonary function tests** would be used to diagnose an obstructive or restrictive pulmonary defect, a **chest radiograph** would be used to rule out pulmonary pathology and a **pulse oximetry or arterial blood gas** would determine whether the patient is oxygenating well.

94. The answer is b. *(McPhee, pp 265-266.)* **Sarcoidosis** is a multisystemic disease of unknown cause. The histologic hallmark of the disease is noncaseating granulomas, and staging is based on chest radiograph findings: bilateral hilar adenopathy alone (stage I), hilar adenopathy with parenchymal reticular or nodular infiltrates (stage II), and parenchymal infiltrates alone (stage III). Lymphadenopathy is found in 70% to 90% of all patients with sarcoidosis. **Pulmonary tuberculosis** is common in immunocompromised patients and those who have been homeless, incarcerated, or in close proximity to an infected person. Patients present with fever, weight loss, night sweats, and cough, often productive of hemoptysis, with infiltrates and lymphadenopathy on chest x-rays. **Berylliosis** causes bilateral hilar adenopathy as well. Patients have a history of occupational exposure to nuclear weapons, fluorescent lights, and ceramics. **Idiopathic fibrosing interstitial pneumonia (formerly known as idiopathic pulmonary fibrosis, or IPF)**. It is the most common interstitial lung disease and the usual age of onset is the fifth or sixth decade of life. Chest radiograph usually reveals fibrosis and there is restrictive physiology on pulmonary function tests. This patient does not have symptoms or signs of **pneumonia**.

95. The answer is d. *(McPhee, p 22.)* The most common causes of chronic, noninfectious cough in adults are **postnasal drip** due to sinusitis or rhinitis (allergic, vasomotor, irritant, perennial nonallergic), **asthma, and gastroesophageal reflux disease (GERD)**. Patients with postnasal drip typically complain of having to clear the throat or a feeling of something dripping in the back of the throat. Physical examination reveals mucopurulent secretions and a **cobblestone** appearance of the mucosa. **Asthma** is more of an episodic disease with wheezing, but occasionally patients complain of only cough. **GERD** must be considered in patients who complain of heartburn or regurgitation. Other causes of chronic cough include bronchitis, postinfectious cough, congestive heart failure, and use of ACE inhibitors (but this patient takes no medications).

96. The answer is c. *(Seidel, p 403.)* This patient has a **pleural effusion** most likely due to tuberculosis. Chest examination of a pleural effusion reveals **distant or absent breath sounds, a pleural friction rub, decreased fremitus, and flatness to percussion**. A pleural friction rub is a raspy, grating sound heard in both inspiration and expiration due to inflamed surfaces rubbing against each other. Occasionally, exaggerated bronchial breath sounds are audible at the edge of the effusion. In **pneumonia,** there is increased fremitus over the infiltrate and there is hyperresonance over the area affected by a **pneumothorax.**

97. The answer is b. *(Fauci, p 1172.)* Based on the patient's risk factors for human immunodeficiency virus (HIV), ***P jiroveci* (formerly *P carinii*) pneumonia (PCP)** is the most likely diagnosis in this patient, but PCP rarely presents with any physical examination findings that distinguish it from other pneumonias. The chest radiograph may reveal **bilateral interstitial infiltrates**, and patients are often **hypoxemic**. **Congestive heart failure** may present with a similar chest radiograph, but patients will have jugular venous distension (JVD) and an S_3 gallop. **Cytomegalovirus** (CMV), **varicella zoster**, and **Kaposi sarcoma** (due to herpesvirus type 8) are other opportunistic infections seen in immunocompromised patients.

98. The answer is b. *(Fauci, pp 1068-1069.)* In young, otherwise healthy patients who present with a localized pneumonia (in this case, right middle lobe) of gradual onset accompanied by dry cough and a predominance of extrapulmonary symptoms (ie, malaise, headache, diarrhea), the most likely diagnosis is atypical pneumonia due to ***C pneumoniae* or *M pneumoniae*.** Patients often complain of a sore throat at the beginning of the illness and a protracted course of symptoms. Physical examination is often unimpressive compared to radiograph findings and the diagnosis is often not made as the course is often indistinguishable from other lower respiratory infections. **Pneumococcal pneumonia** is abrupt in onset, with fever, pleuritic chest pain, and purulent sputum production. ***L pneumoniae*** is an atypical organism, but patients usually have renal and hepatic abnormalities, hyponatremia, and mental status changes. This patient does not give a history to put her at risk for **aspiration** and has no symptoms or physical findings consistent with **pulmonary hypertension**.

99. The answer is d. *(Seidel, p 375.)* In emphysema, there is destruction of alveolar septa and reduced elastic recoil. This causes collapse of the small airways and prolongs the expiratory phase of respiration. During the prolonged expiration, patients will have **rapid and shallow breathing** and **purse their lips** to avoid collapse of the small airways **(this causes auto–positive end-expiratory pressure [auto-PEEP])**. The respiratory rate is increased by having a markedly shortened inspiratory interval. **Kussmaul respirations** are fast and deep respirations to increase the tidal volume and combat the metabolic acidosis seen in patients with diabetic ketoacidosis. **Biot respirations**, seen in patients with increased intracranial pressure, are irregular, unpredictable periods of apnea alternating with periods of noisy hyperventilation. **Cheyne-Stokes respiration** is a rhythmic, gradually changing pattern of apnea and hyperpnea that is cardiac or neurologic in origin. **Apneustic breathing** is characterized by a long period of inspiration or gasping with almost no expiratory phase.

100. The answer is d. *(McPhee, pp 1415-1416.)* The definition of **drowning** is death from suffocation after submersion. Freshwater drowning in swimming pools is actually more common than saltwater drowning. The patient described has **noncardiogenic pulmonary edema,** which is a complication of **near drowning** (survival after suffocation from submersion). This is a result of direct pulmonary injury, loss of surfactant, and contaminants in the water. Respiratory failure, severe hypothermia, and neurologic injury are the three most common threats to life after submersion.

101. The answer is a. *(Fauci, p 2517.)* Patients with severe long bone injuries are at risk for developing widespread **fat embolism syndrome**. Several days after the trauma, patients develop restlessness, hypoxemia, delirium, seizures, retinal and conjunctival hemorrhages, visible fat in the retinal vessels, a petechial chest rash, bilateral interstitial infiltrates, fat globules in the urine, and renal failure. There is no treatment for fat embolism other than supportive care and early diagnosis. Even though the patient has new lung infiltrates while hospitalized, his presentation makes fat embolism far more likely. He has no signs of congestive heart failure and we have no reason to suspect PCP in this patient presenting after a traumatic accident. Mendelsons syndrome is a chemical pneumonitis resulting from aspiration while under anesthesia.

102. The answer is c. *(Fauci, p 1640.)* Patients with emphysema or chronic bronchitis at baseline often have a thin body habitus due to caloric expenditure in excess of intake, increased anteroposterior thickness of the thorax **(barrel chest)**, **clubbing**, **productive cough**, and often employ **pursed-lip breathing** to prolong the expiratory phase of respiration and prevent sudden collapse of the small airways. When these patients have an exacerbation severe enough to warrant possible intubation, they often use **accessory muscles of respiration, assume a "tripod" position** to facilitate the movement of these muscles and may display **nasal flaring and cyanosis** as well.

103. The answer is c. *(McPhee, p 250.)* A **lung abscess** is a thick-walled cavity surrounded by consolidation, usually presenting with an air-fluid level on imaging. Periodontal disease and a history of aspiration, often as a result of loss of consciousness due to seizure, alcoholism, or illicit drug use, predispose to this anaerobic infection. Patients complain of several days or weeks of malaise and fever and eventually develop chills, cough, pleuritic chest pain, and cough productive of putrid sputum. Due to position at the time of loss of consciousness and to the anatomy of the lung, the lung segments most often involved in lung abscesses include **the posterior segment of the right upper lobe** (wide, short, and vertically placed) and the **superior segments of both lower lobes.** The next most likely cause would be a community-acquired pneumonia, but this patient's presentation is not consistent with a plural effusion, lung cancer, or a pneumothorax.

104. The answer is a. *(McPhee, pp 291-293.)* **Acute respiratory distress syndrome (ARDS)** is the most severe form of acute lung injury and leads to acute respiratory failure. One-third of patients present with sepsis, as with this patient, but other risk factors include aspiration, burns, multiple transfusions, near-drowning, and shock. ARDS is due to severe and widespread increased alveolar capillary permeability secondary to injury of the alveolar and capillary epithelium. This leads to the accumulation of protein-rich edematous fluid within the septal walls, followed by escape of the fluid into the alveolar spaces, where it coagulates to form hyaline membranes lining the alveoli. There is marked impairment of gas exchange that causes severe dyspnea, diffuse crackles, tachypnea, hypoxemia, and cyanosis. The cyanosis may be refractory to oxygen therapy. Chest radiograph reveals bilateral infiltrates. This patient's presentation is not typical for **hospital-acquired pneumonia** which occurs at least 48 hours after admission and is usually due to gram-negative pathogens and *S. aureus*. In addition, she does not have evidence of volume overload due to **cardiogenic edema** and does not likely have a **pulmonary embolism** as her V/Q scan is low probability in the setting of, at most, moderate pretest probability.

105. The answer is b. *(McPhee, p 623.)* This patient with cirrhosis has developed the **hepatopulmonary syndrome**, which is a triad of liver disease, intrapulmonary vascular dilations, and increased alveolar-arterial oxygen gradient on room air. While paracentesis will likely improve his symptomatic shortness of breath, it will not address this problem. Patients with this syndrome often have **greater dyspnea (platypnea) and hemoglobin oxygen desaturation in the upright position (orthodeoxia).** An upright position increases perfusion to the lower lobes and worsens V/Q matching.

106. The answer is b. *(McPhee, pp 216-221.)* **Asthma** is an airway disease characterized by a hyperreactive tracheobronchial tree that manifests physiologically as narrowing of the airway passages. **The classic triad of symptoms is dyspnea, cough, and wheezing.** Attacks are usually episodic, may be nocturnal, and often follow exposure to specific allergens, exertion, viral infection, or emotional excitement. Wheezing is described as whistling and is typically an expiratory sound, but may be heard in both inspiration and expiration when severe. The expiratory phase becomes prolonged, and the patient develops tachypnea, tachycardia, and mild systolic hypertension. Accessory muscles of respiration (sternocleidomastoid and intercostals) may be used to improve breathing. If the asthma attack is severe, the patient will develop a **pulsus paradoxus** (an inspiratory drop in systolic blood pressure of more than 10 mm Hg). Patients with **epiglottitis** present with fever, drooling, and dysphagia; lung examination will be normal. Children with **croup** or **laryngotracheobronchitis** present with labored breathing and stridor and use accessory muscles to assist breathing. Children with **tonsillitis** have erythematous, exudative tonsils and are febrile. Those with **pneumonia** present with fever and findings of an infiltrate (increased tactile fremitus, dullness to percussion).

107. The answer is c. *(McPhee, pp 253-254.)* **Health-care workers with a positive (≥ 10 mm) PPD require chemoprophylaxis**, optimally with isoniazid for 9 months. Alternative regimens include a combination of rifampin and pyrazinamide or, if the other drugs are not well-tolerated, rifampin alone. A positive PPD may mean that the patient currently has tuberculosis or may have had tuberculosis in the past. The immune response to a PPD develops up to 10 weeks after tuberculosis infection. A PPD may be a falsely positive due to nontuberculosis *Mycobacterium*. For those over age 55 with a negative test, another PPD is placed 1 week later to boost a response. A negative boost implies the patient is anergic or uninfected. **Anergy testing** is poorly effective and was done in the past to distinguish a true-negative PPD from anergy.

A PPD skin test is classified as positive by the American Thoracic Society and the Centers for Disease Control and Prevention (1995) according to the reaction size and patient population:

≥5 mm: HIV patients or HIV at-risk patients; close contacts of patients with active TB; persons with CXR showing healed TB

≥10 mm: Immigrants; intravenous drug abusers; patients with underlying medical conditions increasing the risk for TB like diabetes and chronic kidney disease; residents and employees of health-care facilities, nursing homes, prisons, and mental institutions

≥15 mm: All other persons

108. The answer is g. *(McPhee, p 261.)* The area between the pleural sacs—the mediastinum—is divided anatomically into the anterior mediastinum, middle mediastinum, and posterior mediastinum. The most common masses found in the **anterior mediastinum** are the **four Ts** = Thymomas, Teratomas, Thyroid masses, and paraThyroid masses. Lymphomas may also be found in the anterior mediastinum. Masses in the **middle mediastinum** include enlarged lymph nodes, lymphomas, vascular masses, pleuropericardial cysts, and bronchogenic cysts. The **posterior mediastinum** is the likely area for neurogenic tumors, lymphomas, pheochromocytomas, myelomas, meningoceles, meningomyeloceles, gastroenteric cysts, and diverticula.

109. The answer is b. *(McPhee, pp 434-437.)* The **early phase of septic shock** is characterized by vasodilation resulting in a warm, flushed patient with a normal or elevated cardiac output. Despite the elevation in cardiac output, however, cardiac function is remarkably abnormal. Fever, agitation, or confusion is often present. In **late septic shock**, patients become obtunded with decreased cardiac output and hypotension that is not reversible by volume replacement. Patients with **cardiogenic shock** have signs of pulmonary vascular congestion (jugular venous distention, S_3 gallop, bilateral lung crackles), increased PCWP, and decreased cardiac output. **Neurogenic shock** follows a spinal cord injury (warm skin, bradycardia, neurologic deficits), and **hypovolemic shock** is characterized by a physical examination consistent with volume depletion (tachycardia; hypotension; cool, clammy skin; poor capillary refill) and decreased PCWP. A mnemonic to remember the causes of shock is **SHOCK: S**epsis, **H**ypovolemia, **O**ther (ie, Addison disease), **C**NS (neurogenic), **K**ardiac causes.

110. The answer is d. *(McPhee, pp 434-435.)* **Bacteremia** is the presence of bacteria in blood culture bottles. **SIRS** is not a diagnosis but a response to a variety of clinical situations (ie, infection, burns, trauma, pancreatitis) and is characterized by two or more of the following: (1) temperature higher than 38°C (> 100.5°F) or less than 36.1°C (< 97°F), (2) heart rate more than 90 beats per minute, (3) respiratory rate more than 20 breaths per minute, (4) $Paco_2$ of less than 32 mm Hg, (5) white blood cell count of more than 12,000/μL or less than 4000/μL or more than 10% immature (band) forms. In **sepsis, patients meet SIRS criteria and there is a definitive source of infection. Severe sepsis** is sepsis associated with organ dysfunction, hypoperfusion, or hypotension (ie, lactic acidosis, oliguria, altered mental status), as in this case. **Septic shock** is sepsis-induced hypotension despite adequate fluid resuscitation. **MODS** is the presence of organ dysfunction in an acutely ill patient such that homeostasis cannot be maintained without intervention.

111. The answer is b. *(McPhee, pp 981-983.)* **Accidental overdose** of opiates may occur in drug addicted patients; they present with pinpoint pupils **(miosis)**, hypothermia, bradycardia, hypotension, and shallow breathing. Treatment involves the immediate reversal of the opiates with **naloxone**. During withdrawal, patients experience yawning, diaphoresis, rhinorrhea, restlessness, anxiety, muscular twitching, vomiting, diarrhea, hypertension, tachycardia, and tachypnea. **Methanol** (methyl alcohol or wood alcohol) is found in "moonshine"; patients present with blindness. **Ethylene glycol** is found in antifreeze; ingestion leads to seizures and coma. Patients develop oxalate crystals in the urine, and deposition may result in renal failure. Both methanol and ethylene glycol overdoses are treated with ethanol to prevent the formation of formic acid (toxic). Patients with **carbon monoxide** poisoning appear cherry red but are hypoxemic. **Cocaine** is a stimulant and can cause symptoms ranging from hyperactivity to full-blown psychoses. On examination patients have dilated pupils **(mydriasis)**, tachycardia, elevated blood pressure, and often confusion.

112. The answer is e. *(McPhee, p 784.)* **Anaphylaxis** may occur several minutes after the introduction of a specific antigen; presenting symptoms may include pruritus, urticaria, angioedema, abdominal pain, nausea, vomiting, diarrhea, respiratory distress, and shock. This life-threatening emergency requires immediate treatment with epinephrine (for α- and β-adrenergic effects resulting in vasoconstriction), antihistamines, β-agonist inhaled treatments for bronchospasm, oxygen, steroids, and vascular and ventilatory support when needed. **Angioedema** may appear, with or without urticaria, and occurs at the mucosal surfaces of the upper respiratory tract. It is characterized by a nonpitting edema of the subcutaneous tissues, and patients are at risk for death due to airway obstruction from laryngeal edema. It would be unlikely for this patient to present for the first time with asthma in his forties and this presentation is not typical for a PE.

113. The answer is a. *(McPhee, p 126.)* **Hereditary angioedema** is an autosomal dominant disease due to a deficiency of **C1 inhibitor (C1INH).** The family history and the lack of urticaria suggest the diagnosis. **Acquired C1 inhibitor deficiency** has the same clinical manifestations as the inherited form but is associated with lymphoproliferative disorders and lacks the family history. **Serum sickness** is due to the deposition of drug-antibody complexes causing complement activation and subsequent urticaria, arthralgias, lymphadenopathy, glomerulonephritis, and cerebritis. **Most cases of serum sickness are due to penicillin. Asthma and cystic fibrosis** are not associated with facial swelling.

114. The answer is b. *(Fauci, pp 2065-2067.)* **Latex anaphylaxis** may occur in patients, like this young girl, who have spina bifida or congenital urologic defects and have undergone repetitive surgeries. Other groups at risk include employees of rubber manufacturers and health-care workers. The diagnosis is confirmed by skin-prick testing for IgE to latex or by radioallergosorbent test (RAST) assay. Patients with latex-induced anaphylaxis must avoid latex during surgical procedures and live in a latex-free environment.

115. The answer is b. *(Fauci, pp 1417-1418.)* **High-altitude sickness** can occur at altitudes greater than 9500 ft, and mountain climbers at extreme altitudes (over 18,000 ft) are susceptible to hypoxemia and physiologic deterioration. Allowing sufficient time to acclimate and avoiding rapid ascent may prevent **acute mountain sickness (AMS)**. AMS is characterized by a severe headache, breathlessness, nausea, vomiting, weakness, and lassitude, but may progress to ataxia, altered mental status, pulmonary edema, cerebral edema, and coma. Funduscopic examination may reveal retinal hemorrhages and venous tortuosity. Descent is the definitive treatment for all forms of AMS but if this is not possible, treatment in hyperbaric chambers or administration of acetazolamide should help ameliorate symptoms. This patient does not have **hypothermia** (defined as core body temperature of less than 35°C [95°F]) or **dehydration** with a normal BP. **Carbon monoxide poisoning** most often occurs indoors from portable heaters and manifests as headache, confusion, and abdominal pain.

116. The answer is b. *(McPhee, p 1433.)* Gasoline engines, paint removers, and the incomplete combustion of wood, coal, or natural gas produce **carbon monoxide (CO)**, which binds preferentially to hemoglobin and decreases the release of oxygen to tissues. It is especially important to exclude this poisoning in the winter because of the furnaces used in heating. Patients develop a cherry-red appearance, headache, dizziness, confusion, visual field defects, blindness, nausea, abdominal pain, syncope, chest pain, heart arrhythmias, seizures, and coma. Pulse oximetry reveals a falsely elevated saturation; therefore, the diagnosis must be confirmed by determining the actual carboxyhemoglobin fraction in an arterial blood gas. **Methemoglobinemia** (from chemicals, antimalarials, and sulfonamides) results in **cyanosis that is unresponsive to oxygen**. Patients have **chocolate-colored blood**, a gray appearance, and a falsely normal saturation.

117 and 118. The answers are 117-a, 118-d. *(Seidel, p 374.)* **Pectus excavatum**, or **funnel breast**, is a congenital, hereditary malformation characterized by depression of the sternum below the clavicular-manubrial junction with symmetric inward bending of the costal cartilages. This may affect pulmonary and heart function. **Pectus carinatum**, or **pigeon breast**, is a deformity where the sternum protrudes from the narrowed thorax. **Kyphosis** is posterior deviation of the spine. **Scoliosis** is lateral deviation of the spine. **Lordosis** is an exaggerated convex curvature of the lumbar spine.

119 and 120. The answers are 119-c, 120-d. *(McPhee, pp 287-289.)* The patient with **obstructive sleep apnea syndrome (OSAS)** presents complaining of disruptive snoring and daytime hypersomnolence. Obesity is a risk factor for OSAS, but many patients with OSAS are not obese. Patients have upper airway narrowing from enlarged soft tissues, and good respiratory effort occurs against the airway obstruction. Diagnosis is best made by overnight **polysomnography** to document the apneic periods (10–15 events per hour of sleep, each event more than 10 seconds in duration). Obesity represents a mechanical load to the respiratory system, since excess weight reduces chest wall compliance. Patients with **obesity hypoventilation syndrome, or pickwickian syndrome**, demonstrate a decrease in central respiratory drive (no respiratory effort), especially during sleep (sleep-induced hypoventilation), since vital capacity is further reduced in the recumbent position. **Depression** may present with excessive sleepiness, but will also be accompanied by depressed mood and anhedonia, among other symptoms. **Narcolepsy** is excessive daytime sleepiness associated with abnormalities in REM sleep. Narcoleptic sleep attacks are brief and may occur during sedentary periods or when the patient is driving, eating, or conversing. **Cataplexy** occurs when strong emotion (ie, laughing or crying) precipitates sudden loss of muscle tone and **somnambulism** is sleepwalking.

121 to 123. The answers are 121-b, 122-a, 123-e. *(Seidel, p 896.)* **Cyanide poisoning** is associated with a **bitter almond** odor elevated venous oxygen saturation because tissues fail to take up arterial oxygen. Patients in **diabetic ketoacidosis (DKA)** often have a fruity breath odor. Hyperpnea refers to respiration, which is deep (increase in tidal volume) as well as rapid **(Kussmaul breathing)**. **Arsenic ingestion** and **parathion poisoning** are associated with a **garlic** odor. **Marijuana** odor is that of **burned rope**, and **rotten egg odor** is associated with poisoning due to hydrogen sulfide **mercaptans**. The odor of **camphor,** along with abdominal pain and hemolysis, is associated with ingestion of **naphthalene (mothballs)**.

Cardiovascular System

Questions

124. A 47-year-old woman presents with chest pain that worsens with inspiration and improves when she bends forward. Pain is relieved when the patient holds her breath. Blood pressure is 140/90 mm Hg. Heart examination reveals coarse, scratchy sounds heard throughout the cardiac cycle. Electrocardiogram (ECG) reveals diffuse ST elevations. Which of the following is the most appropriate next step in management?

a. Intravenous heparin
b. Oral prednisone
c. Fibrinolytics
d. Oral ibuprofen
e. Primary angioplasty
f. Chest radiograph

125. A 47-year-old perimenopausal woman presents for her annual checkup. She denies chest pain, shortness of breath, and palpitations. She has no family history of heart disease and does not smoke cigarettes. She has no past medical history of hypertension or diabetes mellitus. She takes no medications, and she exercises in a fitness center three times a week. Her blood pressure is 110/75 mm Hg and her heart rate is 66 beats per minute and regular. Physical examination reveals no jugular venous distention. Lung examination is normal. A split S_1 best heard over the tricuspid area is now audible but was not present 1 year ago. There is no peripheral edema. Which of the following is the most appropriate next step in diagnosis?

a. Transthoracic echocardiogram
b. Cardiac stress test
c. Cardiac isoenzymes
d. Cardiac catheterization
e. Electrocardiogram

126. A 16-year-old adolescent is found to have an unexpected sound audible in the right side of the neck. The sound is loudest in diastole and with the patient in the sitting position. The sound disappears when the patient is lying down or with the Valsalva maneuver. He has no complaints and is very athletic in school. He has no clubbing or cyanosis. Blood pressure and heart rate are normal. The rest of the physical examination is normal. Which of the following is the most likely diagnosis?

a. Thyroid bruit
b. Venous hum
c. Carotid bruit
d. Arteriovenous (AV) malformation
e. Transmitted murmur

127. A 23-year-old woman presents with a 2-year history of palpitations. She denies chest pain and dizziness. Past medical history is significant for pectus excavatum. Blood pressure and heart rate are normal. Physical examination reveals an apical late systolic crescendo-decrescendo murmur preceded by a midsystolic click that occurs earlier with standing. Which of the following do you expect to find on transthoracic echocardiogram?

a. Aortic stenosis
b. Mitral valve prolapse
c. Mitral stenosis
d. Tricuspid regurgitation
e. Aortic regurgitation

128. You are called to evaluate a 57-year-old man in the emergency room (ER) with diabetes and high cholesterol who complains of pressure-like chest pain that started while he was shoveling snow 45 minutes ago. The pain radiates to the jaw and medial aspect of the left arm. The patient reports no dizziness, nausea, vomiting, or palpitations. He has a past medical history of hypertension and he smokes two packs of cigarettes per day. He has a brother who had a myocardial infarction (MI) that required balloon angioplasty when he was in his forties. On physical examination the patient appears pale and diaphoretic. Blood pressure is 160/100 mm Hg and pulse is 108 beats per minute. His extremities are cool. Heart examination reveals an S_4 gallop. Lungs are normal. Peripheral pulses are palpable and bilaterally equal. He has no peripheral edema. Which of the following should be ideally accomplished in the first 10 minutes of management in the ER?

a. Administration of 160 to 325 mg chewable aspirin
b. Initiation of intravenous nitroglycerin
c. Percutaneous coronary intervention
d. An exercise stress test
e. Thrombolysis

129. A 41-year-old intravenous drug abuser presents with shortness of breath and pleuritic chest pain. He is febrile with a temperature of 39.7°C (103.5°F). He has no skin lesions, and funduscopic examination is negative. He has jugular venous distension that increases with compression of the liver. The liver is pulsatile. The jugular venous pulse shows a prominent *v* wave. The patient has splenomegaly. Heart auscultation reveals a holosystolic murmur heard best at the left lower sternal that increases with inspiration. Which of the following is the most likely diagnosis?

a. Bacterial endocarditis of the tricuspid valve
b. Bacterial endocarditis of the mitral valve
c. Rheumatic fever
d. Pericarditis
e. Acute hepatitis

130. A 58-year-old man with a history of poorly controlled hypertension presents to the emergency room with shortness of breath for 2 days. He admits to drinking heavily over the weekend. He has three-pillow orthopnea and paroxysmal nocturnal dyspnea as well as lower extremity edema. He does not have chest pain, palpitations, dizziness, or cough. His blood pressure is 180/100 mm Hg and his heart rate averages 130 beats per minute. His electrocardiogram is shown in the following figure. Which of the following will never be found in a person with this rhythm?

a. A pulse deficit compared with the central rate
b. Jugular venous distention
c. A third heart sound (S_3)
d. A fourth heart sound (S_4)
e. Lower extremity edema

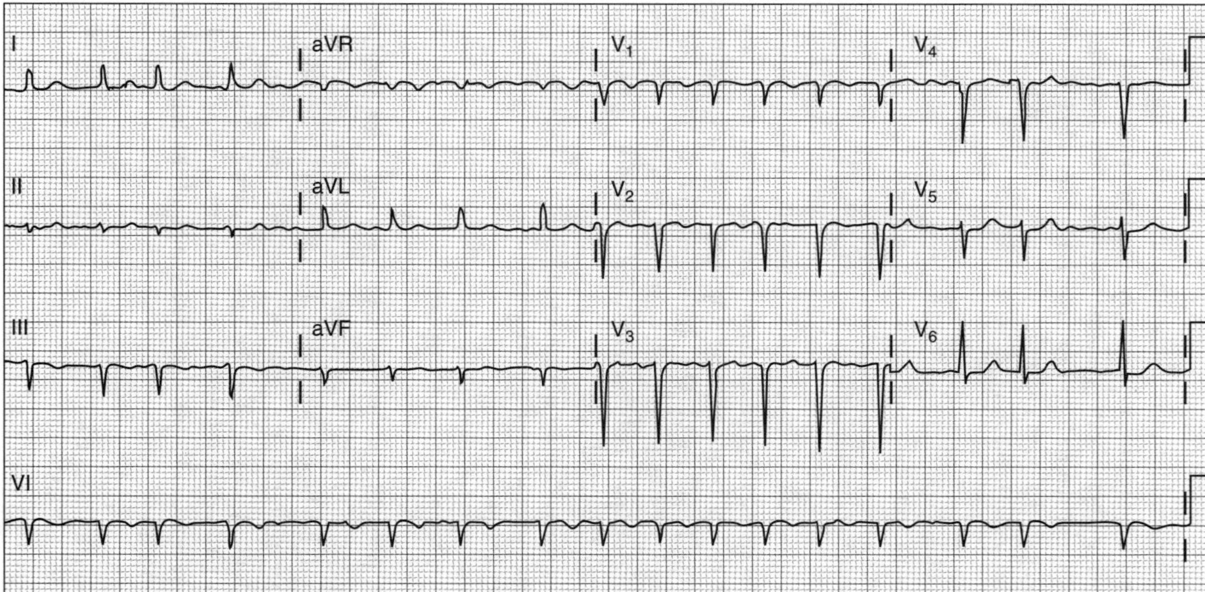

(Reproduced, with permission, from Knoop KJ, Stack LB, Storrow AB, et al. Atlas of Emergency Medicine, 3rd ed. New York: McGraw-Hill; 2009:760. Photo contributor: R. Jason Thurman, MD.)

131. An 18-year-old woman presents 2 weeks after an exudative pharyngitis with fever and arthritis that is asymmetrical and involves more than three joints. The arthritis is migratory, affecting one joint for several days and improving, then affecting another joint. On physical examination, the patient has a macular rash consisting of ring-shaped lesions with clear centers and her cardiac examination reveals an S_3 gallop. Which of the following is the most likely diagnosis?

a. Lyme disease
b. Endocarditis
c. Rheumatoid arthritis
d. Gout
e. Rheumatic fever

132. A 52-year-old man presents to your office complaining of leg pains. He says that he notices the discomfort primarily in his calf when he walks and seems to feel better after he stops to rest for a few minutes. He has smoked since high school. On physical examination, he has diminished popliteal and dorsalis pedis pulses with loss of hair and skin mottling on the anterior tibial surface bilaterally. What is the most appropriate next step in diagnosing this condition?

a. Lower extremity Doppler ultrasound
b. Angiography of the lower extremities
c. Ankle-brachial index
d. Magnetic resonance angiography (MRA)
e. Computed tomographic (CT) angiography

133. A 23-year-old student presents to your office for health clearance to play collegiate sports. He is asymptomatic and exercises daily. On physical examination, his blood pressure is 160/50 mm Hg and his pulse rate is 60 beats per minute with a rapid rise and fall. Heart examination reveals a hyperdynamic apical impulse with an early diastolic rumble at the apex and a high-pitched decrescendo diastolic murmur at the left sternal border. Nail beds reveal capillary pulsations. Which of the following is the most likely diagnosis?

a. Cardiac tamponade
b. Aortic insufficiency (AI)
c. Mitral stenosis (MS)
d. Atrial septal defect (ASD)
e. Tetralogy of Fallot

134. While palpating the pulse of a patient, you note that the pulse wave has two equal peaks during systole. You auscultate the heart and are certain that there is only one heartbeat for each two pulse waves. Which of the following best describes this finding?

a. Pulsus alternans
b. Dicrotic pulse
c. Pulsus parvus et tardus
d. Pulsus bigeminus
e. Pulsus bisferiens

135. A 68-year-old woman with a history of hypertension and diabetes mellitus presents with shortness of breath. She denies chest pain and palpitations. Physical examination reveals a blood pressure of 130/60 mm Hg and a heart rate of 72 beats per minute. The patient's lungs are normal, and heart auscultation reveals an S_4 gallop. She has no jugular venous distention (JVD) and no peripheral edema. Chest radiograph shows a normal size heart, and ECG shows left ventricular hypertrophy. Echocardiogram reveals concentric left ventricular hypertrophy (LVH) with a hyperdynamic left ventricle. Which of the following is the most likely diagnosis?

a. Systolic dysfunction
b. Diastolic dysfunction
c. Left heart failure
d. Right heart failure
e. Normal heart

136. A 50-year-old woman presents with malaise and weight loss. She denies chest pain, shortness of breath, dizziness, and palpitations. Her temperature is 38.3°C (100.9°F), and her heart rate is 80 beats per minute. There is a diastolic sound that is variable from cycle to cycle. Splinter hemorrhages are visible in the fingernails of both hands. Which of the following is the most likely diagnosis?

a. Mitral stenosis
b. Endocarditis
c. Aortic insufficiency
d. Atrial myxoma
e. Tricuspid stenosis

137. A 30-year-old woman presents for a routine checkup. She has no complaints and denies previous medical problems. On heart examination, the patient has a loud S_1. She has a grade 2 low-pitched mid- to late diastolic murmur that is heard best at the apex. Immediately preceding the murmur is a loud extra sound. Which of the following is the most likely diagnosis?

a. Mitral valve prolapse (MVP)
b. Mitral stenosis
c. Ventricular septal defect
d. Aortic insufficiency
e. Atrial septal defect

138. A 16-year-old adolescent comes to your practice for a physical examination to enroll in a sports program. Upon taking his vital signs, you note that his right arm blood pressure is 150/110 mm Hg. On auscultation, a systolic murmur best heard over the middle of the upper back is detected. The report from a chest x-ray done a few months ago, when he had a productive cough and fever, comments on notching of the ribs. Which of the following would most likely confirm your suspicion of the etiology of your findings today?

a. Elevated blood pressure in the legs
b. Unequal arm blood pressures
c. Delayed femoral pulse when compared to the brachial pulse
d. Earlier femoral pulse when compared to the brachial pulse
e. Normal ECG findings

139. A 66-year-old man with a history of lung cancer treated 5 years ago presents with worsening shortness of breath and fatigue. His blood pressure and heart rate are normal. Physical examination is positive for jugular venous distension which does not fall with inspiration, ascites, and peripheral edema. A loud and high-pitched extra sound is heard in early diastole corresponding to early ventricular filling. Which of the following is the most likely diagnosis?

a. Pericardial effusion
b. Pericardial tamponade
c. Dilated cardiomyopathy
d. Constrictive pericarditis
e. Infectious myocarditis

140. A 57-year-old man presents with midsternal pressure-like chest pain that radiates to the left arm accompanied by diaphoresis and nausea. He has a blood pressure of 80/50 mm Hg and neck vein distention with inspiration. The rest of the physical examination is normal. Electrocardiogram reveals ST elevations in leads II, III, and aVf. Which of the following is the most likely diagnosis?

a. Congestive heart failure
b. Pericardial tamponade
c. Right ventricular infarction
d. Anterior wall ST-segment elevation MI
e. Rupture of the papillary muscle

141. A mother brings her 11-year-old son to your office because he easily becomes short of breath while running. She states that he does not seem to be able to play for as long a period of time as his friends. The patient's blood pressure is 140/60 mm Hg, and he has bounding peripheral pulses. On auscultation of the heart, you detect a harsh, loud continuous murmur heard best below the left clavicle. Which of the following is the most likely diagnosis?

a. Cervical venous hum
b. Hepatic venous hum
c. Coarctation of the aorta
d. Patent ductus arteriosus
e. Mammary souffle

142. A 54-year-old man with a 20-year history of chronic obstructive lung disease has a heave that is palpable at the left lower sternal border at the third, fourth, and fifth intercostal spaces. He has no palpable thrill. Which of the following best explains the etiology of the heave?

a. It is probably a displaced point of maximum impulse (PMI).
b. It means the patient has congestive heart failure.
c. It means the patient has aortic stenosis.
d. It means the patient has right ventricular hypertrophy.
e. It means the patient has a pericardial effusion.

143. A 64-year-old man with a history of poorly controlled hypertension presents with sharp midsternal chest pain that occurred suddenly and radiates to his back between his shoulder blades. Blood pressure is 170/110 mm Hg with a normal pulse in his right arm and 90/60 mm Hg with a diminished pulse in his left arm. Heart auscultation reveals a diastolic murmur. He has a tracheal tug sign. ECG is normal. Chest radiograph reveals a widened mediastinum. Which of the following is the most likely diagnosis?

a. Myocardial infarction
b. Pulmonary embolus
c. Aortic dissection
d. Coarctation of the aorta
e. Aortic stenosis

144. An 81-year-old woman presents with syncope. Blood pressure is 120/80 mm Hg and heart rate is 30 beats per minute. There is no jugular venous distension, but cannon *a* waves are visible. Lung and heart examinations are otherwise normal. Her ECG is shown in the following figure. Which of the following is the most likely cause of her syncope?

a. Ventricular tachycardia
b. Complete heart block
c. Atrial flutter
d. Atrial fibrillation
e. Cardiac tamponade
f. Myocardial infarction

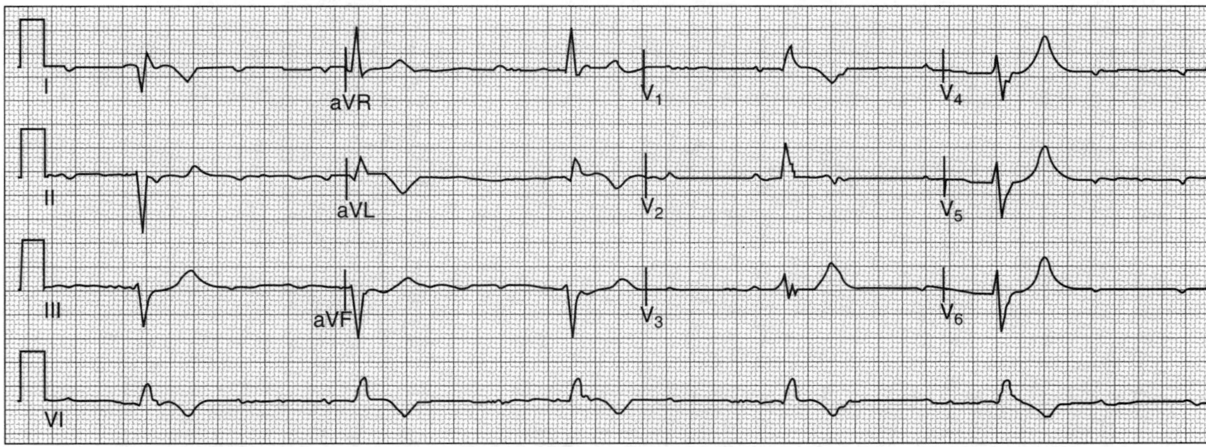

(Reproduced, with permission, from Knoop KJ, Stack LB, Storrow AB, et al. Atlas of Emergency Medicine, 3rd ed. New York: McGraw-Hill; 2009:750. Photo contributor: James V. Ritchie, MD.)

145. A 16-year-old adolescent is referred to your office for a blood pressure of 140/55 mm Hg. He has a well-healed surgical scar about 12-cm long over the medial aspect of his left thigh. On questioning, he states that he acquired the scar 4 years ago by impaling his thigh on a large nail after falling. Auscultation of the scar reveals a bruit, and there is a palpable thrill. Which of the following is the most likely diagnosis?

a. Premature atherosclerosis
b. Arteriovenous fistula
c. Scar tissue compressing the femoral artery
d. Congenital femoral artery bruit
e. Patent ductus arteriosus

146. A 55-year-old woman with diabetes and hypertension comes to your office for a routine checkup. She has no other medical problems and does not smoke. Her father died of an MI at her age. Her blood pressure is 150/90 mm Hg and her physical examination is normal. Upon obtaining a screening fasting lipid profile, what is the goal for her low-density lipoprotein (LDL) cholesterol?

a. LDL <160 mg/dL
b. LDL <130 mg/dL
c. LDL <100 mg/dL
d. LDL <190 mg/dL
e. LDL <40 mg/dL

147. A 51-year-old man is involved in a motor vehicle accident. He was not wearing a seat belt and remembers striking the steering wheel during the collision. On arrival at the emergency room, the patient is complaining of chest pain and shortness of breath. His blood pressure is 120/80 mm Hg but decreases to 90/50 mm Hg at the end of inspiration. He has JVD with distant heart sounds. Lung examination reveals normal breath sounds bilaterally. Which of the following is the most likely diagnosis?

a. Aortic dissection
b. Dilated cardiomyopathy
c. Pneumothorax
d. Congestive heart failure
e. Cardiac tamponade

148. A 71-year-old man complains of occasional lower back pain. His blood pressure is 150/85 mm Hg and his pulse is 80 beats per minute. Cardiac examination reveals an S_4 gallop. Abdominal examination reveals a pulsatile mass approximately 5.0 cm in diameter palpable in the epigastric area. Peripheral pulses are normal. Which of the following is the most appropriate test to order to evaluate this problem?

a. CT scan without contrast
b. Transthoracic echocardiography
c. Abdominal ultrasound
d. Abdominal radiograph
e. Contrast aortography

149. A 47-year-old man has been at home recovering from an anterior myocardial infarction that occurred 10 days ago. He presents to your office complaining of persistent chest pain that is worse on inspiration and that is different from his heart attack pain. The pain radiates to both clavicles. The pain is worse when the patient is lying down and improves with sitting up and leaning forward. The patient has a temperature of 38.4°C (101.2°F) and a normal blood pressure. Heart auscultation reveals a pericardial rub. Lung examination is positive for dullness and diminished breath sounds at the right base. Chest radiograph reveals a small right-sided pleural effusion. Laboratory data reveal that the patient has a mild leukocytosis and an increased erythrocyte sedimentation rate (ESR). Which of the following is the most likely diagnosis?

a. Extension of the myocardial infarction
b. Unstable angina
c. Prinzmetal angina
d. Pulmonary embolus
e. Dressler syndrome

150. A 22-year-old asymptomatic woman has a split second heart sound on physical examination at the upper left sternal border. The split S_2 is audible with deep inspiration and disappears with expiration. Which of the following can you tell her about these physical examination findings?

a. You should tell her that she needs an echocardiogram.
b. You should tell her that she needs an ECG.
c. You can reassure her that she inherited this problem from her parents.
d. You can reassure her that this is perfectly normal.
e. You should tell her that she needs a stress test.

151. An 82-year-old woman presents for her annual physical examination. She has a history of hypertension, for which she takes a calcium channel blocker. She does not smoke cigarettes. Physical examination reveals a blood pressure of 135/85 mm Hg. Heart examination is remarkable for a short systolic murmur that peaks early in systole and does not radiate. The second heart sound is normal in intensity. Which of the following is the most likely diagnosis?

a. Aortic sclerosis
b. Aortic stenosis
c. Mitral regurgitation
d. Tricuspid regurgitation
e. Mitral valve prolapse

152. A 10-year-old boy is brought to the emergency room because of chest pain. He has had a fever for the last 5 days. Physical examination is remarkable for conjunctival injection, strawberry tongue, cervical lymphadenopathy, a diffuse polymorphous rash, and edema of the hands and feet. Electrocardiogram is consistent with a myocardial infarction. Which of the following is the most appropriate next step in management?

a. Intravenous fibrinolytics
b. Percutaneous angioplasty
c. Intravenous steroids
d. Intravenous gamma globulin
e. Coronary artery bypass surgery

153. You are asked to provide a consult on a 13-year-old boy who wishes to join his high school track team. The patient is asymptomatic. Heart examination reveals a grade II, nonradiating systolic ejection murmur heard best at the left sternal border. He also has a physiologic split of S_2. The murmur does not increase with Valsalva maneuver, hand grip, or inspiration. Which of the following is the most appropriate next step in management?

a. No further management is necessary
b. Transthoracic echocardiogram
c. Transesophageal echocardiogram
d. Electrocardiogram
e. Holter monitor
f. Stress test

154. A 73-year-old man with a history of hypertension presents for a blood pressure check. He is compliant with his four antihypertensive medications but thinks that sometimes they make him dizzy. He does not drink alcohol or smoke cigarettes. He walks several miles each day and follows a low-salt diet. His blood pressure in your office is 170/90 mm Hg. The brachial artery is palpable when the sphygmomanometer cuff is inflated above systolic blood pressure. Which of the following is the most appropriate next step in management?

a. Add a fifth antihypertensive medication.
b. Maximize present antihypertensive medication.
c. Measure intraarterial pressure directly.
d. Stress the importance of compliance with medications.
e. No further management is indicated.

155. A 24-year-old man presents to the emergency room after a syncopal episode. He states that before he blacked out he experienced palpitations and the feeling that his heart was racing. He has no known medical problems and does not smoke, drink, or take any medications or illicit drugs. His ECG is shown in the following figure. Which of the following is the most likely etiology of his symptoms?

a. An accessory AV pathway
b. Rapid impulse formation from the sinoatrial node
c. An ectopic focus in the atria
d. Dual pathways within the AV node
e. Increased vagal influence on the normal pacemaker

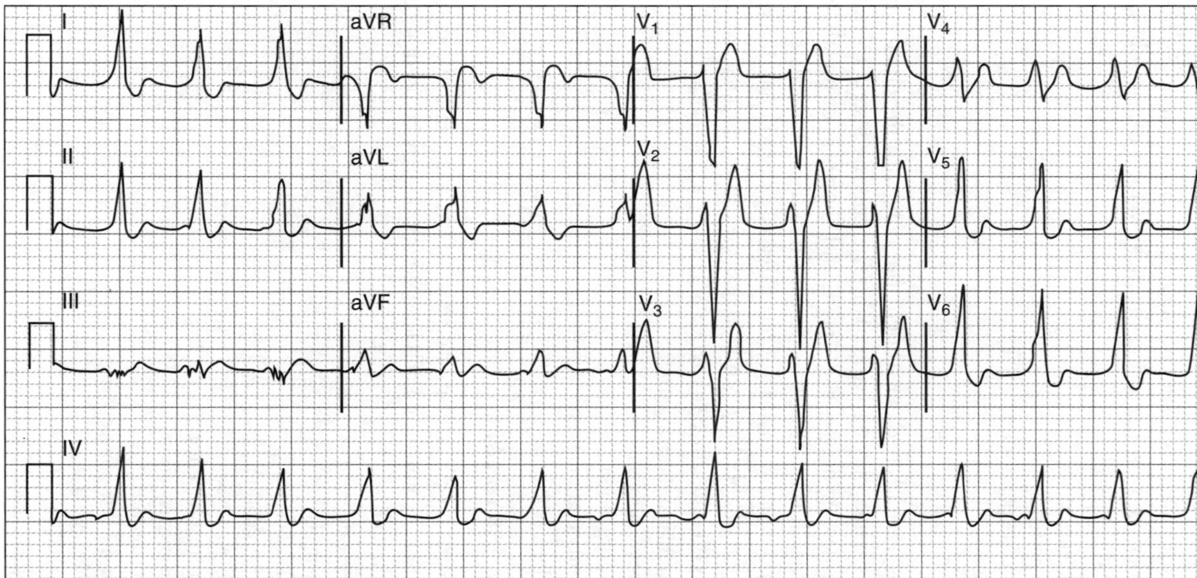

(Reproduced, with permission, from Fauci AS, Braunwald E, Kasper DL, et al. *Harrison's Principles of Internal Medicine*, 17th ed. New York: McGraw-Hill; 2008: Fig. e21-20. http://www.accessmedicine.com.)

156. A 35-year-old pregnant woman presents at 37 weeks of pregnancy with blood pressure measurements on successive visits around 145/95 mmHg. Protein is detected on her urine dipstick. Which of the following is the most likely diagnosis?

a. Prehypertension
b. Chronic hypertension
c. Gestational hypertension
d. Preeclampsia
e. Eclampsia

157. A 23-year-old medical student presents with the chief complaint of palpitations while playing basketball. The episode lasted 15 minutes. He denies dizziness, syncope, chest pain, and shortness of breath. He admits to a sedentary lifestyle but tries to eat three healthy meals per day. He is adopted, and a family history of heart disease is unknown. Physical examination is remarkable for a triple apical precordial impulse. Which of the following is the most likely diagnosis?

a. Hypertrophic cardiomyopathy
b. Pulmonary embolism
c. Aortic regurgitation
d. Right ventricular infarction
e. Atrial septal defect

Questions 158 to 161

For each patient with a heart murmur, select the heart lesion most likely responsible for the murmur. Each lettered option may be used once, multiple times, or not at all.

a. Aortic stenosis
b. Mitral stenosis
c. Aortic insufficiency
d. Mitral regurgitation
e. Pulmonic stenosis
f. Pulmonic insufficiency
g. Tricuspid regurgitation
h. Tricuspid stenosis
i. Hypertrophic cardiomyopathy
j. Mitral valve prolapse
k. Ventricular septal defect
l. Atrial septal defect
m. Idiopathic calcific aortic stenosis

158. A 50-year-old man presents with syncope that occurred while he was dancing at his high school reunion party. His blood pressure is normal but his pulse pressure is narrow. Heart examination reveals a crescendo-decrescendo systolic murmur heard best at the second left intercostal space that radiates to the carotid artery. The patient has a soft S_2 heart sound.

159. A 19-year-old man presents after having a syncopal episode while playing in a college intramural basketball game. His father died suddenly at the age of 30. Physical examination reveals a rapid, brisk carotid upstroke. Heart examination reveals a holosystolic murmur heard best in the left sternal border that radiates to the neck. The murmur increases with Valsalva maneuver.

160. A 14-year-old adolescent experiences shortness of breath while in a gym class. Heart examination reveals fixed splitting of S_2. There is a crescendo-decrescendo systolic murmur heard best in the left second intercostal space.

161. A 56-year-old man is 4 days post–myocardial infarction. A thrill is palpable over the precordium. On heart auscultation, a new holosystolic murmur is heard at the left lower sternal border that radiates to the right of the sternum.

Cardiovascular System

Answers

124. The answer is d. *(McPhee, pp 376-378.)* The pericardium is a double-walled sac that protects the heart; inflammation and roughening of the sac **(pericarditis)**, caused by infection, uremia surgery or cancer, may result in the formation of a **pericardial rub.** The scratchy sound is **triphasic**, representing systole and diastole of the ventricle and atrial systole. The rub results from heart movement against the inflamed pericardium and is best heard with the diaphragm of the stethoscope placed at the left lower sternal border with the patient leaning forward. The characteristic ECG in pericarditis often reveals ST elevation with PR depression early and T-wave inversion later. The first-line treatment for benign pericarditis is **anti-inflammatory agents**, such as nonsteroidals ibuprofen, indomethacin, or aspirin. If these do not work, oral steroids would be an appropriate next therapy. A chest radiograph would not help with definitive diagnosis; a better choice to visualize a pericardial effusion would be an echocardiogram, though in this case, the classic rub and ECG findings are diagnostic. This patient's ST elevations are not the result of ischemia, therefore, there is no need for anticoagulation or angioplasty.

125. The answer is e. *(Seidel, p 437.)* S_1 consists of mitral valve closure followed by tricuspid closure. Splitting of S_1 is seldom heard. In most cases, the valves close together and make a single sound, but if right ventricular contraction is delayed—as in the case of right bundle branch block (RBBB)—closure of the tricuspid valve occurs long after the mitral valve has closed, and a split S_1 is heard. The best test to use to diagnose RBBB is an **ECG**; the other answer choices would not help diagnose this problem.

126. The answer is b. *(Seidel, p 472.)* **Venous hums** are innocent murmurs (occurring in 25% of young adults) caused by turbulent flow through the internal jugular vein and heard best over the **anterior part of the sternocleidomastoid muscle at the medial end of the clavicle**. They are heard best **in the sitting position during diastole** and disappear on lying down, with Valsalva maneuver, or with compression of the ipsilateral jugular vein. In adults, they are present in the setting of anemia, pregnancy, and hyperthyroidism. Venous hums are often confused with **carotid bruits** (usually heard best with the bell in systole) and **precordial murmurs** (such as aortic stenosis) transmitted to the neck, which this patient lacks. **Thyroid bruits** are heard directly over a hyperactive thyroid gland.

127. The answer is b. *(Fauci, p 1472.)* The diagnosis of **mitral valve prolapse (MVP)** is clinical but can be confirmed by echocardiography. It is diagnosed in 10% of all healthy women, usually between their teens and age 30 years. Many are thin, and some have minor chest wall abnormalities. The most important finding on examination is a **mid- or late systolic click**, which may be followed, as in this patient, with a **high-pitched, late systolic crescendo-decrescendo murmur best heard at the apex.** In contrast to all other valvular abnormalities (except hypertrophic cardiomyopathy), anything that decreases left ventricular (LV) volume, such as standing and the strain phase of the Valsalva maneuver, causes the click and murmur to occur earlier. Any maneuvers that increase LV volume move these sounds away from S_1 and diminish them. Most patients with MVP have a benign course, and complications are rare. **Aortic stenosis** results from either a congenital malformation or degenerative or calcific changes and is manifested on physical exam as a crescendo-decrescendo systolic ejection murmur at the right upper sternal border and apex, often radiating to the carotids. It is sometimes accompanied by a systolic ejection click. Patients with **mitral stenosis** have an opening snap following S_2 (during diastole) and a diastolic rumble at the apex. **Tricuspid regurgitation** murmurs are holosystolic and best heard at the left sternal border during inspiration. **Aortic regurgitation or insufficiency (AI)** is a high-pitched decrescendo diastolic murmur sometimes accompanied by a mid- or late diastolic low-pitched mitral murmur (Austin Flint murmur). Patients with AI often have a wide arterial pulse pressure, as well as other interesting findings like a Corrigan or water hammer pulse (with a rapid rise and fall), Quincke pulses (nail-bed capillary pulsations), Duroziez sign (to and fro murmur over the femoral artery) and Musset sign (head bob with each pulse).

128. The answer is a. *(McPhee, pp 330-336.)* This patient with multiple cardiac risk factors and a fairly classic angina presentation should be assumed to have an **acute myocardial infarction (AMI)** until proven otherwise. Myocardial infarction occurs when an atherosclerotic plaque ruptures or ulcerates. Cardiac risk factors for this patient include male gender, positive family history, hypertension, diabetes mellitus, tobacco use, and hyperlipidemia. Patients may demonstrate the **Levine sign** (clenching of the fist over the sternum to demonstrate the severity of the pain). In addition to performing a good history and physical examination, within 10 minutes of presenting to the ER, physicians should administer to patients a **chewable aspirin or other antiplatelet agent**, **sublingual nitroglycerin every 5 minutes for three doses**, and **intravenous morphine sulfate** to control the chest pain. In addition, **IV access** should be established, **supplemental oxygen** should be given for an oxygen saturation below 90%, **serum cardiac isoenzymes** should be drawn and **electrocardiograms** should be repeatedly obtained. If sublingual nitroglycerin is not controlling the pain, an **IV drip of nitroglycerin** may be administered. A person having an AMI should not undergo a **stress test** while unstable. For patients with an ST-elevation MI, primary **percutaneous coronary intervention (PCI)** should be performed within 90 minutes (as long as it is within 12 hours of symptom onset) or **thrombolysis** within 30 minutes.

129. The answer is a. *(McPhee, pp 1303-1307.)* **Intravenous drug abusers** like this patient are at risk for developing acute endocarditis of the **tricuspid valve** due to ***Staphylococcus aureus*** bacteria. Other signs of bacterial endocarditis include splinter hemorrhages (subungual streaks), **Roth spots** (oval retinal hemorrhages with a pale center), **Osler nodes** (tender nodes on finger or toe pads), **Janeway lesions** (small nontender hemorrhages on the palms and soles), clubbing, and splenomegaly. The increased venous return of inspiration (which can be accomplished with the **Müller maneuver**, sucking in with the nares held closed) increases murmurs of the right side of the heart, and expiration increases murmurs of the left side of the heart. A useful way to remember this is **RIght (Right Inspiration) and LEft (Left Expiration)**. The murmur of **tricuspid regurgitation**, found in this patient, is a holosystolic murmur heard best at the left lower sternal border that increases with inspiration. Other findings in tricuspid regurgitation include distended neck veins, prominent *v* waves, hepatomegaly, pulsatile liver, edema, and a positive **Pasteur-Rondot sign** or **hepatojugular reflux** (pressure applied over the liver causes increased distension of the neck veins). **Rheumatic heart disease** and mitral valve prolapse predispose patients to endocarditis; in this situation, the organism is often *Streptococcus viridans,* and the **mitral valve** is most commonly involved. **Pericarditis** presents with a pericardial friction rub. **Acute hepatitis** results from infectious and autoimmune causes, among others, but would not present with a murmur, as seen in this case.

130. The answer is d. *(McPhee, pp 346-349.)* This patient has new-onset **atrial fibrillation** (irregularly irregular rhythm) with a rapid ventricular rate and decreased filling time, leading to volume overload. This patient's risk factors for developing this rhythm are his hypertension and acute alcohol excess, sometimes called "holiday heart." A useful mnemonic for causes of atrial fibrillation is **PIRATES: P**-pericarditis, pulmonary disease, pulmonary embolism; **I**-ischemia, infarction, infection, and inflammation; **R**-rheumatic heart disease; **A**-atrial septal defect; **T**-thyrotoxicosis; **E**-elevated blood pressure, ETOH excess and withdrawal; **S**-sleep apnea, surgery (cardiothoracic). Patients with atrial fibrillation will have a "**pulse deficit,**" or a higher apical than peripheral pulse rate, because not all ventricular beats are conducted effectively enough to produce a peripheral pulse. **You will not find an** S_4, which is associated with effective atrial contraction, in patients with atrial fibrillation. Because this patient is in volume overload, **you will expect to find pulmonary rales, an elevated jugular venous pulsation, an** S_3 **(indicating impairment of ventricular function) and lower extremity edema**. Rate control and diuresis would be the first steps in management of this patient, followed by anticoagulation.

131. The answer is e. *(McPhee, pp 374-376.)* **Rheumatic fever** is due to group A streptococci and often presents with a migratory polyarthritis, as in this patient. Patients have a history of sore throat 2 weeks prior to presentation. Rheumatic fever is often diagnosed using the **Jones criteria** (A helpful mnemonic is **"FEAR CASES"**). The diagnosis of rheumatic fever requires demonstration of previous streptococcal infection and either two **major or one major and two minor criteria** with evidence of previous group A streptococci. **Minor = FEAR =** **F**ever, prolonged PR interval on **E**lectrocardiogram, **A**rthralgia, blood results indicating an elevated acute-phase **R**eactant. **Major = CASES =** **C**arditis, migratory poly**A**rthritis involving large joints, **S**ydenham chorea (involuntary movements of the tongue, face, and arms), **E**rythema marginatum (ring-shaped macules with clear centers), and Subcutaneous nodules (almost exclusively seen in children). **Aschoff bodies** (histiocytes) are found histologically in rheumatic fever. The characteristic rash of **Lyme disease** is erythema migrans. A chronic arthritis may develop in up to 10% of untreated patients infected with *Borrelia burgdorferi,* but this arthritis is usually monoarticular or oligoarticular, affecting the knees, ankles, hips, elbows, and wrists (large joints). **Endocarditis** presents with a left-sided murmur (right in the setting of IV drug use) and possibly evidence of septic emboli. **Rheumatoid arthritis** is a systemic inflammatory disease characterized by symmetric synovitis, almost always involving the hands, with morning stiffness and often rheumatoid nodules on the extensor tendinous surfaces and in the heart and lungs. **Gout** is an inflammatory arthritis due to uric acid crystal deposition in joints such as the first MTP joint (**podagra**), the knee, and the wrists, among others.

132. The answer is c. *(McPhee, pp 416-417.)* This **smoker** has classic symptoms of **intermittent claudication**, which is indicative of arterial occlusive disease in the lower extremity, usually involving the superficial femoral artery. Patients complain of **exertional calf pain,** relieved by rest and on examination have diminished or absent distal pulses in the leg, as well as coolness, pallor, thin and mottled skin, and loss of hair. A helpful mnemonic for arterial occlusion is **"the Ps"**: **P**allor, **P**ain, **P**ulselessness, **P**aresthesia (with major artery occlusion), and (rarely) **P**aralysis. The best first step in diagnosis is to perform the **ankle-brachial index (ABI)**, the ratio of the systolic blood pressure at the ankle to the highest arm systolic pressure. A resting ABI less than 0.9 is abnormal and one less than 0.3 corresponds to rest pain and critical ischemia. If revascularization is needed, **angiography, CTA, and MRA** will localize the obstruction. A **Doppler ultrasound** will reveal deep venous thrombosis, which presents with unilateral leg swelling.

133. The answer is b. *(McPhee, pp 311-313.)* The patient has physical findings consistent with **aortic insufficiency (AI)**. Etiologies may include dissecting aorta, Marfan syndrome, bicuspid aortic valve, rheumatic heart disease, ankylosing spondylitis, endocarditis, and syphilis. Associated signs of AI (all due to the large stroke volume with fast runoff) include a **wide arterial pulse pressure** and a **diastolic rumble** (from the aortic regurgitant flow displacing the mitral valve, often called the **Austin Flint murmur**), **Musset sign** (head bobbing with the heartbeat), **water-hammer pulse or Corrigan pulse** (rapidly rising and collapsing pulse), **Hill sign** (an increase of > 40 mm Hg in femoral artery systolic BP compared to brachial artery BP), **Quincke pulse** (nail-bed capillary pulsations), **pistol-shot pulse** (booming sound heard over the femoral arteries), and **Duroziez sign** (bruit auscultated over the femoral artery when compressed). None of the other cardiac abnormalities listed fit the presentation given.

134. The answer is e. *(Seidel, pp 470-471.)* **Pulsus bisferiens (bisferious pulse)**, with two strong systolic peaks, is found in AI and in hypertrophic cardiomyopathy (HCM). In the latter, the first wave or percussion wave is due to the rapid flow rate of initial contraction, and the second wave, or tidal wave, is due to the slower rate of continued contraction. The **dicrotic pulse** has two palpable pulses, but one is in systole and the other is in diastole. **Pulsus bigeminus** results from a smaller premature contraction following a normal pulsation, in rapid succession. **Pulsus alternans** involves alternation between large- and small-amplitude pulsations and is usually seen with severe left ventricular decompensation and cardiac tamponade. **Pulsus parvus et tardus** (small and slow rising) is seen in aortic stenosis (AS) and represents a delayed systolic peak due to obstruction to left ventricular ejection.

135. The answer is b. *(Fauci, p 1552.)* When a patient's left ventricular ejection fraction is diminished, he or she has **systolic dysfunction**. Patients (especially older ones like this) with hypertension and diabetes mellitus are predisposed to **diastolic dysfunction** (inability of the ventricle to relax for filling) and typically have an S_4 gallop, elevated filling pressures, and a hyperdynamic ventricle (ejection fraction > 50%). Patients with **left heart failure** present with pulmonary congestion (ie, crackles); patients with **right heart failure** present with JVD, an S_3 gallop, hepatomegaly, ascites, and peripheral edema.

136. The answer is d. *(McPhee, pp 382-383.)* **Atrial myxomas** are benign tumors of the heart that may embolize systemically. Patients present with fever, malaise, weight loss, leukocytosis, and emboli. If the tumor is large, signs of low cardiac output may result. A "**tumor plop**" is the hallmark sound of atrial myxoma; it is **a diastolic sound that is variable from cycle to cycle** (related to the motion of the tumor) and represents the diastolic prolapse of the myxoma through an opened mitral or tricuspid valve. The other answer choices do not fit this presentation.

137. The answer is b. *(Seidel, p 446.)* **Mitral stenosis (MS)** is characterized by an **opening snap** closely following P_2 and just prior to a low-pitched, rumbling diastolic murmur. **Aortic insufficiency** is characterized by a high-pitched diastolic decrescendo murmur. **MVP** consists of a midsystolic click with a late systolic murmur. A **VSD** causes a harsh, holosystolic murmur at the left lower sternal border while an **ASD** is characterized by a systolic murmur and a fixed-split S_2.

138. The answer is c. *(McPhee, pp 296-297.)* **Coarctation of the aorta** is narrowing of the aorta usually just distal to the origin of the ductus arteriosus and subclavian artery and should be considered as a cause of **secondary hypertension in young patients. Blood pressure is elevated in the arms, but normal in the legs. Absent, delayed, or markedly diminished femoral pulses** may also be found. **Late systolic ejection murmurs** can be heard best over the spine posteriorly. Chest radiograph in coarctation shows **rib notching** secondary to the dilated collateral arteries and may also have a "**3**" sign along the aortic shadow from the narrowed area of coarctation and the postenotic dilation of the descending aorta. The electrocardiogram usually shows **left ventricular hypertrophy**.

139. The answer is d. *(McPhee, pp 379-380.)* **Constrictive pericarditis** may be idiopathic (60% of cases) or due to tuberculosis, mediastinal irradiation (as in this patient), or cardiac surgery. Inflammation causes the pericardium to thicken and become fibrotic, thereby restricting diastolic filling. Patients present in right heart failure, as in this case. On examination, a **pericardial knock**, a higher pitched S_3, may be heard in early diastole and patients may have **Kussmaul sign**, where the jugular venous pulsation does not fall as it should with inspiration. The diagnosis is confirmed by showing a thickened pericardium on CT scan or MRI. The treatment is pericardiectomy. It is often hard to distinguish this diagnosis from **restrictive cardiomyopathy**, which also presents with right-sided failure but in the latter, ventricular interaction increases with inspiration. Often, the patient with restrictive cardiomyopathy presents with other signs of the systemic illness. Patients with **dilated cardiomyopathy** often present with left-sided failure symptoms and signs. **Infectious myocarditis** often follows an upper respiratory infection and manifests as chest pain or heart failure. In patients with large **pericardial effusions, cardiac tamponade** may result and be diagnosed by detecting **pulsus paradoxus** (systolic pressure decline of greater than 10 mm Hg during inspiration) on examination.

140. The answer is c. *(McPhee, p 338.)* This patient with cardiac chest pain symptoms and ECG **changes in the inferior leads (II, III, and aVf)** is suffering an inferior infarction. **Right ventricular (RV) infarction is seen in up to 30% of inferior wall infarctions**; patients usually present with hypotension, clear lungs and elevated venous pressure. **Kussmaul sign** (inspiratory distension of the neck veins) is seen in right ventricular infarction, right heart failure, constrictive pericarditis, superior vena cava syndrome, and tricuspid stenosis. Inspiration normally generates a negative intrapleural pressure, which sucks blood into the heart, but with the aforementioned diseases, there is impairment of right heart filling and blood cannot enter the heart, causing venous pressure to rise. In these patients, venous pressure will not fall normally, or may even rise, with inspiration. Therapy for RV infarction includes **volume expansion** to maintain adequate RV preload and improve left ventricular function. Kussmaul sign is **never** seen in uncomplicated pure **cardiac tamponade**. In **congestive heart failure**, patients usually have other findings on physical examination like elevated jugular venous pressure, lower extremity edema and an enlarged, displaced apical impulse. In an **anterior MI,** there would be ECG changes in leads V_1, V_2, and V_3. **Rupture of a papillary muscle** is a rare complication of an acute anterior or inferior infarction and is diagnosed by a new systolic murmur and pulmonary edema.

141. The answer is d. *(McPhee, pp 301-302.)* The ductus arteriosus, which is patent in the fetal circulation, may fail to close at birth. Patients with **patent ductus arteriosus (PDA)** may be asymptomatic or may complain of dyspnea, palpitations, and exercise intolerance. The pulse pressure is usually widened and pulses are bounding due to the runoff of blood through the ductus. The classic late systolic **continuous machinery murmur** of PDA is best heard in the first and second intercostal spaces below the left clavicle. Other **continuous murmurs** include the **cervical venous hum** (due to increased blood flow in the internal jugular vein; disappears with compression of the vein), the **hepatic venous hum** (disappears with compression of epigastrium), and the **mammary souffle** (heard over the breast, due to increased blood flow in pregnancy).

142. The answer is d. *(Seidel, p 430.)* The left parasternal border at the third, fourth, and fifth intercostal spaces should be palpated for a **right ventricular lift** or **heave**. It is a nondiagnostic finding and results from any etiology of right ventricular hypertrophy. A **heave** that is palpable at the apex is consistent with LVH. A **precordial thrill** is a palpable murmur that may accompany heart disease. It is always considered pathologic and may be felt during systole (ie, AS, VSD, MR, PDA, tetralogy of Fallot) or diastole (ie, AI, MS). The presence of a thrill characterizes a murmur as at least grade 4 in intensity.

143. The answer is c. *(McPhee, pp 426-427.)* **Dissection of the aorta** occurs when the intima is interrupted so that blood enters the wall of the aorta and separates its layers, forming a second lumen. **Type A** dissections occur proximal to the left subclavian and are surgical emergencies. **Type B** dissections occur in the proximal descending aorta and, if stable, may be managed medically by controlling the blood pressure and heart rate to prevent extension of the dissection. Anything that weakens the media can lead to dissection, but **hypertension** is the most common risk factor. Aortic dissection is a major cause of morbidity and mortality in Marfan syndrome. Other etiologies of dissection include cystic medial necrosis (described in patients with bicuspid aortic valves), syphilis, Ehlers-Danlos syndrome, trauma, and bacterial infections. Patients often have **diastolic murmurs due to aortic insufficiency** from a proximal dissection into the valve. A **tracheal tug** is considered positive if the pulsating aorta is felt when the trachea is pulled upward, a sign that the expanding aorta is contacting the left mainstem bronchus. **Aortic stenosis** would cause a crescendo-decrescendo murmur at the right upper sternal border that radiates to the carotid. **Coarctation of the aorta** would present with elevated blood pressure in both arms with normal leg pressures. Patients also have delayed or diminished femoral pulses.

144. The answer is b. *(McPhee, p 355.)* The ECG shows **complete heart block (also called third-degree block)**, in which atrial and ventricular electrical activities are dissociated, but the P-P and R-R intervals remain constant. Occasionally the P waves are hidden in the QRS complex. The ventricular rate is usually slower than 45 beats per minute. **Exaggerated *a* waves** of the **jugular venous pulsation** are called **cannon waves** and are due to the right atrium contracting against increased resistance (ie, PS, tricuspid stenosis [TS], complete heart block). The activity of the right side of the heart is transmitted normally through the jugular veins as a visualized pulse. See following figure.

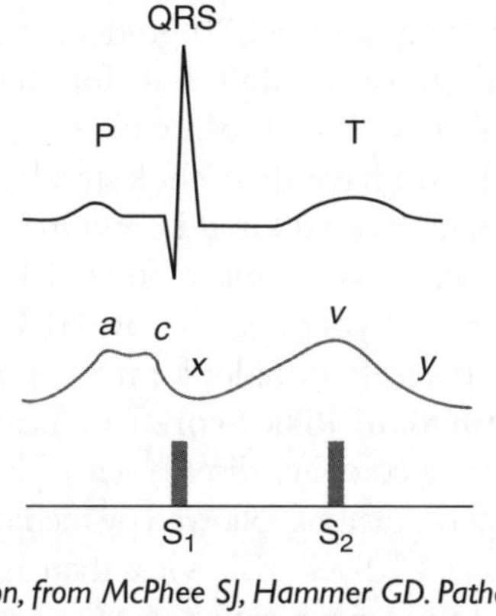

(Reproduced, with permission, from McPhee SJ, Hammer GD. Pathophysiology of Disease: An Introduction to Clinical Medicine, 6th ed. New York: McGraw-Hill; 2010:265.)

The ***a* wave** is due to venous distension caused by atrial contraction. It is the most dominant wave, especially during inspiration. The *a* wave is not present during atrial fibrillation. The **c wave** of the venous pressure curve occurs as a result of ventricular contraction, which forces the tricuspid valve (TV) back toward the atrium. For that reason, it is simultaneous with the carotid pulse. If the TV is incompetent, the *c* wave will be increased. The *v* wave is the result of atrial filling while the AV valves are closed. The **v wave** becomes large with TR. The downward **x slope** is caused by atrial filling, and the **y slope** is caused by the open TV and the rapid filling of the ventricle. The *y* descent is abolished in cardiac tamponade.

A **myocardial infarction** would present with ST elevation in a vascular distribution, which is absent here. **Ventricular tachycardia** is a wide complex tachycardia; **atrial fibrillation** is an irregularly irregular rhythm often accompanied by a rapid ventricular rate, while **atrial flutter** often causes a regular tachycardia of 100 to 150 beats per minute with a "sawtooth pattern" of atrial activity.

145. The answer is b. *(Seidel, p 486.)* An acquired **arteriovenous fistula** may be diagnosed by the presence of a continuous murmur and a palpable thrill over an area of previous trauma. The large pulse pressure is an indication that a large portion of the cardiac output is bypassing the systemic vascular resistance through the fistula.

146. The answer is c. *(McPhee, pp 1126-1129.)* According to the National Cholesterol Education Program (NCEP) guidelines, patients with **known coronary disease and those at high risk for developing it, like this patient with diabetes**, as well as those with peripheral vascular disease and carotid plaques, should have their cholesterol strictly controlled. As a result, the LDL goal is less than **100 mg/dL** and may even be pushed lower than 70 mg/dL. Those with two or more other risk factors for developing coronary disease (smoking, hypertension, low HDL, family history of premature heart disease and age 45 or older for men or 55 or older for women) should undergo **Framingham Risk Score** stratification to determine their 10-year risk for developing coronary disease. Lifestyle modification is always first-line therapy for hyperlipidemia, followed by medication. For patients with risk factors, if the calculated 10-year risk is less than 10%, the LDL goal is less than 130 mg/dL, with drug therapy commencing at greater than 160 mg/dL; for those with a greater than 10% risk, the goal is still less than 130 mg/dL, but therapy should commence if the LDL is greater than this goal at all. For patients with one or fewer risk factors, the LDL goal is less than 160 mg/dL.

147. The answer is e. *(Fauci, pp 1490-1492.)* **Cardiac tamponade** is the accumulation of fluid in the pericardial sac in amounts sufficient to cause obstruction of blood flow back to the heart. Cardiac tamponade may follow trauma or surgery and also may be a complication of malignancy (ie, lung, breast, lymphoma), chronic renal failure, or hypothyroidism. The three classic features of cardiac tamponade, or the **Beck triad**, are **hypotension, soft or absent heart sounds, and JVD with a prominent *x* descent but absent *y* descent.** The patient has other classic signs of cardiac tamponade, including **pulsus paradoxus**, an inspiratory drop (from expiration) in systolic blood pressure of more than 10 mm Hg (normal <10 mm Hg). Pulsus paradoxus may also be seen in severe asthma and constrictive pericarditis. ECG in tamponade may show low voltage and **pulsus alternans**. Chest radiograph may show enlargement of the cardiac shadow (globular-shaped). **Aortic dissection** would cause unequal blood pressures when checked in both arms and a **pneumothorax** would result in absent breath sounds over the area where the lung no longer is expanded. While **CHF** (sometimes resulting from a **dilated cardiomyopathy**) might cause JVD, it would not cause the pulsus paradoxus of this case.

148. The answer is c. *(McPhee, pp 423-424.)* **Abdominal aortic aneurysms (AAAs)** are usually due to atherosclerosis and the vast majority originates below the renal arteries. The aneurysms are typically asymptomatic until they rupture, but patients may complain of lower back or hypogastric pain. Normal diameter of the aorta is less than 2 cm. When the diameter of the AAA is more than 5.5 cm, repair is generally suggested. Risk of rupture is 1% to 2% over 5 years when the AAA is less than 5 cm, but 20% to 40% when the AAA reaches 6 cm in diameter. The best method of evaluating this patient's AAA is by **ultrasound** initially (and to follow size) or with a **CT scan with contrast or MRI** when the diameter is nearing 5.5 cm. **Abdominal radiography will miss three-quarters of cases** as it can only pick up the calcified outline of an aneurysm. **Contrast aortography** is *not* a first-line diagnostic test as it carries a risk of complications such as bleeding, allergic reactions, and atheroembolism. **Transthoracic echocardiography** is an appropriate way to assess thoracic aortic aneurysms.

149. The answer is e. *(McPhee, p 339.)* This patient has **post–myocardial infarction syndrome**, or **Dressler syndrome**, an autoimmune complication of myocardial infarction. It occurs from 3 days to 6 weeks after the infarction and usually responds quickly to salicylates. The fever, pericarditis, leukocytosis, elevated ESR, and pleural effusion are all part of the autoimmune process. None of the other choices would result in pain exacerbated by position change or the presence of a pericardial rub.

150. The answer is d. *(Seidel, p 436.)* This patient has a **physiologically split S_2** and you can reassure her that **this is perfectly normal.** A normal S_2 consists of closure of the aortic valve (A_2) followed by closure of the pulmonic valve (P_2). It is best heard at the **base** of the heart, in the left second intercostal space, where it is louder than S_1. **Inspiration** (increases venous return and decreases thoracic pressure) **normally** increases the split of S_2 by two mechanisms. First, there is delayed pulmonic valve closure, which is due to prolonged right ventricular ejection time from increased stroke volume. Second, inspiration increases the compliance of the pulmonary vasculature and thereby decreases the return of blood to the left heart and shortens its ejection time by the same mechanism.

151. The answer is a. *(Seidel, p 458.)* **Aortic sclerosis** is found in 65% of patients over the age of 65. Approximately 20% of these will progress to significant aortic stenosis. Degenerative valve disease is more common in men, in smokers, and in patients with hypertension. When compared with the murmur of aortic stenosis, the murmur of aortic sclerosis is more likely to be short, occurs at midsystole, and **does not radiate to the carotids**. The **intensity of the second heart sound is normal** in patients with aortic sclerosis, while a loud S_2 is present in aortic stenosis. **Mitral and tricuspid regurgitation** cause holosystolic murmurs, with the MR murmur radiating to the axilla. **MVP** presents with a mid-systolic click and a mid to late systolic crescendo-decrescendo murmur at the apex.

152. The answer is d. *(Seidel, p 490.)* The patient has **Kawasaki disease** (mucocutaneous lymph node syndrome), an acute illness of uncertain etiology that affects young males more than females; Asian children are at higher risk. Patients present with fever, conjunctival injection, cervical lymphadenopathy, **strawberry tongue**, rash, and edema. Cardiac involvement may include myocardial infarction, coronary artery aneurysms, or generalized vasculitis of the small vessels of the heart. The treatment is **gamma globulin**. Steroids may worsen aneurysmal dilatation.

153. The answer is a. *(Seidel, p 442.)* The patient has a **functional or innocent heart murmu**r. These are nonpathologic murmurs generated by flow abnormalities (systolic ejection), not structural heart abnormalities. Innocent murmurs are extremely common in children, adolescents, and young athletes, and are the most common kinds of murmurs encountered by physicians. No further workup is necessary at this time.

154. The answer is c. *(McPhee, p 394.)* The patient has a positive **Osler sign** (a palpable brachial or radial artery when the cuff is inflated above systolic pressure). Older patients may have noncompressible vessels and falsely elevated blood pressure readings by sphygmomanometry. In those, like this patient, who may not tolerate increasing medication, it may be necessary to **measure intra-arterial pressure** before increasing or adding blood pressure medication.

155. The answer is a. *(McPhee, pp 345-346.)* This patient has **Wolff-Parkinson-White syndrome**, as evidenced by his symptoms (palpitations and syncope) coupled with the classic ECG findings of a **shortened PR interval with a delta wave**, the slurred upstroke of a widened QRS complex. This finding indicates preexcitation due to early depolarization of the ventricle adjacent to **an accessory pathway or bypass tract** between the atria and the ventricle, causing an AV reentrant tachycardia. Up to one-third of patients will develop atrial flutter or atrial fibrillation with a rapid ventricular response. **Digoxin, beta blockers, and calcium channel blockers should be avoided** as they decrease the refractory time of the accessory pathway and may increase ventricular rates.

156. The answer is d. *(Fauci, pp 44-45.)* Hypertension in pregnancy comes in several forms. Pregnant patients with preexisting hypertension, those with blood pressure elevations before 20 weeks gestation with no preexisting diagnosis, and those in whom blood pressure elevations in pregnancy do not normalize postpartum have **chronic hypertension**, of which **prehypertension** is a milder form. Women with chronic hypertension, diabetes, advanced maternal age (> 35 years) and obesity, among other factors, are at higher risk for developing **preeclampsia**, or new-onset hypertension after 20 weeks gestation that is associated with proteinuria, as in this patient. Patients with this diagnosis are at high risk for developing seizures, signaling transition to **eclampsia**, which carries a high fetal and maternal mortality risk. The definitive treatment for preeclampsia is delivery of the fetus. Patients who experience blood pressure elevations without proteinuria for the first time during pregnancy, and in whom blood pressure normalizes by 12 weeks postpartum, are retrospectively diagnosed with **gestational hypertension**.

157. The answer is a. *(Fauci, pp 1484-1485.)* This patient has **hypertrophic cardiomyopathy (HCM)**, which is often detected on physical examination by the presence of a harsh, **diamond-shaped midsystolic murmur** at the left sternal border and apex, a **bisferiens carotid pulse**, as well as a **loud S_4** and a **double or triple apical impulse**, resulting from a prominent atrial filling wave and early and late systolic impulses.

158 to 161. The answers are 158-a, 159-i, 160-l, 161-k. *(Seidel, pp 446-449, 455-456.)* Patients with **aortic stenosis (AS)** may present with symptoms of angina, syncope, dyspnea, or congestive heart failure. The etiologies of AS include rheumatic fever and congenital bicuspid valve. The typical AS murmur is **midsystolic crescendo-decrescendo** and **radiating toward the carotid**, with a **soft or absent S_2**. **Hypertrophic obstructive cardiomyopathy (HOCM or HCM)** is the most common cause of sudden cardiac death in young adults. Patients may be asymptomatic, and over half have a positive family history of sudden death. A loud systolic murmur along the left sternal border radiates to the neck. Squatting to **standing and the Valsalva maneuver** both decrease right ventricular filling and decrease venous return, thereby **increasing the murmurs of HCM and MVP**. Standing decreases venous return because of pooling of the blood in the lower extremities caused by gravity. The Valsalva maneuver decreases cardiac output and increases heart rate. **Standing decreases all other murmurs. ASD** is a common anomaly in adults and is classically diagnosed with **fixed splitting of S_2**, as well as a high-pitched diamond-shaped murmur heard best at the upper left sternal border, possibly accompanied by a thrill. **VSD** may be a congenital anomaly or a **complication of myocardial infarction**; on physical examination patients have a coarse **holosystolic murmur** best heard between the third and fifth intercostal spaces along the left sternal border, often associated with a thrill or heave. Over time, both defects may cause a left-to-right shunt, which may lead to pulmonary hypertension (loud S_2) and pulmonary obstruction **(Eisenmenger syndrome)**.

Gastrointestinal System

Questions

162. A 22-year-old college student with a 7-year history of Crohn disease presents to her gastroenterologist with a 2-month history of numbness and tingling of her feet and fingertips. Her past surgical history is significant for several previous bowel resections. On physical examination, there is loss of vibration and position sense of the hands and feet. Motor and cerebellar examinations are normal. Deep tendon reflexes are intact. Which of the following is the most likely diagnosis?

a. Vitamin D deficiency
b. Vitamin E deficiency
c. Vitamin A deficiency
d. Vitamin B_{12} deficiency
e. Vitamin K deficiency

163. A 52-year-old man is 48 hours postlaryngectomy for malignancy. On physical examination, he has inflammation around the surgical incision, which prevents him from swallowing easily. He has no abdominal pain, nausea, vomiting, or diarrhea. Abdominal examination reveals normal bowel sounds and no tenderness. Which of the following is the most appropriate method of feeding this patient?

a. Enteral formula nutrition
b. Pureed soft food diet
c. Total parenteral nutrition
d. Intravenous dextrose
e. Peripheral alimentation

164. A 42-year-old woman presents to the emergency room complaining of the sudden onset of right upper abdominal pain. Her pain started after she ate a hamburger for lunch. She is nauseated and vomited twice at home. She denies diarrhea. Her temperature is 39°C (102.2°F), blood pressure is 140/90 mm Hg, and pulse is 110 beats per minute. She appears anxious and distressed. She is not jaundiced. Abdominal examination reveals normal bowel sounds. While you are palpating under her right costal margin, the patient abruptly halts her inspiration and pulls away because of sharp pain. Which of the following is the best test to diagnose the cause of her pain?

a. Abdominal radiograph
b. Ultrasound of the abdomen
c. Dimethyl iminodiacetic acid (HIDA) scan
d. Magnetic resonance imaging (MRI) of the abdomen
e. Upper endoscopy

165. A 16-year-old adolescent presents to the emergency room with a history of a football injury to the left flank earlier that day while at practice. He reports that at the time of the injury he only had the wind knocked out of him and he recovered in a few minutes. About 1 hour later he began to experience pain in the left upper quadrant and left shoulder. He also feels dizzy and lightheaded on standing. Physical examination demonstrates orthostatic changes in blood pressure and heart rate. His chest wall is nontender and his heart and lung examinations are normal. Abdominal auscultation reveals normal bowel sounds, but the patient complains of tenderness when palpating the left upper quadrant. Rectal examination and urinalysis are normal. Which of the following is the most likely diagnosis?

a. Dislocation of the left shoulder
b. Left rib fracture
c. Left pneumothorax
d. Ruptured spleen
e. Contusion of the left kidney

166. A 71-year-old Asian American man presents to your office with the chief complaint of a 40-lb weight loss over the last 4 months. He has anorexia, dyspepsia, and generalized weakness. Abdominal examination is positive for a scaphoid abdomen, a supraclavicular lymph node on the left and a palpable nodule found in the area of the umbilicus. Which of the following is the most likely cause of the physical examination findings?

a. Gastric cancer
b. Lung cancer
c. Hepatocellular cancer
d. Renal cell carcinoma
e. Hodgkin lymphoma

167. A 40-year-old man presents to the emergency room complaining of 3 days of severe abdominal pain that radiates to his back, accompanied by several episodes of vomiting. He drinks alcohol daily. On physical examination, the patient is found on the stretcher lying in the fetal position. He is febrile and appears ill. The skin of his abdomen has an area of bluish periumbilical discoloration. There is no flank discoloration. Abdominal examination reveals decreased bowel sounds. The patient has severe midepigastric tenderness on palpation and complains of exquisite pain when your hands are abruptly withdrawn from his abdomen. Rectal examination is normal. Which of the following is the most likely diagnosis?

a. Acute cholecystitis
b. Pyelonephritis
c. Necrotizing pancreatitis
d. Chronic pancreatitis
e. Diverticulitis
f. Appendicitis

168. A 60-year-old man with a history of appendectomy 30 years ago presents to the emergency room complaining of abdominal pain. He describes the pain as colicky and crampy and feels it builds up, then it improves on its own. He has vomited at least 10 times since the pain started this morning. He states that he has not had a bowel movement for 2 days and cannot recall the last time he passed flatus. The abdomen is slightly distended. Abdominal auscultation reveals high-pitched bowel sounds and peristaltic rushes. Percussion reveals a tympanic abdomen. The patient is diffusely tender with palpation but has no rebound tenderness. Rectal examination reveals the absence of stool. Which of the following is the most appropriate first test to confirm your diagnosis?

a. Thick barium upper gastrointestinal series
b. MRI of the abdomen
c. HIDA scan
d. Spiral CT scan
e. Abdominal radiograph

169. A 3-year-old boy is accompanied by his mother to your office. She describes an almost year-long history of him having loose bowel movements that often float on the water of the toilet bowl, along with excessive gas and weight loss. He is short for his age. On examination, he has abdominal distention with hyperactive bowel sounds. Over his trunk, neck, and scalp he has a papulovesicular skin rash. What would be the next appropriate step in diagnosis?

a. Endoscopic mucosal biopsy
b. Hydrogen breath test
c. IgA endomysial antibody test
d. Flat and upright abdominal x-ray
e. No further diagnostic testing is needed

170. A 51-year-old woman presents to the emergency room complaining of right upper quadrant and epigastric pain for 5 hours, which improves when she leans forward. She has nausea and vomiting but does not have hematemesis or melena. She is a smoker and admits to drinking several beers daily. She is afebrile, but you note icterus of her eyes and sublingual area. On abdominal examination you feel a nontender mass in her right upper quadrant. Which of the following is the most likely diagnosis?

a. Cholelithiasis
b. Acute cholecystitis
c. Cirrhosis of the liver
d. Carcinoma of the pancreas
e. Acute viral hepatitis

171. A 32-year-old man presents with severe abdominal pain, which he describes as sharp and diffuse. He does not drink alcohol or take any medications. He has a medical history significant for peptic ulcer disease over 5 years ago. He has stable vital signs and has no orthostatic changes. You observe that the patient is lying very still on the emergency room stretcher. On physical examination, he has a rigid abdomen and decreased bowel sounds. He has localized left upper quadrant guarding and rebound tenderness. He has referred rebound tenderness on palpation of the right upper quadrant. Rectal examination is fecal occult blood test (FOBT) negative. Which of the following is the best method of confirming the diagnosis in this patient?

a. Barium swallow
b. Leukocytosis
c. Upper endoscopy
d. Upright abdominal radiograph
e. Colonoscopy

172. A 74-year-old man presents with the abrupt onset of pain in the left lower abdomen, which has been progressively worsening over the last 2 days. He states that the pain is unremitting. He has some diarrhea but no nausea or vomiting. He has no dysuria or hematuria. His temperature is 38.9°C (102°F). Bowel sounds are decreased. The patient has involuntary guarding. There is tenderness and rebound tenderness when the left lower quadrant is palpated. The referred rebound test is positive. There is no costovertebral angle (CVA) tenderness. Rectal examination reveals brown stool, which is fecal occult blood test (FOBT) positive. Blood work demonstrates a leukocytosis. Which of the following is the most likely diagnosis?

a. Colon cancer
b. Diverticulitis
c. Pancreatitis
d. Pyelonephritis
e. Appendicitis

173. A 32-year-old man presents with fever, vomiting, and diffuse abdominal pain. On physical examination, his temperature is 39.4°C (103°F) and his heart rate is 120 beats per minute. He reports worsening of his abdominal pain when hitting bumps in the car on the way to the emergency room and on examination, has severe pain when palpating one-third of the way along a line drawn from the right anterior superior iliac spine to the umbilicus. He has a positive Rovsing sign. Which of the following is the most appropriate next step in diagnosis?

a. CT of the abdomen
b. Ultrasound of the abdomen
c. Surgical intervention
d. Paracentesis
e. Plain film of the abdomen

174. A 71-year-old woman with a history of a previous myocardial infarction presents to her family physician for a routine checkup. The physician notices that she has lost 20 lb since her last visit 6 months ago. When questioned, the patient gives a history of intermittent periumbilical pain that begins 30 minutes after eating and lasts for 2 to 3 hours. She claims the pain is worse after large meals, so she has begun to eat less out of fear of precipitating the pain. Her physical examination is unremarkable. Which of the following is the most likely diagnosis?

a. Pancreatitis
b. Mesenteric ischemia
c. Cholecystitis
d. Small-bowel obstruction
e. Peptic ulcer disease

175. A patient with a long history of cirrhosis presents with asterixis. He is alert and oriented to person, place, and time. His breath is positive for fetor hepaticus. His abdomen is significant for caput medusae and a positive fluid wave. He has no focal neurologic deficit. His wife states that the patient is very functional at home but is moderately confused and drowsy. Which is the most helpful test to confirm the diagnosis in this patient?

a. Serum lactate level
b. Serum ammonia level
c. Serum iron level
d. Serum alkaline phosphatase level
e. Serum sodium level

176. A 24-year-old HIV-positive patient who has had AIDS for 3 years presents with painful swallowing and dysphagia to solids and liquids. He has no previous history of heartburn or reflux disease. His CD4 count is 41/μL, and he recently required 3 weeks of antibiotics for *Pneumocystis jirovecii* pneumonia. Examination of the pharynx reveals no oral thrush. Barium swallow demonstrates multiple nodular filling defects of various sizes that resemble a cluster of grapes. Which of the following is the most likely diagnosis?

a. *Candida* esophagitis
b. Gastroesophageal Reflux disease
c. Barrett esophagus
d. Achalasia
e. Plummer-Vinson syndrome
f. Schatzki ring

177. A 47-year-old woman admits to excessive alcohol use on a thorough history. What finding on physical examination can be attributed to her alcohol use?

a. Palmar creases
b. Increased body hair
c. Tympany of the abdomen
d. Splenomegaly
e. Livedo reticularis

178. A 70-year-old woman with a 25-year history of diabetes mellitus presents with early satiety, bloating, and nausea after meals. She has had previous surgery for gallbladder stones and appendicitis. Her diabetes is complicated by retinopathy and peripheral neuropathy. On physical examination, bowel sounds are normal. A succussion splash is audible. The abdomen is tympanic, and there is no hepatosplenomegaly. There is no tenderness. Rectal examination is normal. Serum glucose is 310 mg/dL. Which of the following is the most likely diagnosis?

a. Celiac sprue
b. Whipple disease
c. Gastroparesis
d. Gluten-sensitive enteropathy
e. Tropical sprue

179. A 23-year-old man presents with mild, persistent jaundice. His serum bilirubin is always less than 5 mg/dL and is primarily unconjugated bilirubin. The jaundice is exacerbated by fasting, surgery, fever, infection, and alcohol ingestion. Which of the following is the most likely diagnosis?

a. Dubin-Johnson syndrome
b. Rotor syndrome
c. Crigler-Najjar type 1 syndrome
d. Crigler-Najjar type 2 syndrome
e. Gilbert syndrome

180. A 42-year-old morbidly obese woman complains of a nonproductive cough for 8 months. She reports regurgitation after eating, and when she does, it has a sour taste. She has been on a proton pump inhibitor for 3 months without relief. Abdominal examination is normal. Rectal examination is FOBT negative. Which of the following is the most appropriate next step in diagnosis?

a. Barium esophagography
b. Upper endoscopy
c. Esophageal manometry
d. Esophageal pH monitoring
e. Bernstein test

181. A 16-year-old adolescent has had lifelong constipation. He requires suppositories and, often, enemas to initiate bowel movements. His abdomen is distended. Palpation reveals a tubular mass in the left lower quadrant. Rectal examination reveals no stool in the vault. Barium enema reveals a dilated colon above a normal-appearing rectum. Which of the following is the most likely diagnosis?

a. Colon carcinoma
b. Gardner syndrome
c. Peutz-Jeghers syndrome
d. Hirschsprung disease
e. Volvulus

182. A 49-year-old patient presents with altered mental status. His wife states that over the last week her husband has been taking several over-the-counter pills every few hours for some headache and abdominal discomfort. He uses no illicit drugs but drinks four to five beers daily. Over the last 24 hours, the patient has become progressively lethargic. Vital signs reveal a temperature of 36.1°C (97°F), blood pressure of 100/70 mm Hg, heart rate of 120 beats per minute, and respiratory rate of 26 breaths per minute. The patient is jaundiced with right upper quadrant (RUQ) abdominal tenderness on palpation. He has no rebound tenderness or splenomegaly but has an enlarged liver. There is no ascites or peripheral edema. Heart and lung examinations are normal. The patient responds to painful stimuli and has asterixis. He has no focal neurologic deficit. Which of the following is the most likely diagnosis?

a. Alcohol intoxication
b. Alcohol withdrawal
c. Delirium tremens
d. Acetaminophen toxicity
e. Wilson disease

183. A 19-year-old woman attending school in Massachusetts presents with the chief complaint of bloody diarrhea for 2 months. She has abdominal discomfort and feels she has lost some weight. She also complains of tenesmus. Abdominal examination is normal. Rectal examination reveals stool containing blood and pus. Which of the following is the most likely diagnosis?

a. Irritable bowel syndrome
b. Ulcerative colitis
c. Giardiasis
d. Hemorrhoids
e. Diverticulosis

184. A 50-year-old man has a 10-year history of chronic active hepatitis from the hepatitis C virus. He is brought to the emergency room because of cachexia and disturbed mental status. On physical examination, the patient has palmar erythema and clubbing. He is jaundiced with massive ascites. He has asterixis. Laboratory data reveal severe hypoalbuminemia and hyperbilirubinemia. Which of the following is used to determine prognosis in this patient with end-stage liver disease?

a. International normalization ratio (INR)
b. Unconjugated bilirubin
c. Presence of jaundice
d. Presence of hepatomegaly
e. Serum blood urea nitrogen

185. A 44-year-old man with a history of Roux-en-Y gastric bypass surgery 1 year ago presents with fatigue, paresthesias in his feet and hands, and some difficulty with balance. Which of the following is the most likely etiology of his symptoms?

a. Dumping syndrome
b. Bacterial overgrowth
c. Gastric carcinoma
d. Gastritis
e. Malabsorption

186. A 21-year-old woman presents with jaundice and hepatomegaly. She has nausea, vomiting, and diarrhea. She recalls eating raw oysters 1 to 2 months ago. She has not traveled recently and denies drug use or unprotected sexual intercourse. She has no history of blood transfusion. Which of the following is the most likely viral etiology?

a. Hepatitis A
b. Hepatitis B
c. Hepatitis C
d. Hepatitis D
e. Hepatitis E
f. Hepatitis G

Questions 187 to 189

For each patient with a gastrointestinal bleed, select the most likely diagnosis. Each lettered option may be used once, multiple times, or not at all.

a. Gastric cancer
b. Erosive gastritis
c. Dieulafoy lesion
d. Mallory-Weiss tear
e. Gastrinoma
f. Esophageal varices

187. A 38-year-old man arrives at the emergency room with the chief complaint of hematemesis for 3 hours. He spent the previous night vomiting approximately 10 to 12 times after eating some "bad chicken."

188. A 44-year-old man with a history of heavy alcohol use for years presents to the emergency room with the acute onset of hematemesis. He appears jaundiced and has some mild ascites.

189. A 51-year-old man has massive coffee ground emesis and melena. He has been taking nonsteroidal anti-inflammatory medications daily because of arthritis pain.

Questions 190 and 191

For each description for detection of ascites, select the appropriate named sign. Each lettered option may be used once, more than once, or not at all.

a. Shifting dullness
b. Fluid wave
c. Puddle sign
d. Bulging flanks
e. Flank dullness

190. The patient is on his back, and with a push from one side of the abdomen, fluid is felt on the opposite side.

191. The border of dullness moves to the dependent side and tympany moves toward the top when the patient turns to the side from the supine position.

Questions 192 to 197

For each patient with liver disease, select the most likely disorder. Each lettered option may be used once, more than once, or not at all.

a. Hemochromatosis
b. Primary biliary cirrhosis
c. Sclerosing cholangitis
d. Hepatocellular carcinoma
e. Zollinger-Ellison syndrome
f. Alcoholic hepatitis
g. Wilson disease
h. α_1-Antitrypsin deficiency
i. Metastatic carcinoma of the liver
j. Budd-Chiari syndrome

192. A 54-year-old woman presents with generalized pruritus that keeps her awake at night. Liver size by percussion in the midclavicular line is 17 cm. There is no splenomegaly. Serum alkaline phosphatase level is three times the normal value.

193. A 44-year-old man with a 20-year history of ulcerative colitis presents with fever and RUQ pain. Physical examination reveals jaundice and RUQ tenderness with palpation. Endoscopic retrograde cholangiopancreatography (ERCP) shows multifocal strictures of the extrahepatic biliary tree.

194. A 41-year-old woman has a history of recurrent duodenal ulcer disease. She takes no medications and has no evidence of *Helicobacter pylori* infection. Her serum gastrin level is 800 pg/mL.

195. A 53-year-old alcoholic presents with mild RUQ tenderness and jaundice. Liver function tests reveal an elevated aspartate aminotransferase (AST) and alanine aminotransferase (ALT) level, but the AST is two times greater than the ALT.

196. A 39-year-old man presents with jaundice and ascites. He has a history of diabetes mellitus and was recently diagnosed as having heart disease. On physical examination, he has a bronze appearance to his skin, arthritic changes of the fingers, and testicular atrophy.

197. A 43-year-old man presents with cirrhosis. Slit-lamp examination reveals a yellow-brown ring in the limbus of the cornea. The patient has recently developed an unsteady gait, tremors, and involuntary chorea-like movements.

Questions 198 and 199

For each patient with infectious diarrhea, choose the most likely etiology. Each lettered option may be used once, more than once, or not at all.

a. *Clostridium difficile*
b. *Giardia lamblia*
c. Enterotoxigenic *Escherichia coli*
d. *Bacillus cereus*
e. *Escherichia coli* O157:H7
f. *Cryptosporidium*
g. *Entamoeba histolytica*
h. *Shigella*

198. A 51-year-old woman complains of 10 soft and watery, but nonbloody, stools per day. She was recently treated for pneumonia.

199. A 6-year-old boy ate a hamburger at a fast food restaurant and 2 days later developed fever, abdominal pain, and bloody diarrhea. He was subsequently admitted to the hospital and diagnosed with acute renal failure, microangiopathic hemolytic anemia, and thrombocytopenia.

Gastrointestinal System

Answers

162. The answer is d. *(McPhee, pp 445-446.)* The patient in the question presents with symptoms consistent with **vitamin B_{12} deficiency**. Patients with a history of previous bowel resection are susceptible to malabsorption of the essential nutrients. Since the vitamin B_{12}–intrinsic factor complex is absorbed in the ileum, vitamin B_{12} must be replaced in patients with terminal ileum resection. Other signs of vitamin B_{12} deficiency include megaloblastic anemia, altered cerebral function, neuropsychiatric changes, and difficulty with balance (posterior columns). Ileal resections also cause deficiency in bile salts, which are essential for the absorption of the **fat-soluble vitamins (A, D, E, and K)**. Patients with **vitamin A deficiency** present with night blindness, keratomalacia, scaling of the skin, increased intracranial pressure, and depressed immunity. **Osteomalacia** and **rickets** are a result of **vitamin D** deficiency. **Vitamin E deficiency** is rare; patients may present with neuropathy, ophthalmoplegia, and ataxia; hemolysis may occur in infants. Clotting times are prolonged in patients with **vitamin K deficiency**.

163. The answer is a. *(McPhee, pp 1147-1148.)* It is always preferential to use the gut for feeding when possible. The indications for **enteral tube feeding** include poor appetite or anorexia, inability to ingest food due to dysphagia or injury to the head and neck (as in this patient), gastroparesis, and maldigestion. **Peripheral parenteral nutrition (PPN)** is reserved for patients who require short-term parenteral nutrition and are not hypermetabolic or fluid restricted. PPN patients must have suitable peripheral venous access. **Central total parenteral nutrition (TPN)** is indicated in patients with poor peripheral venous access or in those who require long-term nutrition (> 7 days). This patient would not be able to tolerate a **pureed diet** at this point and **intravenous dextrose** will not meet the patient's nutritional requirements for healing over days to weeks.

164. The answer is c. *(McPhee, pp 635-637.)* This patient with fever and **Murphy sign**, the finding of an inspiratory halt with palpation of the right upper quadrant (RUQ) after a fatty meal, has acute **cholecystitis**. The liver and gallbladder move inferiorly as the diaphragm descends on deep inspiration, so the inflamed gallbladder becomes compressed against the inverted wall, and the patient experiences sharp pain abruptly halting inspiration. Cholecystitis risk factors are the **four F's** (Fat, Forty, Female, and Fertile). Other risk factors include diabetes, a positive family history, and medications such as oral contraceptives. Cholecystitis is associated with gallstones in 90% of cases. The **most sensitive test for detecting gallstones and cholecystitis is the HIDA scan** (98% sensitive and 81% specific for cholecystitis). It shows obstruction of the cystic duct (the primary cause of cholecystitis). **Abdominal ultrasound**, which is **usually the first-line test to detect gallstones,** only has a sensitivity of 67% and a specificity of 82% for detection of cholecystitis by seeing gallbladder wall thickening. **Plain films** detect gallstones in only 15% of cases. **MRI of the abdomen** would not be the best choice to visualize an inflamed gallbladder and **upper endoscopy** is best used to examine the esophagus and stomach for inflammation or ulcers.

165. The answer is d. *(Fauci, pp 93-94.)* The clinical picture is most consistent with a **ruptured spleen**. Intense pain in the left upper quadrant that radiates to the top of the left shoulder **(Kehr sign)** is due to diaphragmatic irritation, in this case by blood from the ruptured spleen. The spinal levels supplying most of the sensory fibers of the diaphragm **(C3-C5 and the phrenic nerve)** are the same levels as for some of the sensory supply to the shoulder. Therefore, diaphragmatic irritation is sometimes perceived as shoulder pain. Of all of the answer choices, only blood loss from the spleen causes signs of shock, including hypotension and orthostatic changes. This patient would also lack full range of motion of his left arm with a **dislocation of his shoulder** and he would have tenderness of his rib cage if he had **a rib fracture**. In the case of a **pneumothorax** he would have absent breath sounds and a **contusion of his kidney** would cause hematuria but none of the other findings in this case.

166. The answer is a. *(McPhee, pp 1470-1471.)* The patient has a **Virchow node** (left supraclavicular node) as well as a metastatic nodule of the umbilicus often referred to as a **Sister Mary Joseph nodule**. These findings, coupled with his dyspepsia and weight loss (as well as, in some patients, early satiety, melena, and postprandial vomiting) are indicative of **metastatic gastric carcinoma**. Because of its vascular and embryologic connections, the umbilicus is a susceptible site for metastatic disease. The primary sites likley to metastasize to the umbilicus are the **stomach, ovary, colon, rectum, and pancreas** (in descending order). A **scaphoid abdomen** in this patient implies malnourishment; the abdomen appears hollow or concave. *Scaphoid* may also refer to the normal boatlike appearance of the abdomen seen in thin patients. None of the other answer choices lead to these specific findings.

167. The answer is c. *(McPhee, pp 641-645.)* The two most common causes of acute pancreatitis are excessive alcohol ingestion and passage of a gallstone, though medications, trauma, and hyperlipidemia may result in pancreatic inflammation as well. This patient who excessively drinks alcohol most likely has **necrotizing pancreatitis**, which is a complication of acute pancreatitis. Other complications of pancreatitis include pseudocyst, abscess, and phlegmon. The periumbilical discoloration **(Cullen sign)** suggests a hemoperitoneum. Ecchymoses of the flanks would be a positive **Grey Turner sign**. When the patient experiences pain as the hands of the examiner are abruptly withdrawn from the abdomen, he or she is said to have **rebound tenderness** (a sign of peritonitis). Decreased or absent bowel sounds and **involuntary guarding** are other signs of peritonitis. An abdominal radiograph in acute pancreatitis might show a **sentinel loop** (air-filled small intestine in the LUQ) and **colon cutoff sign** (air in the transverse colon). Patients with **chronic pancreatitis** present with bouts of abdominal pain and signs of pancreatic insufficiency (weight loss, steatorrhea, and diabetes). The abdominal radiograph in patients with chronic pancreatitis demonstrates **calcifications in the pancreas** (pathognomonic). **Acute cholecystitis** would likely be associated with gallstones and a positive Murphy's sign in the right upper quadrant. **Pyelonephritis** would present with urinary symptoms and costovertebral angle tenderness. **Diverticulitis** causes left lower quadrant pain and **appendicitis** leads to right lower quadrant pain.

168. The answer is e. *(Fauci, pp 1912-1914.)* The patient has a past medical history of appendectomy, which predisposes him to adhesions that often cause **small-bowel obstruction (SBO)**. Other etiologies for SBO include incarcerated hernia, stricture, and malignancy. The hallmarks of intestinal obstruction are paroxysmal abdominal pain, distension, vomiting, and obstipation. The high-pitched bowel sounds, peristaltic rushes, and tympany with percussion are physical findings when air is under pressure in viscera and intestinal fluid is present (ie, obstruction). **Abdominal radiographs** are the appropriate first test as they may reveal **dilated loops** of fluid- and gas-filled bowel in a ladderlike pattern and **air-fluid levels**. **CT scan** (not spiral) may differentiate partial and complete obstructions. Thin barium may be used for this purpose as well, but **thick barium should be avoided** in any SBO considered high grade or complete and in any colonic obstruction. **MRI** would not be the first test to order and a **HIDA scan** is best used to detect gallstones, not an SBO.

169. The answer is c. *(McPhee, pp 559-560.)* This young patient with short stature, diarrhea, steatorrhea, and flatulence has classic symptoms of **celiac disease**, the result of an immunologic response to gluten in the diet that damages the small intestinal mucosa, causing malabsorption. Classic symptoms often occur in infants, while the majority of cases appear with atypical symptoms (depression, fatigue, delayed puberty) in later childhood or adulthood, making it hard to diagnose. This patient also has **dermatitis herpetiformis**, a characteristic skin rash occurring in less than 10% of patients with celiac disease, though almost all patients with this rash have a positive intestinal mucosal biopsy. The first step to diagnosis in patients suspected of having celiac disease is to obtain the **IgA endomysial antibody test and IgA tTG antibody test**—negative tests virtually exclude the diagnosis. In patients with positive serologic testing, **endoscopic biopsy of the intestinal mucosa will confirm the diagnosis**, showing blunting of intestinal villi and infiltration of the lamina propria with lymphocytes and plasma cells. These abnormalities resolve on a gluten-free diet. The **hydrogen breath test** is used to confirm the diagnosis of lactase deficiency. An **abdominal x-ray** will not aid diagnosis.

170. The answer is d. *(McPhee, pp 1461-465.)* This patient's symptoms and signs, including the presence of the **Courvoisier sign**, a palpable nontender gallbladder in this patient with painless jaundice, are almost assuredly due to **cancer of the biliary tract or head of the pancreas**. The majority of patients present with vague abdominal pain, though painless jaundice should move pancreatic cancer to the top of any differential diagnosis. **Cholelithiasis, acute viral hepatits, and acute cholecystitis** would lead to right upper quadrant pain and often fever and jaundice, but no mass. Patients with **cirrhosis** present with a nonpalpable fibrotic liver and signs of portal hypertension and often ascites, not jaundice or a mass.

171. The answer is d. *(McPhee, p 555.)* This patient likely has a perforated peptic ulcer, as his physical examination findings—guarding, rigidity, absent, or diminished bowel sounds, rebound and referred rebound tenderness, and lying perfectly still—are all signs of **peritonitis**. A **plain film of the abdomen** in this patient with a probable perforated ulcer might show **free intraperitoneal air under the diaphragm** (in up to 75% of patients). The free air establishes the diagnosis, and no further studies are needed. **Barium studies** are contraindicated in perforation.

172. The answer is b. *(McPhee, pp 588-589.)* The patient most likely has **diverticulitis**, an acute inflammatory process caused by bacteria in a diverticulum (outpouching of the mucosa or submucosa). It may occur in up to 50% of patients with diverticulosis. Diverticulitis is **usually left-sided**, since the diameter of the sigmoid colon is the smallest of the colon and higher wall tension and intraluminal pressure in this area result in diverticular formation. Peritonitis often results in **involuntary guarding** (abdominal rigidity due to reflex muscle spasm from the peritoneal irritation). Decreased bowel sounds may be heard in peritonitis or in any condition that causes an **ileus** (absence of peristalsis). Tenderness upon abrupt withdrawal of the hand **(rebound tenderness or Blumberg sign)** occurs because when the abdominal wall passively springs back into place, it carries with it the inflamed peritoneum. The **referred rebound test** is conducted in the same way, but the patient will experience pain a site away from where the test is performed. **Colon cancer** may present with hematochezia or signs of obstruction but not infection or peritonitis. **Pancreatitis** causes epigastric pain, **pyelonephritis** results in dysuria and back pain with CVA tenderness, and **appendicitis** most often causes right lower quadrant pain.

173. The answer is a. *(McPhee, pp 567-568.)* On examination, this patient has pain at **McBurney point**, located 1.5 to 2 in from the anterior spinous process of the ileum on a straight line drawn from the process to the umbilicus, the spot on the abdomen that overlies the anatomic position of the appendix. **Rovsing sign** is one of the many signs that may indicate **appendicitis** and occurs when palpation of the left lower quadrant (LLQ) causes **referred rebound pain** in the right lower quadrant (RLQ). The pain the patient describes on the drive over may be reproduced by **Markle sign**, or the **heel jar test**; the patient stands on his or her toes, and then allows his or her heels to hit the floor, thus jarring the body and causing abdominal pain in the setting of peritonitis. Other signs specific for appendicitis include the **obturator sign** (pain occurring when the right leg, flexed at the hip and knee, is rotated laterally and medially) and the **iliopsoas** sign which produces RLQ pain when the patient flexes at the hip and raises the right leg against the examiner's resistance on the thigh. A patient with appendicitis may also have pain on rectal examination if the posterior appendix is involved. The next best step for the patient who presents with clinical appendicitis is to confirm the diagnosis and rule out other causes of lower quadrant pain with **imaging with CT or ultrasound of the abdomen,** though **CT scanning is more accurate**. Once the diagnosis is confirmed, **surgical intervention** is needed. **Plain films** will not reveal the inflammation of the appendix and **paracentesis** is used to remove ascites.

174. The answer is b. *(McPhee, p 421.)* This patient has chronic **mesenteric, or intestinal ischemia** characterized by preexisting vascular disease and the symptom triad of **postprandial pain 30 minutes to 3 hours after eating** (often referred to as **abdominal angina), anorexia** to avoid pain from eating, and resultant **weight loss**. The classic acute presentation is often of steady, severe epigastric, and midabdominal **pain out of proportion to physical examination findings**. The acute catastrophic event can cause rectal bleeding, peritonitis, and shock. The diagnosis may be confirmed by angiography; embolectomy or surgery is required in selected cases. **Pancreatitis and cholecystitis** would result in tenderness on examination and **small-bowel obstruction** would cause nausea and vomiting without bowel movements. While **peptic ulcer disease** would present similarly to this case, she likely would experience some relief with antacids and have epigastric tenderness on palpation.

175. The answer is b. *(McPhee, pp 622-623.)* This patient's clinical presentation is consistent with **hepatic encephalopathy. Asterixis**, also referred to as liver flap or flapping tremor, is a nonrhythmic, asymmetric lapse in a sustained position of an extremity. It is nonspecific for cirrhosis and may be seen in other metabolic derangements (ie, renal disease and metabolic acidosis). **Fetor hepaticus** (due to mercaptans) is a musty odor of the breath and urine and is part of the encephalopathy. **Caput medusae** are the dilated periumbilical veins (ie, **reopened umbilical veins**) seen in patients with portal hypertension. **Serum ammonia** is representative of toxin build-up from liver failure in patients with encephalopathy but is not solely responsible for the altered mental status. None of the other choices would confirm the diagnosis.

It is often helpful to stage the hepatic encephalopathy to follow the course of the illness:

Stage 1: euphoria/depression, **mild confusion**, slurred speech, disordered sleep, +/−asterixis
Stage 2: **lethargy**, moderate confusion, + asterixis
Stage 3: **marked confusion**, incoherent speech, sleeping but arousable, + asterixis
Stage 4: **comatose**, −asterixis

176. The answer is a. *(McPhee, p 535.)* **Odynophagia** (painful swallowing) is the most common presenting symptom of infectious esophagitis. In an HIV-positive patient, especially one recently on antibiotics, ***Candida albicans*** is the most common organism, but only three quarters of patients have concomitant oral thrush. Diagnostic tests can be delayed to see if the patient responds to **empiric antifungal therapy**. If not, **upper endoscopy** should be employed to rule out other organisms, including cytomegalovirus and herpes simplex virus. **Gastroesophageal reflux disease** may cause a noninfectious esophagitis, but it is less likely in this patient. **Barrett esophagus** (premalignant lesion for adenocarcinoma of the esophagus) is replacement of the squamous epithelium by columnar epithelium from chronic reflux of gastric acid. **Dysphagia**, or difficulty swallowing may be the result of several problems. Patients with **achalasia**, failure of the lower esophageal sphincter to relax (motor disorder of smooth muscle), complain of progressive dysphagia to liquids and solids. Patients with **cancer** typically present with dysphagia to solids, which progresses to include liquids, accompanied by weight loss. Middle-aged women with **Plummer-Vinson syndrome (hypopharyngeal web)** present with dysphagia to solids and iron-deficiency anemia. **Schatzki ring** is a weblike constriction near the lower esophageal sphincter (LES) that produces intermittent dysphagia to solids.

177. The answer is d. *(McPhee, p 619.)* There are several common physical examination findings resulting from excessive alcohol use. On the abdominal examination, patients may have **caput medusa** (engorged periumbilical veins), **hepatomegaly** (or a small, contracted liver in the case of cirrhosis) **and ascites** which can be detected using the **fluid wave or shifting dullness**

tests. **Splenomegaly** is present in up to half of patients due to portal hypertension. Dermatologically, patients develop **palmar erythema and spider angiomata** (lacy spider veins on the upper half of the body) as well as **diminished body hair**. On the musculoskeletal examination they may have **Dupuytren contractures** and signs of wasting, as well as peripheral edema. On chest examination they may have **gynecomastia** or exhibit **signs of heart failure** (jugular venous distention, S_3, inferiorly and laterally displaced apical impulse) if they develop alcoholic cardiomyopathy. On genitourinary examination, males will have **testicular atrophy**. In addition, if they develop encephalopathy, they may have **altered mental status and asterixis** (flapping of the hands with dorsiflexion, like "stopping traffic,") at the wrist. **Livedo reticularis** is a mottled purple discoloration of the skin associated not with alcohol use, but rather with antiphospholipid antibody syndrome, polyarteritis nodosa, and Disseminated Intravascular Coagulation (DIC), among other conditions.

178. The answer is c. *(McPhee, p 566.)* Diabetic patients, especially those with poor control, may develop autonomic dysfunction which results in delayed gastric emptying **(gastroparesis)**. Often, patients will have a **succussion splash** (a splash is heard with the stethoscope when shaking the patient, due to the air-fluid interface). Diagnosis is made by a **gastric emptying study**. Patients with **celiac sprue** (also called **gluten-sensitive enteropathy**) present with bloating, diarrhea, and excessive flatus. They typically have signs of malabsorption, such as hypoalbuminemia, iron-deficiency anemia, hypocholesterolemia, and decreased carotene level. The diagnosis is made by small-bowel biopsy, and the treatment is a wheat-free diet. **Whipple disease** is a multisystemic disorder characterized by arthralgias, abdominal pain, fever, weight loss, lymphadenopathy, heart disease, and neurologic disease. Finding **periodic acid–Schiff (PAS) positive-staining foamy macrophages** in tissues makes the diagnosis, and treatment for this previously fatal disease is antibiotics (for *Tropheryma whippelii*). **Tropical sprue** often responds to antibiotics and may occur months or even years after a patient returns from the tropics.

179. The answer is e. *(McPhee, p 599.)* **Gilbert disease** is the most common cause of benign, asymptomatic, hereditary jaundice. It is found in up to **10%** of the population and is due to a **partial deficiency of glucuronyl transferase**, resulting in mild unconjugated hyperbilirubinemia which worsens after a fast. Patients with **Dubin-Johnson syndrome** develop jaundice with stress, but it is primarily conjugated bilirubin. Hepatocytes have brown pigment and the gallbladder is not seen on oral cholecystography. **Rotor syndrome** is similar to Dubin-Johnson syndrome, but in this case there is no pigment in the liver and the gallbladder is visible. **Crigler-Najjar type 1 syndrome** (predominance of unconjugated bilirubin) is severe (absence of glucuronosyltransferase), and patients typically have bilirubin levels of more than 20 mg/dL. **Crigler-Najjar type 2 syndrome** is a relatively benign disorder due to partial deficiency of glucuronosyltransferase; patients present as adolescents with bilirubin levels of 6 to 20 mg/dL.

180. The answer is b. *(McPhee, pp 530-534.)* This patient has symptoms consistent with **gastroesophageal reflux disease (GERD)**. Risk factors include obesity, pregnancy, scleroderma, and diet (caffeine, alcohol, nicotine, chocolate, fatty foods). The most common etiology of GERD is transient LES relaxation, but it may also be due to hiatal hernia and acidic gastric contents. The sour taste of GERD is often referred to as **water brash**. Atypical symptoms of GERD may include asthma, chronic cough, chronic laryngitis, sore throat, and chest pain. Patients with uncomplicated initial symptoms may be treated empirically with H_2 blockers or proton-pump inhibitors. In patients in whom 8 weeks of antacid therapy is inadequate or who have accompanying dysphagia, odynophagia, weight loss, or iron deficiency, further evaluation with **upper endoscopy** is warranted to look for tissue damage and complications such as Barrett esophagus or strictures. **Barium swallows** are used in patients with severe dysphagia to identify abnormalities such as strictures and **esophageal manometry and pH monitoring** are used to evaluate patients with negative endoscopic findings who have persistent symptoms on medication. The **Bernstein test** was an old way of diagnosing GERD by reproducing symptoms through dropping acid into the esophagus.

181. The answer is d. *(McPhee, pp 507-508.)* **Hirschsprung disease** (aganglionic megacolon) is a disorder characterized by the absence of enteric neurons in the submucosal and myenteric plexuses. The contracted segment of bowel is unable to relax, and a mass may become palpable. Patients describe lifelong constipation. **Peutz-Jeghers syndrome** is autosomal dominant (AD) and is characterized by hamartomatous polyps in the small intestine and perioral melanin deposits. **Gardner syndrome** (also AD) is familial adenomatous polyposis syndrome. Gardner syndrome and Peutz–Jeghers syndrome are risk factors for **colon cancer**, which often presents with rectal bleeding. **Volvulus** (malrotation that leads to gangrene) is usually seen in the first year of life; infants present with bilious vomiting, bloody stools, rigid and discolored abdomen, and shock.

182. The answer is d. *(McPhee, p 1428.)* This patient with alcohol abuse and likely underlying liver disease probably has **fulminant hepatitis** from **acetaminophen toxicity**. Because of his alcohol use, he has insufficient glutathione stores and induced P450 enzymatic activity and is at greater risk for developing toxicity. Patients who survive the complication of fulminant hepatic failure will begin to recover over the following week, but some require liver transplantation. A serum acetaminophen level should be obtained, and immediate treatment with **N-acetylcysteine (NAC)**, which provides cysteine for glutathione synthesis, is indicated. Signs of **alcohol intoxication** include euphoria, dysarthria, ataxia, labile mood, lethargy, coma, respiratory depression, and death. Patients experiencing **alcohol withdrawal** present with a hyperexcitable state (ie, hypertension, tachycardia, flushing, sweating, and mydriasis) and have tremors, disordered perceptions, seizures, and delirium tremens. **Delirium tremens** occurs 2 to 4 days after alcohol abstinence and is characterized by hallucinations that may lead to dangerous, combative, and destructive behavior. **Wilson disease** is an autosomal recessive disorder characterized by excessive copper deposition in the brain and liver; patients present before age 40 with hepatitis, splenomegaly, hemolytic anemia, portal hypertension, and psychiatric or neurologic abnormalities.

183. The answer is b. *(McPhee, pp 582-587.)* It is often difficult to distinguish clinically between **ulcerative colitis (UC)** and **Crohn disease (CD)**. Patients like this with UC experience bloody diarrhea and mucus, fecal urgency, and lower abdominal cramping. Barium enema showing **involvement of the colon** supports UC. Patients with CD usually have less rectal bleeding and rarely have tenesmus. Typically, patients with CD have skip lesions and rectal sparing. Patients with **irritable bowel syndrome** complain of abdominal pain with altered frequency or consistency of stool but have no weight loss or bleeding. More than half of patients with irritable bowel syndrome have psychiatric disorders. Patients with **diverticulosis** (saclike protrusions of the mucosa through the muscularis) are usually older and asymptomatic; hemorrhage occurs in a small percentage of patients. **Giardiasis** may be found in immunocompromised patients, day-care workers, male homosexuals, individuals who drink untreated water (hikers and campers), and international travelers (especially to Russia). Patients with **hemorrhoids** present with rectal bleeding and pain.

184. The answer is a. *(Fauci, pp 1922-1923.)* Until recently, the **Child-Pugh classification** has been used to clinically stage severity of cirrhosis and is a reliable predictor of survival and complications in patients with end-stage liver disease.

CHILD-PUGH CLASSIFICATION

	A	B	C
Bilirubin (mg/dL)	<2.0	2.0-3.0	>3.0
Albumin (g/dL)	>3.5	3.0-3.5	<3.0
Ascites	None	Easily controlled	Not controlled
Neurologic	None	Minimal	Advanced (coma)
Nutrition	Excellent	Good	Wasting

This system has been replaced with the model for end-stage liver disease, or **MELD, score**. Calculated using **the international normalization ratio (INR), serum bilirubin, and serum creatinine**, it helps establish priority listing for liver transplantation in the United States.

185. The answer is e. *(Fauci, pp 472-473.)* Bariatric surgery can be performed on patients with severe obesity (BMI $\geq$ 40 kg/m^2) or moderate obesity (BMI > 30 kg/m^2) with concomitant medical issues. Restrictive procedures limit the amount of food the stomach can hold. The **Roux-en-Y gastric bypass** combines restriction with selective malabsorption. Some patients with a history of **restrictive-malabsorptive gastric bypass procedures** develop deficiencies **of iron, folate, calcium, vitamin D, and vitamin B_{12}**. This patient's symptoms are consistent with vitamin B_{12} deficiency, thereby necessitating supplementation.

186. The answer is a. *(McPhee, pp 601-602.)* Hepatitis A, C, D, E, and G are all RNA viruses, while hepatitis B is a DNA virus. This patient likely has **hepatitis A (HAV)** which is almost exclusively transmitted via the fecal-oral route and is spread from person to person. Outbreaks have been traced to contaminated food, water, milk, and undercooked shellfish. **Hepatitis B (HBV)**

is transmitted sexually, perinatally, and through blood products. **Hepatitis C (HCV)** is transmitted primarily via blood products. Perinatal transmission and sexual transmission of HCV is less than 5%. HCV is the most common cause of chronic hepatitis in the United States. **Hepatitis D (HDV)** is endemic in patients with HBV in the Mediterranean countries, but in the United States it is confined to blood products. HDV was probably introduced into the United States by intravenous drug abusers. **Hepatitis E (HEV)** resembles HAV (fecal-oral route) but is found primarily in India, Africa, Asia, and Central America. **Hepatitis G (HGV)** is blood borne, and its mode of transmission parallels that of HCV.

187 to 189. The answers are 187-d, 188-f, 189-b. *(McPhee, pp 544-545.)* **Mallory-Weiss** tears are longitudinal tears in the mucosa of the gastroesophageal junction due to prolonged and violent retching or vomiting. **Esophageal varices** are dilated submucosal veins that develop in patients with portal hypertension, such as alcoholics with cirrhosis. Bleeding varices have the highest morbidity and mortality rate of all causes of gastrointestinal bleeding. Overuse of NSAIDs may cause a bleeding **peptic ulcer (gastric or duodenal)** or just **erosive gastritis**. Both often cause hematemesis and if the blood has been retained in the stomach, the digestive processes change the hemoglobin to a brown or black pigment commonly referred to as **coffee ground emesis**. **Gastric cancer** is often asymptomatic until it is advanced, when it presents as dyspepsia, early satiety, weight loss and often signs of gastrointestinal bleeding. A **Dieulafoy lesion** is an aberrantly large artery in the submucosa of either the stomach or the duodenum that bleeds. It is a rare lesion that is often missed at endoscopy; multiple endoscopies may be required to make the diagnosis. **Gastrinomas (Zollinger-Ellison syndrome)** are gastrin-secreting tumors that cause peptic ulcers.

190 and 191. The answers are 190-b, 191-a. *(Seidel, p 549.)* Patients with ascites may have **dullness to percussion at the flanks**, but **shifting dullness** and a **positive fluid wave** are the best physical examination findings for diagnosing ascites. In patients with ascites, the border of dullness shifts to the dependent side as the fluid resettles with gravity when the patient rolls to the side. A **fluid wave** occurs when a sharp tap at one end of the abdomen pushes the ascitic fluid so that its "wave" is felt on the other side. The patient places his or her hand in the middle of the abdomen to stop the transmission through adipose tissue. Asking the patient to go into the uncomfortable position of being on all fours and percussing the umbilicus for dullness is the **puddle sign** (low sensitivity and specificity). **Bulging flanks** (flanks are pushed outward) are seen in obese patients as well as in patients with ascites.

192 to 197. The answers are 192-b, 193-c, 194-e, 195-f, 196-a, 197-g. *(McPhee, pp 556-557, 614-616, 625-630, 640-641.)* Patients (like the 54-year-old woman) with **primary biliary cirrhosis (PBC)** often present with generalized pruritus, asymptomatic cholestasis, or an isolated alkaline phosphatase level. It occurs most frequently in women, and antimitochondrial antibodies (AMAs) are present in over 90% of affected patients. **Sclerosing cholangitis** is a complication of ulcerative colitis; patients have fibrosing inflammation of the intrahepatic and extrahepatic bile ducts that is best diagnosed by ERCP. Seventy percent of patients present with the **Charcot triad** of fever, jaundice, and RUQ pain. The **Reynolds pentad** is the Charcot triad with the addition of shock and altered mental status. Sclerosing cholangitis is a life-threatening illness requiring emergency bile duct decompression. **Zollinger-Ellison syndrome** should be considered in patients with a history of recurrent duodenal ulcer disease. In this condition gastrinomas may be single or multiple, and up to two-thirds are malignant. Twenty-five percent of gastrinomas are associated with multiple endocrine neoplasia (MEN) type 1 and may be found in the pancreas or duodenum. Serum gastrin levels are typically elevated (>150 pg/mL). Patients who drink heavily may develop **alcoholic hepatitis**, which is characterized by abdominal pain, jaundice and AST elevated by twice as much as ALT because alcohol inhibits ALT synthesis more than AST synthesis. Patients with **hemochromatosis** present with suntan-like pigmentation **("bronze diabetes")**, degenerative arthritis of the hands and fingers proximal interphalangeal joints (PIPs), impotence, amenorrhea, testicular atrophy, cardiac disease, liver disease, and glucose intolerance. Hemochromatosis is diagnosed by an elevated serum iron level, an elevated ferritin level, and an elevated transferrin saturation (>55%). Patients with **Wilson disease** have **Kayser-Fleischer rings** (yellow-brown) in the Descemet membrane and neurologic symptoms. Wilson disease is diagnosed by a low ceruloplasmin level. **α_1-Antitrypsin deficiency** is characterized by liver disease and emphysema. **Budd-Chiari syndrome** is occlusion of the inferior vena cava or hepatic veins. The most common malignancy of the liver is **metastatic** (from primary sites, in order of decreasing frequency: colon, pancreas, breast, and lung) though **hepatocellular carcinoma** may arise in patients with cirrhosis from alcohol or hepatitis C, among other associations.

198 and 199. The answers are 198-a, 199-e. *(Fauci, pp 247-248.)* Patients with diarrhea have more than three bowel movements a day that are often liquid in consistency. Acute onset of symptoms that lasts fewer than 2 weeks is most likely infectious or drug-induced. The first patient, who has recently been treated with antibiotics and has multiple watery stools daily, most likely has ***C. difficile* infection**. *Clostridium difficile* overgrowth results from disruption of normal gastrointestinal flora by almost any antibiotic, especially clindamycin, ampicillin, and second- and third-generation cephalosporins. It secretes toxins that cause diarrhea and pseudomembranous colitis. The second patient has diarrhea due to ***E. coli*** O157:H7, which is associated with eating undercooked ground beef and can be followed by **hemolytic uremic syndrome** (acute renal failure, microangiopathic hemolytic anemia, and thrombocytopenia) in the very young and the elderly. Many tourists to endemic areas of Latin America, Asia, and Africa develop watery traveler's diarrhea, accompanied by abdominal pain and vomiting, frequently due to water or food contaminate with **enterotoxigenic *E. coli***. Campers and swimmers in wilderness areas are at increased risk for contracting infection up to a week later with ***G lamblia***. Bloody diarrhea associated with abdominal pain and fever following eating chicken at a picnic or restaurant, or through day-care contact, suggests severe inflammation due to infection with ***Shigella***. ***Salmonella*** causes watery or bloody diarrhea from ingesting infected mayonnaise or raw eggs and may cause traveler's diarrhea as well. Immunocompromised patients are at high risk for opportunistic infection with protozoans like ***Cryptosporidium***.

Renal and Genitourinary System

Questions

200. A 24-year-old man presents with a painless testicular mass. He does not recall any trauma, has no other medical issues and has no family history of cancer. He does not smoke, drink alcohol, or use illicit drugs. Physical examination reveals a 3-cm mass in the right scrotum that is hard and tender. The mass cannot be transilluminated. There is no lymphadenopathy and the rest of his physical examination is normal. The serum alpha-fetoprotein level is elevated. Which of the following is the most likely diagnosis?

a. Seminoma
b. Nonseminoma
c. Hematoma
d. Leydig cell tumor
e. Sertoli cell tumor

201. An 18-year-old man presents with a mass in the right inguinal area. When the examining finger is inserted into the lower part of the scrotum and carried along the vas deferens into the inguinal canal to inspect for herniation, the mass (viscus) strikes the tip of the examining finger when the patient is asked to cough. When the right inguinal area medial to the internal ring is compressed, and the patient is asked to cough again, the examining finger does not sense any mass striking it. Which of the following best describes the hernia?

a. This type of hernia almost always resolves spontaneously before puberty.
b. If the hernial sac extends into the scrotum, then this is a true surgical emergency.
c. Inguinal hernias are more common in women than men.
d. The appendix may be found in the hernial sac.
e. This type of hernia is frequently present in elderly women.

202. A 19-year-old male student presents for a precollege screening visit. On physical examination, the patient is tall, has a scant beard (he states that he needs to shave only every other month), and gynecomastia. His testes are firm and measure less than 2 cm each. The patient states that he functions as a normal man sexually, although he feels his libido is diminished compared to that of his friends. Which of the following is the most likely diagnosis?

a. Turner syndrome
b. Klinefelter syndrome
c. Ambiguous genitalia
d. Delayed puberty
e. Normal male

203. A 29-year-old man presents with his wife as part of a work-up for infertility. She has already been evaluated and no cause has been identified. The man describes normal sexual function and is completely asymptomatic. When you have him stand to perform the testicular examination, you visualize a scrotal swelling and on palpation feel a mass similar to a bag of worms. Which of the following is the most likely diagnosis?

a. Varicocele
b. Spermatocele
c. Inguinal hernia
d. Hematocele
e. Hydrocele

204. A 48-year-old diabetic man presents with peripheral edema. He has been physically active all of his life. His family history is unremarkable. His blood pressure is normal. On physical examination, the patient is noted to have anasarca. Kidneys are not palpable. Urinalysis reveals a moderate amount of proteinuria, and "grape clusters" are seen under light microscopy. Which of the following would you expect to find associated with this disorder?

a. Serum albumin of 4 g/dL
b. Urine protein excretion of 1 g/1.73 m^2 in 24 hours
c. Hyperlipidemia
d. Hematuria
e. Normal urine under polarized light

205. While examining the genitalia of an uncircumcised patient, you are unable to retract the foreskin. There is no evidence of erythema. Which of the following is the most likely diagnosis?

a. Balanitis
b. Phimosis
c. Escutcheon
d. Smegma
e. Priapism

206. A 34-year-old married man complains of lumps in his scrotal skin. He has no fever, penile discharge or other complaints. On physical examination, the lesions are small and mobile. An oily material can be extruded from the lesions. Which of the following is the most likely diagnosis?

a. Scrotal edema
b. Scrotal carcinoma
c. Epidermoid cysts
d. Molluscum contagiosum
e. Condyloma acuminatum

207. A 41-year-old man complains of soft, raised, flesh-colored growths or projections on his glans penis, prepuce, and penile shaft. Several excisional biopsies are done to look for malignancy. Which of the following is the most likely diagnosis?

a. Genital herpes
b. Condyloma acuminatum
c. Molluscum contagiosum
d. Condylomata lata
e. Peyronie disease

208. A 21-year-old man who recently recovered from the mumps presents to the emergency room complaining of a swollen and painful left testicle. Physical examination reveals testicular tenderness. Which of the following is the most likely diagnosis?

a. Orchitis
b. Epididymitis
c. Testicular tumor
d. Varicocele
e. Spermatocele

209. A 32-year-old woman comes to the emergency room complaining of bilateral flank pain and bloody urine. Family history reveals that her mother and one sibling have renal failure and receive hemodialysis. The patient's blood pressure is 170/100 mm Hg. Physical examination is normal except her kidneys are easily palpated bilaterally and are 20 cm each. Which of the following is the most likely diagnosis?

a. Horseshoe kidney
b. Polycystic kidney disease
c. Bilateral hydronephrosis
d. Kidney carcinoma
e. Medullary sponge kidney

210. A 34-year-old man presents to the emergency room complaining of protracted penile erection. The erection is not associated with sexual desire but is associated with severe pain. He denies any recent illicit drug or medication use. He has a past medical history significant for sickle cell disease. Which of the following is the appropriate next step in management?

a. Narcotics
b. Hydroxyurea
c. Folic acid
d. Exchange transfusion
e. Oxygen by nasal cannula

211. A 34-year-old firefighter presents to the emergency room complaining of the sudden onset of severe right-sided flank pain that radiates to the right groin and genitalia. He is unable to lie still on the stretcher. He denies any history of trauma. He denies any dysuria, frequency, nocturia, or fever. Examination of the genitalia is normal. Abdominal and rectal examinations are normal. There is positive right costovertebral angle (CVA) tenderness. Urinalysis reveals blood. Which of the following is the most likely diagnosis?

a. Pyelonephritis
b. Renal calculi
c. Testicular torsion
d. Strangulated hernia
e. Acute prostatitis

212. A 68-year-old man presents for his annual checkup. On a thorough review of symptoms, you find that he has urgency, difficulty starting his stream and nocturia. He has no past medical history and takes no medications. He does not smoke cigarettes or drink alcohol. Physical examination is normal except for the rectal examination, which is positive for an enlarged nontender prostate and a 3-mm prostatic nodule. Which of the following is the most appropriate next step in management?

a. Magnetic resonance imaging (MRI) of the prostate
b. Prostate-specific antigen (PSA) level
c. Transrectal ultrasound-guided prostate biopsy
d. Creatinine level
e. Blood urea nitrogen

213. A 10-year-old boy with no history of trauma presents to the emergency room with a 14-hour history of a painful scrotum. Elevation of the scrotum does not relieve the pain. He also complains of nausea and vomiting. Examination reveals an enlarged, tender, erythematous scrotum that does not transilluminate. The testicle is in a transverse (horizontal) position. Cremasteric reflex is absent on the side of the swelling. Which of the following is the most likely diagnosis?

a. Spermatocele
b. Hydrocele
c. Epididymitis
d. Varicocele
e. Testicular torsion

214. A 24-year-old uncircumcised male presents to the emergency room complaining of pain and difficulty on attempting to retract the foreskin of his penis. He has a history of diabetes with recurrent episodes of candidal balanitis. Which of the following is the most likely diagnosis?

a. Hypospadias
b. Phimosis
c. Paraphimosis
d. Priapism
e. Epispadias

215. A 49-year-old woman with multiple myeloma presents with glucosuria, hypophosphatemia, hypouricemia, aminoaciduria, and proteinuria. Further analysis of the electrolytes reveals the patient has a hyperchloremic metabolic acidosis. The urine pH is less than 5.5. Which of the following is the most likely diagnosis?

a. Fanconi syndrome
b. Type 1 renal tubular acidosis
c. Diabetic ketoacidosis
d. Type 4 renal tubular acidosis
e. Kimmelstiel-Wilson disease

216. A 16-year-old boy complains of gradually worsening scrotal pain and swelling with fever and dysuria. On physical examination, the scrotum is edematous and erythematous. There is exquisite tenderness when palpating posterolaterally to the testicle. When you elevate the testicle, the scrotal pain is relieved. Which of the following is the most likely etiology of his symptoms?

a. *Escherichia coli* infection
b. *Chlamydia trachomatis* infection
c. Testicular torsion
d. Varicocele
e. Hydrocele

217. A 19-year-old woman presents with severe right-sided flank pain accompanied by fever, shaking, chills, dysuria, and frequency. She is sexually active with one partner and always uses condoms. Her last menstrual period was 5 days ago. On physical examination, her temperature is 39.9°C (103.8°F) and her heart rate is 120 beats per minute. Blood pressure and respirations are normal. Abdominal examination reveals suprapubic tenderness with palpation. The patient complains of pain when percussion is performed with the ulnar surface of the fist over the right costovertebral angle (CVA). Pelvic examination is normal. Which of the following is the most likely diagnosis?

a. Diverticulitis
b. Acute cystitis
c. Renal calculi
d. Pyelonephritis
e. Appendicitis

218. A 64-year-old woman with congestive heart failure treated with multiple medications, including diuretics and an ACE inhibitor, is admitted after a syncopal episode. Her diuretic dose was recently increased due to volume overload in the clinic. She reports having felt dizzy prior to the episode and is orthostatic on examination. On review of her laboratory results, she is noted to have acute renal failure, with a blood urea nitrogen (BUN) of 42 mg/dL and a creatinine of 2 mg/dL. Her urine sediment reveals hyaline casts. Which of the following is the most likely cause of her acute kidney injury?

a. Acute tubular necrosis
b. Postrenal obstruction
c. Acute glomerulonephritis
d. Acute interstitial nephritis
e. Prerenal azotemia

219. A 52-year-old mother of three children complains of leakage of urine when she coughs or laughs. She is on no medications and has no other medical issues. She works full-time and exercises every other day. On physical examination she leaks urine with vigorous coughing and has a negligible postvoid residual. What is the first step in management of her incontinence?

a. Teach her pelvic floor muscle (Kegel) exercises.
b. Teach her scheduled voiding.
c. Start antimuscarinic drug therapy.
d. Prescribe an alpha agonist.
e. Refer her for surgery.

220. A 56-year-old man with diabetes, hypertension, and stable angina controlled with insulin, a beta-blocker, an ACE-inhibitor and sublingual nitroglycerin comes for routine follow-up. He has been under a lot of stress after losing his job, but does not smoke, drink, or use recreational drugs. At the very end of the visit, he tells you that he is concerned because he is now unable to sustain an erection enough to have sexual intercourse. He states that he does not even have morning erections anymore. On physical examination, he is a circumcised male with normal testes. His lower extremity neurologic examination is within normal limits and his pedal pulses are 2+. Which of the following is a contraindication to prescribing oral phosphodiesterase inhibitors to this patient?

a. His diabetes
b. His angina
c. His use of nitroglycerin
d. His use of an ACE-inhibitor
e. His use of a beta-blocker

221. A 23-year-old man presents complaining of hematuria for 1 day following a recent upper respiratory infection. He has no other symptoms but states that the hematuria started after he played in a fast-paced basketball game. He takes no medications and does not drink alcohol or use illicit drugs. He has no family history of renal disease. Physical examination is normal. Urinalysis reveals erythrocytes and erythrocyte casts. Which of the following is the most likely diagnosis?

a. Bladder carcinoma
b. IgA nephropathy
c. Poststreptococcal glomerulonephritis
d. Alport syndrome
e. Minimal change disease

227. A 39-year-old man with a 12-year history of human immunodeficiency virus (HIV) presents with 3+ pitting edema of the lower extremities. He denies fever, polyuria, frequency, nocturia, and hematuria. He does not drink alcohol, smoke cigarettes, or use illicit drugs. He has no past medical history of hypertension or diabetes mellitus. He is compliant with his HIV medication. Blood pressure is 120/80 mm Hg; heart, lung, and abdominal examinations are normal. Serum albumin is 2.8 mg/dL (normal = 3.5-5.7 mg/dL), and 24-hour urine protein is 3800 mg/dL (normal < 150 mg/dL). The patient has significantly elevated lipid (predominantly LDL) levels. Which of the following is the most likely cause for the lipid abnormalities?

a. A defect in the LDL receptor resulting in an increase in lipid levels
b. A defect in the VLDL receptor resulting in an increase in lipid levels
c. Increased lipoprotein clearance of lipids from the blood by lipoprotein lipase
d. Decreased lipoprotein clearance of lipids from the blood by lipoprotein lipase
e. Decreased hepatic synthesis of proteins

Questions 228 and 229

For each patient with hematuria, select the most likely diagnosis. Each lettered option may be used once, multiple times, or not at all.

a. Prostate cancer
b. Renal cell carcinoma
c. Bladder cancer
d. Carcinoma of the ureter
e. Nephrolithiasis

228. A 55-year-old man presents with hematuria, flank pain, and fever. Physical examination reveals the presence of an abdominal mass.

229. A 57-year-old man with a history of smoking presents with hematuria. He has owned and operated a chain of dry cleaners for over 30 years.

Renal and Genitourinary System

Answers

200. The answer is b. *(McPhee, pp 1492-1494.)* The vast majority of primary testicular tumors, the most common tumors in men between 20 and 35 years of age, are **germ cell tumors** and are slightly more often found on the right side than the left. These can be **divided into seminomas and nonseminomas** primarily, with the remainder being nongerminal neoplasms like Leydig and Sertoli cell tumors. The most common symptom is **painless enlargement of the testis.** A man who presents with a testicular mass and an **elevated serum alpha-fetoprotein (AFP) level** most likely has **nonseminomatous testicular cancer.** The elevated AFP implies yolk sac or nonseminomatous elements. Patients with pure **seminomas** (more common than nonseminomas) often **have elevations in human chorionic gonadotropin (hCG) rather than in AFP.** All germ cell tumors, even if advanced, are curable with chemotherapy. **Leydig and Sertoli cell tumors** tend to produce estrogen, causing gynecomastia and impotence. With no history of trauma, a **hematoma** is unlikely. Swellings containing serous fluid transilluminate; those containing blood and tissue do not. **Testicular lymphoma** is the most common bilateral testicular tumor.

201. The answer is d. *(Seidel, p 657.)* The digital examination described is consistent with an **indirect hernia** (a hernia that lies **within** the inguinal canal and passes through the internal inguinal ring, often exiting the external ring into the scrotum), which is the most common of all hernias. This type of hernia often affects children and young males and requires eventual surgical repair. A **direct hernia** bulges anteriorly through Hesselbach triangle, thus it is felt on the medial side of the finger on digital examination. The **appendix**—or, for that matter, any visceral organ—**may be found in a hernial sac. All hernias** except femoral hernias **are more common in males** than in females. Hernias become **surgical emergencies if they become incarcerated** and irreducible, compromising the circulation to the bowel.

202. The answer is b. *(Seidel, p 664.)* **Klinefelter syndrome,** the most common (1 in 500) disorder of sexual differentiation, is associated with XXY chromosomal inheritance. Boys appear normal before puberty, but thereafter those with this disorder are characterized by tall stature, hypogonadism or a small scrotum with pea-sized testes (normal testes are 5 cm long), a female distribution of pubic hair, and gynecomastia. Newborns require prompt chromosomal studies if born with **ambiguous genitalia** (small penis with hypospadias or enlarged clitoris). Patients with gonadal dysgenesis or **Turner syndrome** are 45, X0; the syndrome is characterized by primary amenorrhea, short stature, webbed neck, and multiple congenital abnormalities. A male with **delayed puberty** may not complete his growth or not have testicular development by age 20.

203. The answer is a. *(Seidel, pp 661-662.)* **Varicoceles** are dilation of veins within the spermatic cord, causing a "**bag of worms**" found almost exclusively on the **left side**, usually palpated when the patient is standing. It is a well-recognized cause of decreased testicular function. **Spermatoceles** are cystic swellings of the epididymis which transluminate and lie superior and posterior to the testis. On palpation, a **hydrocele**, clear intraperitoneal fluid accumulating in the tunica vaginalis, is a **soft, nontender fullness that transluminates.** The testis can be felt posterior to the fluid collection, which often enlarges with standing. Abdominal trauma, as from a car seat belt, can disrupt intra-abdominal contents, and the blood can migrate through a patent processus vaginalis. The scrotal blood will not transilluminate and will be gravity dependent **(hematocele). Indirect inguinal hernias** often pass into the scrotum and are reducible.

204. The answer is c. *(McPhee, pp 838-840.)* This patient has **nephrotic syndrome**, which often presents as peripheral edema or **anasarca,** generalized body edema. One-third of patients with nephrotic syndrome have a systemic disease such as diabetes mellitus or systemic lupus erythematosus (SLE), and two-thirds have either (1) membranous nephropathy due to hepatitis C, SLE, syphilis, or medications; (2) minimal change disease; (3) focal glomerular sclerosis (associated with HIV or heroin use); or (4) membranoproliferative glomerulonephritis. On laboratory analysis, patients have **urine protein excretion of greater than 3.5 g/1.73 m^2 per 24 hours, serum albumin less than 3 g/dL**, and over half have **hyperlipidemia.** The "**grape clusters**" seen in this patient under light microscopy are lipid deposits or oval fat bodies in sloughed tubular epithelial cells that appear as **Maltese crosses** under polarized light.

205. The answer is b. *(Seidel, p 648.)* **Phimosis** is the condition in which the foreskin in an uncircumcised patient cannot be retracted; this may occur normally in the first 6 years of life. Phimosis is usually congenital but may be due to recurrent infections or balanoposthitis (inflammation of the glans penis and prepuce). **Balanitis** is inflammation of the glans penis due to candida fungal infection and occurs in uncircumcised persons. **Escutcheon** is the hair pattern associated with genitalia. **Smegma** is a white, cheeselike material that collects around the glans penis in an uncircumcised man. **Priapism** is a painful, prolonged penile erection, which most often occurs in patients with sickle cell disease, sickle cell trait, or leukemia.

206. The answer is c. *(Seidel, p 649.)* **Epidermoid or sebaceous cysts** appear as small lumps in the scrotal skin, which may enlarge and discharge oily material. **Molluscum contagiosum** appears as pearly white, umbilicated, dome-shaped papules caused by a poxvirus. **Condylomata acuminata** are warts caused by the human papillomavirus (HPV). **Scrotal edema** causes thickening and pitting of the scrotal skin. **Scrotal carcinoma** often presents as ulcerating or fungating lesions and is associated with environmental or industrial carcinogens.

207. The answer is b. *(Seidel, p 659.)* The lesions of **condyloma acuminatum,** or venereal warts, are soft, flesh-colored (may also be pink or red) growths or projections that are found on various parts of the penis or anus. The etiologic agent is human papillomavirus (HPV), sexually transmitted with an incubation period of 1 to 6 months. HPV is often associated with dysplasia, and the warts may degenerate to squamous cell carcinoma of the penis or anus. **Condylomata lata** are the soft, flat-topped, moist, pale nodules and papules of secondary syphilis that appear 2 to 6 months after the primary chancre. These contagious lesions may be seen anywhere on the body, including the palms and soles. **Molluscum contagiosum** is caused by a poxvirus and presents as pearly white, umbilicated, dome-shaped papules. **Peyronie disease** is unilateral deviation of the penis caused by a fibrous band in the corpus cavernosum. It results in deviation (and often pain) of the penis during erection. **Genital herpes** is a sexually transmitted disease characterized by a painful group of vesicles on an erythematous base.

208. The answer is a. *(Seidel, p 662.)* **Orchitis** is an uncommon occurrence except as a sequela of infection with mumps in young males. It is most often unilateral, and testicular atrophy occurs in half of cases. **Epididymitis** results from sexually transmitted infections or bacteria causing urinary tract infections and causes tenderness on palpation of the epididymis and scrotal erythema. **Testicular tumors** are the most common neoplasms in men between the ages of 15 and 30 years. The tumors are nontender, are fixed to the testicle, and do not transilluminate. **Varicoceles** are dilation of veins within the spermatic cord, causing a "**bag of worms**" while **spermatoceles** are cystic swellings of the epididymis that lie superior and posterior to the testis and transluminate.

209. The answer is b. *(McPhee, pp 847-848.)* The kidneys normally extend from T12 to L3 (11 cm long). The right kidney is lower than the left kidney due to the liver above it. Bilaterally enlarged kidneys suggest polycystic kidney disease or bilateral hydronephrosis. **Polycystic kidney disease (PKD)** is one of the most commonly inherited disorders in the United States and may be autosomal dominant (ADPKD) due to a defect on the short arm of chromosome 16. Patients present with **abdominal or flank pain and microscopic or gross hematuria.** The presence of a **palpable kidney in the setting of hypertension** should suggest the diagnosis. Over half of patients will progress to end-stage renal disease by age 60. Extrarenal manifestations of ADPKD include mitral valve prolapse, berry aneurysms of the circle of Willis, diverticulosis, diverticulitis, and liver cysts. **Medullary sponge kidney** is a benign condition seen in older patients (40-50 years) that almost never leads to renal failure. **Horseshoe kidney** is a kidney that can be palpated crossing the midline. **Renal carcinoma** often presents as a hard mass. Patients with **bilateral hydronephrosis** typically have a cause for obstruction and signs of infection, such as fever, hematuria, and dysuria.

210. The answer is d. *(McPhee, pp 637-639.)* **Priapism** is protracted erection associated with pain but not associated with sexual desire. Local abnormalities such as malignancy or inflammatory diseases of the shaft may cause priapism. Priapism may also be secondary to systemic illness, such as leukemia and sickle cell disease. While the other answer choices are all appropriate to treat a sickle cell crisis, this patient who presents with priapism may benefit from **exchange transfusion**.

211. The answer is b. *(McPhee, pp 857-860.)* **Renal colic**, due to **nephrolithiasis**, is severe episodic pain localized to the flank that often radiates to the groin and genitalia and is often accompanied by nausea and vomiting. Patients often constantly move (in contrast to an acute abdomen from peritonitis, where patients stay very still) in an effort to find a more comfortable position. Urinalysis reveals microscopic or gross **hematuria** and urine pH can be used to help determine the makeup of the stone. The most common composition of stones is **calcium oxalate** (radiopaque on plain abdominal film). **Noncontrast spiral CT** is the first-line radiologic study employed to diagnose kidney stones. Patients with **acute bacterial prostatitis** present with fever, dysuria, urgency, frequency, and pain (suprapubic, perineal, and sacral). Rectal examination reveals a warm and exquisitely tender prostate gland. **Pyelonephritis** is unlikely without fever or urinary symptoms. The normal genitalia examination makes the other choices unlikely.

212. The answer is c. *(McPhee, pp 1484-1485.)* This patient presents with symptoms of benign prostatic hypertrophy (BPH), but the nodule found on his examination is not consistent with this diagnosis and must be evaluated to rule out **prostate cancer.** The standard evaluation of a nodule begins with referral to an urologist who will perform a **transrectal ultrasound-guided biopsy.** Serum **prostate-specific antigen (PSA),** although widely used as a screening test for adenocarcinoma of the prostate, is not specific for cancer, and there is an overlap of values in those with cancer and those with BPH. While in this patient evaluation is diagnostic, screening for prostate cancer remains controversial as it may not result in decreased mortality rates. The PSA measurement is more reliable than digital rectal examination (DRE) for detection of prostate cancer and the combined use of PSA and DRE affords a more complete evaluation. PSA levels of more than 10 ng/mL are considered high, results lower than 4 ng/mL are considered normal, and results between 4 and 10 ng/mL are considered borderline. Of note, 20% of patients with prostate cancer will have a normal PSA level. Given the ease of obtaining an ultrasound, **MRI** is not needed for diagnosis. **BUN and creatinine levels** will only reveal renal function, not help diagnose the cause of a prostate nodule.

213. The answer is e. *(Seidel, p 663.)* The tunica vaginalis normally attaches the posterolateral surfaces of the testicle to the scrotum, thereby anchoring it and preventing rotation. When these attachments are missing, the testicle is free to rotate around the spermatic cord and the critical vascular pedicle. This is known as intravaginal **torsion** and is most common in patients between 10 and 20 years of age. Classically, in the case of torsion the testicle will lie transversely within the scrotum, known as the **bell-clapper relationship.** The onset of pain is sudden, and there are no urinary complaints. The pain may be accompanied by nausea and vomiting. Many feel that the initiating factor may be contraction of the cremaster muscle, since **loss of the cremasteric reflex** (normally the testicle and scrotum rise on the side where the inner thigh is stroked with a blunt instrument or finger) is almost invariably found in torsion. None of the other causes listed presents in this classic fashion.

214. The answer is b. *(Seidel, p 648.)* **Phimosis** is the inability to retract the foreskin. It can be seen in young males or in those with recurrent inflammation or infection of the head of the penis (often due to poor hygiene), as in this patient with recurrent balanitis. **Paraphimosis** occurs when the foreskin cannot be returned to the extended position. It may lead to gangrene of the glans penis. **Hypospadias** is a congenital abnormality in which the urethra is situated on the ventral surface of the shaft of the penis. **Epispadias** is a congenital defect in which the urethral meatus appears on the dorsum of the penis. **Priapism** is painful protracted erection associated with malignancy, inflammatory diseases of the shaft or systemic diseases such as sickle cell anemia.

215. The answer is a. *(McPhee, p 810.)* **Renal tubular acidoses (RTAs)** are hyperchloremic acidoses with a normal anion gap. Patients with multiple myeloma often have renal tubular damage from overload by light chains, resulting in the adult **Fanconi syndrome, a type 2 (proximal) RTA** in which the kidney cannot acidify (resorb bicarbonate) or concentrate the urine and there is a loss of glucose and amino acids. It may also be secondary to amyloidosis or heavy metal toxicity. **Type 1 RTA (distal)** causes a metabolic acidosis with an alkaline (pH > 5.5) urine pH and low potassium. In addition, the urine calcium loss coupled with alkaline urine often results in nephrolithiasis. **Type 4 (hyporeninemic hypoaldosteronemic) RTA** causes hyperkalemia and is due to inadequate aldosterone production from diabetes mellitus, sickle cell disease, obstructive uropathy, or medication use (heparin, nonsteroidal anti-inflammatory drugs, ACE inhibitors). Diabetic patients may develop a specific kind of nephropathy (glomerulosclerosis) in which **Kimmelstiel-Wilson** lesions are found histologically (nodules that stain periodic acid–Schiff positive and are deposited in the periphery of the glomerulus).

216. The answer is b. *(McPhee, p 856.)* This patient has **epididymitis**, which in sexually active males under age 40 is most likely caused by infection with ***C. trachomatis* or *Neisseria gonorrhoeae*.** In older men, **gram-negative rods like *E. coli*** are the most likely etiology. The epididymis is located on the posterolateral surface of the testis and should be smooth, discrete, nontender, and larger cephalad. When inflamed, there is tenderness of the posterolaterally positioned epididymis with a normal testicle palpated anteriorly. **Prehn sign** is positive when the patient experiences relief from pain on elevation of the testicle. This sign is not reliable, however, and **testicular torsion** must still be ruled out. **Varicoceles** are dilation of veins and **hydroceles** are usually asymptomatic swellings that can be transilluminated.

217. The answer is d. *(McPhee, pp 852-853.)* The patient presents with **pyelonephritis**, which is an infection of the kidney and renal pelvis. It is characterized by flank pain, fever, dysuria, and frequency. Patients often experience suprapubic and CVA tenderness. Patients with **acute cystitis** may present with dysuria, frequency, urgency, and suprapubic tenderness, but typically the patient is afebrile and the physical examination is normal. The organisms responsible for urinary tract infections are **SEEK PP** = ***S**erratia marcescens,* ***E**scherichia coli,* ***E**nterobacter cloacae,* ***K**lebsiella pneumoniae,* ***P**roteus mirabilis,* and ***P**seudomonas aeruginosa.* **Renal calculi** may cause severe flank pain radiating anteriorly and hematuria. **Diverticulitis** causes left lower quadrant pain and fever while patients with **appendicitis** are febrile with right lower quadrant pain.

218. The answer is e. *(McPhee, pp 819-825.)* Causes of **acute renal failure (ARF)** can be divided into three categories: **prerenal, intrinsic renal, and postrenal.** The BUN:Cr ratio, urinary sediment, and the fractional excretion of sodium (F_ENa) are helpful in differentiating causes of ARF. The calculation for the F_ENa is

$$F_ENa = \frac{Una \times PCr}{UCr \times PNa} \times 100\%$$

This patient has likely been overdiuresed in the setting of treatment with an ACE inhibitor (which decreases the GFR through preventing efferent arteriolar constriction), leading her to become volume depleted and thus reducing effective renal arterial blood flow. Her **BUN:Cr ratio of more than 20:1** and **benign urine sediment** further corroborate that **prerenal azotemia** is the likely cause of her symptoms. Patients with prerenal azotemia have a fractional excretion of sodium less than 1 while those with many intrinsic causes like **acute tubular necrosis (ATN)**, **glomerulonephritis and acute interstitial nephritis** have a **F_ENa greater than 1**. In ATN, spinning down the urine reveals **muddy brown casts.** Patients with interstitial nephritis present with fever, rash, and serum eosinophilia usually caused by drugs such as nonsteroidal anti-inflammatory agents (NSAIDs), infections or immunologic disorders. Glomerulonephritis is rare and presents as hypertension and edema with hematuria, proteinuria and red cell casts on urine examination. The least common cause of ARF is **postrenal obstruction** which causes kidney parenchymal damage (leading to red and white cells in the urine) and a decreased GFR.

219. The answer is a. *(McPhee, pp 70-72.)* Many older adults, especially postmenopausal females, experience **urinary incontinence.** There are three main types of incontinence. The most common type, **urge incontinence**, is due to detrusor muscle overactivity causing an intense urge to urinate and leakage. Management of urge incontinence involves scheduled voiding, relaxation techniques, and treatment with medication such as tolterodine and oxybutynin. If these modalities fail, surgery is the definitive treatment of urge incontinence. Urethral incompetence leads to **stress incontinence**, or loss of urine with laughing, coughing, and sneezing, as in this patient. The best first step is to advice limitation of caffeine and to **teach pelvic floor muscle (Kegel) exercises. Overflow incontinence** is a result of detrusor underactivity—patients complain of frequent urination and leakage of urine. Men with benign prostatic hypertrophy often experience overflow incontinence from urinary retention. Augmented voiding techniques, indwelling catheters, surgical decompression, and treatment with alpha blockers are appropriate treatment options, depending on the cause of overflow. A good mnemonic for the etiologies of incontinence is **DIAPPERS**—**D**elirium, **I**nfection, **A**trophic urethritis or vaginitis, **P**harmaceuticals (diuretics, anticholinergics, opioids, etc.), **P**sychological factors, **E**xcess urinary output, **R**estricted mobility, **S**tool impaction.

220. The answer is c. *(McPhee, pp 862-864.)* This patient complains of **erectile dysfunction**, which can be due to organic as well as psychological problems. His inability to sustain an erection may be a result of his diabetes, hypertension, or possible peripheral vascular disease, as well as from effects of his medications for these issues. The stress he is experiencing may also play a role. Depending on the etiology of his erectile dysfunction, there are many treatment options available, such as behavioral therapy, oral phosphodiesterase inhibitors, vaccum constriction devices, prostaglandin injections, testosterone replacement, and even a penile prosthesis. However, he is **not eligible for treatment with oral phosphodiesterase inhibitors** as their combined effect with the **nitrates** he takes for chest pain may lead to dangerous hypotension.

221. The answer is b. *(McPhee, pp 834-836.)* **IgA nephropathy (Berger disease)** is the most commonly encountered form of focal glomerulonephritis worldwide, and patients will often have microhematuria. It may follow an upper respiratory tract infection, flu-like illness or physical exertion. **Bladder cancer** is a common cause of asymptomatic microhematuria but is usually found in patients over the age of 50. Risk factors for bladder neoplasia include aniline, rubber, other organic solvents, industrial dyes, and tobacco use. **Poststreptococcal glomerulonephritis** occurs 1 to 3 weeks after the group A streptococcal pharyngitis or impetigo and presents with hematuria and proteinuria. **Minimal change disease** almost always presents with severe proteinuria, and erythrocyte casts are not seen in **rhabdomyolysis.** Patients with **Alport syndrome** have nephritic syndrome and hearing loss.

222. The answer is f. *(McPhee, p 830.)* As this patient's condition improved with treatment, there is no need for emergent dialysis. Indications for dialysis are easily remembered with the vowel mnemonic of **A, E, I, O, U**, or **A**cidosis (pH < 7.20) unresolved with bicarbonate treatment, **E**lectrolyte abnormality (refractory hyperkalemia or with ECG changes), fluid **O**verload unresponsive to diuretics, and **U**remic symptoms (pericarditis, encephalopathy, or coagulopathy). The **I** in the mnemonic is a reminder that ingestion of certain drugs (barbiturates, bromide, chloral hydrate, ethanol, ethylene glycol, isopropyl alcohol, lithium, methanol, procainamide, theophylline, salicylates, and heavy metals) is treatable with dialysis.

223. The answer is c. *(McPhee, pp 390-392.)* In patients like this, presenting with hypertension at an early age or those resistant to multiple antihypertensive medications, **secondary causes of hypertension** (as opposed to primary or **essential hypertension**) must be entertained. **Renal artery stenosis** (**RAS**) accounts for less than 5% of hypertension (HTN) cases. The most common cause is atherosclerosis, but in young women the etiology is often fibromuscular dysplasia. Patients may present with a high-pitched abdominal bruit. While renal arteriography is the gold standard diagnostic test, use of noninvasive magnetic resonance or CT angiography is an appropriate first step to diagnosis. Patients with **pheochromocytoma** often present with sudden episodes of hypertension, headache, profuse sweating, anxiety, and palpitations. The diagnosis is made by 24-hour urine collection for catecholamines or metanephrines. Patients with HTN due to **coarctation of the aorta** present with delayed or absent femoral pulses and complain of claudication. Patients with **primary hyperaldosteronism (Conn syndrome)** usually due to bilateral adrenal hyperplasia) present with HTN, fatigue, polyuria, and muscle weakness due to potassium depletion.

224. The answer is b. *(McPhee, p 855.)* **Prostatodynia** is a noninflammatory disorder that affects young and middle-aged men. Patients present complaining of a lifelong history of difficulty voiding. The prostate is normal, and urinalysis is negative for bacteria and leukocytes. Prostatic secretions show a normal number of leukocytes. Treatment consists of alpha-blocking agents. Patients present acutely with **acute bacterial prostatitis** (due to urinary gram-negative bacteria or STIs) and **nonbacterial prostatitis** (due to *Chlamydia, Mycoplasma, Ureaplasma,* and viruses). In these conditions, they will have increased numbers of leukocytes in prostatic secretions with a negative culture if nonbacterial and a positive one if there is a bacterial etiology. Patients with **chronic bacterial prostatitis** will have positive prostatic secretion leukocytes and a positive culture. **Expressing prostatic secretions in patients with acute bacterial prostatitis is contraindicated**.

225. The answer is e. *(Tierney, pp 839–842.)* The patient presents with euvolemic hyponatremia secondary to **primary polydipsia** (compulsive water consumption). Since the hyponatremia developed gradually in the absence of neurologic symptoms (ie, seizures), it should not be corrected rapidly. The appropriate rate of correction should be 12 mEq every 24 hours to prevent **central pontine myelinolysis (CPM)**, which is an osmotically induced demyelination due to overly rapid correction of serum sodium. Patients like this one whose hyponatremia is corrected too rapidly develop paraplegia, quadriplegia, and coma.

226. The answer is c. *(McPhee, pp 724-725.)* Up to 8% of pregnant women have **asymptomatic bacteriuria.** Whereas in other asymptomatic patients, bacteria in the urine do not need to be treated, in pregnancy, it has been associated with preterm labor and carries a risk of progression to pyelonephritis. As a result, this patient **should be treated** with oral antibiotics as an outpatient and another urine culture should subsequently be obtained to insure clearance of the infection. There is no indication for any imaging at this time.

227. The answer is d. *(McPhee, pp 838-840.)* The patient with edema, proteinuria, hypoalbuminemia, and hyperlipidemia has **nephrotic syndrome** secondary to HIV disease. Hyperlipidemia occurs because of increased hepatic protein synthesis and **reduced lipoprotein clearance from the blood by lipoprotein lipase.** Patients have elevations of low-density lipoprotein (LDL), very-low-density lipoprotein (VLDL), and triglycerides (TGL). High-density lipoprotein (HDL) may be normal or decreased. Dietary cholesterol should be limited in these patients (< 300 mg/d); pharmacological therapy is often required.

The **severity of edema** is characterized by a grading system, which is as follows:

1+: a slight pitting edema (2 mm deep) with no distortion on release of finger
2+: a 4-mm-deep pit whose detectable distortion disappears in 10 to 15 seconds
3+: a 6-mm-deep pit that lasts more than 1 minute on release of finger
4+: an 8-mm-deep pit that lasts 2 to 5 minute on release of finger

228 and 229. The answers are 228-b, 229-c. *(McPhee, pp 1489-1492.)* Ninety-five percent of tumors of the kidney are **renal cell carcinomas.** Patients present with hematuria and the presence of an abdominal mass. Causal factors have been implicated in the development of renal cell carcinoma, but cigarette smoking and obesity are the strongest associations.

Bladder cancer, usually presenting as gross or microscopic hematuria and irritative voiding symptoms, is strongly associated with cigarette smoking and chemical compounds (aromatic hydrocarbons). Chimney sweepers and dry cleaners are also at risk for bladder cancer (up to 25% of all bladder cancer is occupationally related). **Prostate cancer** is usually asymptomatic and detected as focal nodules on digital rectal examination or with an elevated serum PSA. **Cancer of the ureter** (transitional cell as found in the bladder) is associated with chronic phenacetin use, cigarette smoking, and hydrocarbon chemical exposure. Patients with **nephrolithiasis**, or kidney stones, present with acute, severe back or flank pain radiating to the groin, with microscopic or gross hematuria and occasionally fever. An easy mnemonic to address hematuria is "If your doctor does not know how to work up hematuria, you should **SWITCH GPS**":

S = stones, sickle cell disease, sickle cell trait, scleroderma, SLE, sulfonamides
W = Wegener granulomatosis
I = infections, instrumentation, iatrogenic, interstitial nephritis
T = trauma, TB, tubulointerstitial disease, tumor, thrombocytopenic thrombotic purpura (TTP)
C = cryoglobulinemia, cyclophosphamide
H = hemolytic-uremic syndrome, hypercalciuria, hemophilia, Henoch Schönlein purpura
G = Goodpasture disease, glomerulonephritis
P = papillary necrosis, polycystic kidney disease, polyarteritis nodosa
S = schistosomiasis, sponge disease (medullary sponge disease)

Endocrinology

Questions

230. A 41-year-old woman with no previous medical problems presents with the chief complaint of generalized weakness. The patient states that she has been irritable lately and finds it difficult to concentrate at work. She has been amenorrheic for 12 months and feels her symptoms might be related to early menopause. On physical examination, her blood pressure is 160/90 mm Hg. The patient has a "moon face" and a "buffalo hump." She is hirsute. Abdominal examination reveals purple striae. Her extremities appear to be atrophied. Which of the following is the best first test to confirm the diagnosis?

a. Blood glucose level
b. Dexamethasone suppression test
c. Spot urine free cortisol level
d. MRI of the pituitary
e. CT scan of the abdomen

231. A 42-year-old man presents to your office for a checkup. He has been in excellent health except for a recent diagnosis of mild hypertension and bilateral carpal tunnel syndrome. On physical examination, the patient is tall, with large and doughy hands. His facial features are coarse, and he has a prominent mandible with wide-spaced teeth. His voice is deep, and he has macroglossia. Heart examination reveals the apical impulse to be displaced 2 cm laterally. His family history is unremarkable. Which of the following is the most likely diagnosis?

a. Acromegaly
b. Gigantism
c. Hypothyroidism
d. Familial prognathism
e. Amyloidosis

232. A 21-year-old woman presents to the emergency room with palpitations. She also notes that she has been losing weight. Physical examination reveals an anxious and highly energetic patient. Her heart rate is 120 beats per minute. She has bilateral exophthalmos with lid retraction. Thyroid examination reveals a diffusely enlarged, nontender thyroid with an audible bruit. The patient also has fine tremors and hyperreflexia. Which of the following is the most appropriate first step in the diagnosis?

a. Free thyroxine
b. Thyroid-stimulating hormone (TSH) level
c. Thyroid resin uptake
d. Thyroxine (T_4)
e. Triiodothyronine (T_3)

233. A 44-year-old man with adult-onset diabetes mellitus comes to the emergency room. He has been out of his insulin for a week. He is drowsy and reports abdominal pain, polyuria, and polydipsia. On physical examination he is hypotensive and tachycardic, but afebrile. His breath has a "fruity" smell to it. His examination is otherwise normal except mild diffuse abdominal tenderness to palpation without rebound or guarding. On his serum chemistries, his sodium is 132 mEq/L (normal is 145 mEq/L), potassium is normal at 4 mEq/L, and glucose reads 450 mg/dL. His venous pH is 7.25, and a urine dipstick reveals ketones. Which of the following is the proper management of his condition at this point?

a. He should be administered bicarbonate.
b. Fluid resuscitation should begin with 0.45% normal saline.
c. He should be started on potassium repletion.
d. He should be given long-acting insulin.
e. He can be treated as an outpatient.

234. A 52-year-old woman presents to her physician with the chief complaint of hoarseness. She sings in her church choir, and her friends have noticed a voice change. Her past medical history is significant for heart arrhythmias, which have been well controlled for 3 years with amiodarone. Physical examination reveals a woman with coarse hair and skin. Her fingernails are thick, and her eyes appear puffy. The thyroid gland is normal and nontender. Her muscle strength is excellent, but the relaxation phase of her ankle reflex is prolonged. Which of the following is the most likely diagnosis?

a. Cushing disease
b. Acromegaly
c. de Quervain thyroiditis
d. Amiodarone-induced hypothyroidism
e. Cretinism

235. You suspect that a 26-year-old woman presenting with galactorrhea and infertility has a large pituitary tumor. If your hunch is correct, which of the following is the most likely visual field defect you will find on physical examination?

a. Bitemporal hemianopsia
b. Left homonymous hemianopsia
c. Right homonymous hemianopsia
d. Right homonymous inferior quadrantanopsia
e. Left homonymous inferior quadrantanopsia

236. A 51-year-old woman is seen in your office several weeks after a parathyroidectomy for a parathyroid adenoma. She is complaining of paresthesias. Physical examination reveals contraction of the right facial muscles when you tap lightly over the right side of the patient's face. Which of the following is the most likely diagnosis?

a. Hypokalemia
b. Hypercalcemia
c. Hyperkalemia
d. Hypocalcemia
e. Hyponatremia

237. A 43-year-old male construction worker is experiencing polyuria and polydipsia, as well as fatigue. He has a strong family history for diabetes mellitus. His physical examination is completely normal except for prehypertension and obesity. You note that a serum chemistry done before the visit reveals a random plasma glucose of 220 mg/dL. Which of the following would confirm a diagnosis of diabetes?

a. A 2-hour plasma glucose on oral glucose tolerance test of 160 mg/dL
b. A 2-hour plasma glucose on oral glucose tolerance test of 180 mg/dL
c. A hemoglobin A_{1c} level of 6%
d. A random plasma glucose of 180 mg/dL
e. A fasting plasma glucose of 130 mg/dL

238. A 37-year-old woman who recently was diagnosed a year ago with hypothyroidism presents with a chief complaint of weakness and a 20-lb weight loss. Her most recent TSH was within normal limits on supplemental thyroxine. On physical examination, the patient has increased skin pigmentation over even nonexposed skin, most prominently over her elbows, knees, and palmar creases. She is afebrile. Her blood pressure is 90/60 mm Hg supine and 70/50 mm Hg standing. The rest of her physical examination is normal. Laboratory data reveal hyponatremia, hyperkalemia, and a metabolic acidosis. Which of the following is the best test to diagnose her condition?

a. Repeat serum TSH
b. Serum DHEA levels
c. Plasma renin
d. Cosyntropin stimulation test
e. Fasting blood glucose

239. A 49-year-old man presents with a compression fracture of his sixth thoracic vertebra. He is a tobacco and alcohol user and has taken oral corticosteroids on and off since childhood for asthma and now for COPD. Which of the following is the most likely diagnosis?

a. Osteomalacia
b. Osteoporosis
c. Scleromalacia
d. Paget disease
e. Multiple myeloma

240. A 46-year-old man with lung cancer is brought to the emergency room with confusion. He is lethargic and oriented to person but not to place or time. An electrocardiogram reveals a shortened QT interval. Which of the following should be the initial step in management?

a. Intravenous corticosteroids
b. Intravenous bisphosphonates
c. Intravenous normal saline
d. Oral hydrochlorothiazide
e. Subcutaneous calcitonin

241. A 22-year-old woman presents with the chief complaint of hirsutism. She has had irregular periods since menarche at the age of 13. She has a normal body weight and her facies is normal. Physical examination reveals excess back and chest hair. Pelvic examination is normal. The luteinizing hormone (LH) value is normal. Serum 17-OH progesterone concentrations are highly elevated. Which of the following is the most likely diagnosis?

a. Cushing syndrome
b. Congenital adrenal hyperplasia
c. Adrenal tumor
d. Idiopathic hirsutism
e. Polycystic ovary disease

242. A 13-year-old adolescent is worried that he is growing breasts and complains that the breasts are often painful, but he has no other complaints. He states that he has been growing taller this past year. On physical examination, you note some acne on the patient's face. His testes and phallus are appropriate for his age, and his scrotum is reddened, with some thinning of the skin. He has fine, sparse pubic hair. Which of the following is the most likely diagnosis?

a. Gonadal tumor
b. Pituitary tumor
c. Adrenal tumor
d. Normal puberty
e. Klinefelter syndrome

243. A 19-year-old collegiate football player is sent to your office by the team's coach because of occasional outbursts of anger and hostility. The patient is otherwise asymptomatic, has no past medical history and denies using tobacco, alcohol, or illicit drugs. Physical examination reveals a blood pressure of 140/90 mm Hg. The patient has gynecomastia and testicular atrophy. He states that his libido and sexual performance are adequate. His urine drug test is negative. Which of the following is the most likely diagnosis?

a. Prolactinoma
b. Kallman syndrome
c. Anabolic steroid use
d. Chronic cocaine use
e. Diabetes mellitus

244. A 17-year-old woman presents with amenorrhea for 3 months. She states that she has had irregular periods since her menarche at the age of 12 years. She has no other symptoms or past medical history. Her physical examination is unremarkable, except breast examination reveals breast engorgement and tenderness. Which of the following should be the first test you order?

a. Serum prolactin
b. Serum FSH
c. Serum hCG
d. Serum LH
e. Serum TSH

245. A 46-year-old woman complains of headache, sweating, and diaphoresis that occur on a daily basis or sometimes twice a day while she is at work. She has gone to the company nurse during these episodes and was told that her blood pressure was elevated. Aside from that, the nurse could not find any other problem. Physical examination is normal, including blood pressure, which is 130/80 mm Hg. Which of the following is the most likely diagnosis?

a. Carcinoid syndrome
b. Thyroid storm
c. Pheochromocytoma
d. Conn syndrome
e. Glucagonoma

246. A 63-year-old woman has a large retroclavicular goiter. Whenever she elevates her arms over her head, she experiences facial plethora and dizziness. Which of the following is the most likely diagnosis?

a. Chronic obstructive lung disease
b. Bilateral vocal cord paralysis
c. Spinal cord compression
d. Superior vena cava syndrome
e. Congestive heart failure

247. A 47-year-old woman presents to your office complaining of fatigue and bone pain. She has a past medical history significant for kidney stones and hypertension treated with a beta blocker. Routine laboratory studies reveal an elevated serum calcium and hypophosphatemia. Which of the following is the most likely diagnosis?

a. Underlying malignancy
b. Vitamin D intoxication
c. Familial hypocalciuric hypercalcemia
d. Osteitis fibrosa cystica
e. Primary hyperparathyroidism

248. A 15-year-old adolescent has noticed the descent of his scrotum. His penis has enlarged in length, and he has developed curly, pigmented hair around the base of the penis. Which of the following would best describe his Tanner stage of development?

a. Tanner stage 1
b. Tanner stage 2
c. Tanner stage 3
d. Tanner stage 4
e. Tanner stage 5

249. The family members of a 70-year-old woman with a 20-year history of diet-controlled diabetes mellitus bring her to the emergency room because she has been confused. They state that the patient recently had a hip fracture and has been recuperating at home where she lives alone. The blood pressure is 90/60 mm Hg and the pulse is 120 beats per minute. The patient is lethargic but follows commands. Pupils are 3 mm bilaterally and reactive to light and accommodation. Neurologic examination reveals no focal deficits. Finger stick glucose is higher than 800 mg/dL, and arterial blood gas reveals a pH of 7.36. Which of the following is the most likely diagnosis?

a. Nonketotic hyperosmolar state
b. Glucagonoma
c. Barbiturate overdose
d. Impaired glucose tolerance
e. Diabetic ketoacidosis

250. A 52-year-old woman with a 20-year history of insulin-dependent diabetes mellitus presents complaining of a rash that has developed on her legs and ankles. Physical examination reveals several oval-shaped plaques with demarcated borders and a glistening yellow surface located on the anterior surface of the lower legs and dorsum of the ankles. Which of the following is the most likely diagnosis?

a. Peripheral neuropathy
b. Peripheral vascular disease
c. Eruptive xanthomas
d. Acanthosis nigricans
e. Necrobiosis lipoidica diabeticorum

251. A 24-year-old man is referred to your practice for elevated cholesterol level. The patient has a father and two siblings with high cholesterol levels who are on medications. His 31-year-old brother recently had a myocardial infarction. On physical examination, the patient has bilateral arcus senilis. His extremities are remarkable for diffuse and nodular thickenings of the Achilles tendon. Which of the following is the most likely diagnosis?

a. Hypothyroidism
b. Nephrotic syndrome
c. Liver disease
d. Type IIA hyperlipoproteinemia
e. Type III dysbetalipoproteinemia

252. A 44-year-old woman with a 20-year history of poorly controlled diabetes mellitus presents with headache and unilateral proptosis. The patient is febrile and appears toxic. Her serum glucose level is 640 mg/dL. An urgent CT scan of the head reveals a retro-orbital abscess and severe opacification of the frontal and ethmoid sinuses. Which of the following organisms is most likely responsible for this infection?

a. *Cryptococcus neoformans*
b. Mucormycosis
c. *Mycobacterium tuberculosis*
d. *Staphylococcus epidermis*
e. *Listeria monocytogenes*

253. A 41-year-old woman presents with amenorrhea for 9 months. She is found to have a prolactin-secreting pituitary adenoma. Laboratory data reveal a serum calcium level of 12.0 mg/dL and hypoglycemia (serum glucose of 49 mg/dL). Which of the following is the most likely diagnosis?

a. MEN-1 syndrome
b. MEN-2A syndrome
c. MEN-2B syndrome
d. Sipple syndrome
e. Kallman syndrome

254. A 42-year-old nursing student presents to the emergency room with confusion, diaphoresis, and dizziness. She is tremulous and tachycardic. Her serum glucose level is found to be 20 mg/dL, and she responds immediately to intravenous dextrose infusion. The patient states that she has been eating well. After the hypoglycemia is corrected, the physical examination is normal. Blood work reveals that insulin levels are high but C-peptide level is low. The rest of the laboratory data are normal. Which of the following is the most likely diagnosis?

a. Insulinoma
b. Surreptitious insulin injection
c. Hypopituitarism
d. Adrenal insufficiency
e. Glucagon deficiency

255. A 15-year-old adolescent has noticed that she has developed straight, barely pigmented hair along the medial border of her labia and her breasts are slight mounds. Which of the following would best describe her Tanner stage of development?

a. Tanner stage 1
b. Tanner stage 2
c. Tanner stage 3
d. Tanner stage 4
e. Tanner stage 5

256. A 49-year-old man with a 25-year history of diabetes mellitus presents with a painful right foot. He denies a history of trauma. On physical examination, the patient has loss of pain and vibration in both feet. His Achilles deep tendon reflexes are absent bilaterally. Peripheral pulses are palpable, and there are no skin lesions. The right foot is erythematous with some edema. The patient's gait reveals a limp due to foot pain. Radiograph of the ankle reveals osteopenia and multiple fractures of the tarsal bones. Which of the following is the most likely diagnosis?

a. Somogyi effect
b. Dawn phenomenon
c. Charcot triad
d. Charcot joint
e. Mature-onset diabetes of the young (MODY)

257. A 60-year-old man is involved in a head-on motor vehicle accident and sustains significant head trauma. He is awake and oriented to person, place, and time but complains of dizziness. Physical examination reveals normal vital signs, no orthostasis, and no neurologic findings. Heart and lung examinations are normal. Overnight in the surgical intensive care unit, the patient develops excessive thirst, polydipsia, and polyuria. He develops orthostatic changes on physical examination. His serum sodium rises to 160 mEq/L (normal is 145 mEq/L), and his serum glucose is normal. Which of the following is the most likely diagnosis?

a. Impaired glucose intolerance
b. Nephrogenic diabetes insipidus
c. Central diabetes insipidus
d. Syndrome of inappropriate antidiuretic hormone secretion (SIADH)
e. Iatrogenic saline infusion

258. A 21-year-old man presents to your office for a preemployment physical examination. He is 6 ft 3 in tall and weighs 70 kg. Heart examination reveals a midsystolic click and systolic murmur that increases with Valsalva maneuver. The patient has an arm span that exceeds his height and has long, slender fingers. When he makes a fist with his thumb inside, the thumb protrudes beyond the ulnar margin of the hand. Which of the following is the most likely diagnosis?

a. Klinefelter syndrome
b. Turner syndrome
c. Ehlers-Danlos syndrome
d. Marfan syndrome
e. Noonan syndrome

Questions 259 and 260

For each man with erectile dysfunction (ED), select the most likely mechanism causing the symptoms. Each lettered option may be used once, multiple times, or not at all.

a. Neuropathic impotence
b. Vascular impotence
c. Psychogenic impotence
d. Retrograde ejaculation
e. Premature ejaculation

259. A previously healthy 42-year-old man presents with impotence. He takes no medications and does not smoke, drink alcohol, or use illicit drugs. He attains nocturnal erections but is impotent with his sexual partner.

260. A 53-year-old diabetic man with a history of gastroparesis and peripheral neuropathy presents with erectile dysfunction.

Endocrinology

Answers

230. The answer is b. *(McPhee, pp 1050-1053.)* This patient's presentation is consistent with **Cushing syndrome, which results from excess corticosteroids**, either from exogenous ingestion of corticosteroids, nonpituitary neoplasms (ie, small cell carcinoma of the lung), adrenal adenomas, adrenal carcinomas, or bilateral adrenal nodular hyperplasia. **Cushing disease** is a subset of the syndrome and refers to hypercortisolism due to adrenocorticotropic hormone (ACTH) hypersecretion by the pituitary gland, usually because of a small (< 1 cm) benign pituitary microadenoma. Symptoms include central obesity, striae, hirsutism, easy bruisability, proximal myopathy, osteoporosis, amenorrhea, hypertension, glucose intolerance, and hypokalemia. Patients will have glucose intolerance, leukocytosis, and hypokalemia, but these findings are nonspecific. **The best screening test for Cushing syndrome is the dexamethasone suppression test**: dexamethasone is given at 11 PM and an AM cortisol is obtained the next morning. **A cortisol under 5 mcg/dL excludes Cushing syndrome.** If the suppression test is abnormal, a **24-hour urine for free cortisol** and creatinine will help confirm the diagnosis. If hypercortisolism exists, a **serum ACTH level** should be drawn. **MRI of the pituitary** may be appropriate to rule out a pituitary lesion or a **CT scan of the abdomen** might reveal an adrenal abnormality.

231. The answer is a. *(McPhee, pp 997-1000.)* This patient has **acromegaly** (hypersecretion of growth hormone after closure of the epiphyses) which is almost always caused by a pituitary adenoma (benign 99% of the time) secreting excess growth hormone. Patients present with tall stature, large hands, large feet, prominent mandible, prognathism, coarse facial features, wide tooth spacing, deep voice, macroglossia, and carpal tunnel syndrome. Patients may have headache, visual field defects, hypertrophy of the laryngeal tissue causing obstructive sleep apnea, hypertension, cardiomegaly, multiple skin tags, premalignant colonic polyps, and diabetes mellitus. **Gigantism** occurs before the closure of the epiphyses.

Amyloidosis is a group of disorders characterized by infiltration of various organs (kidney, heart, intestine, endocrine) by protein fibrils. Patients with amyloidosis may have macroglossia and carpal tunnel syndrome. Macroglossia and carpal tunnel syndrome may also be seen in **hypothyroidism,** in addition to cold intolerance, constipation, hoarseness, weight gain, and other features. Coarse features may also run in families **(familial prognathism)**.

232. The answer is b. *(McPhee, pp 1008-1010.)* This patient with symptoms of thyrotoxicosis, accompanied by **exophthalmos and a thyroid bruit**, most likely has **Graves disease,** which is the most common cause of **hyperthyroidism**. Patients with Graves disease may also have **heat intolerance**, atrial fibrillation, menstrual irregularity, and **pretibial myxedema**. The disease presents between the ages of 20 and 40, and women are affected far more than men. The disorder is due to antibodies that bind to the TSH receptor, causing it to stimulate the thyroid gland to hyperfunction. **Serum TSH** assay is the **most sensitive test** for primary hyper- (and hypo-) thyroidism. TSH will be depressed in Graves disease, while serum T_3, T_4, free thyroxine, and thyroid resin uptake are all usually increased.

233. The answer is c. *(McPhee, pp 1111-1115.)* This patient has **diabetic ketoacidosis**, manifested by extremely elevated blood glucose, metabolic acidosis with a low serum bicarbonate and ketosis (from lack of insulin) detected in the urine and blood. Patients often present with fatigue, nausea, and vomiting, abdominal pain, evidence of dehydration from osmotic diuresis, a **"fruity" odor** of acetone on the breath and rapid deep breathing **(Kussmaul respirations)**. This patient is at least moderately ill and warrants **inpatient** treatment in a step-down or intensive care unit. The mainstay of initial therapy is volume resuscitation and insulin therapy to clear the hyperglycemia and ketoacidosis. Aggressive volume expansion to restore normal perfusion should **begin with 0.9% saline solution** ("normal saline") and should be changed to 0.45% saline ("half-normal saline") when the serum sodium is greater than 150 mEq/L, and eventually to fluids containing 5% dextrose when the blood glucose falls below 250 mg/dL. **Only regular (short-acting) insulin**, either as a continuous drip or hourly intramuscular injection, should be administered until the ketosis clears. Despite overall body deficits, **serum potassium on initial presentation is usually normal or even elevated** due to the acidosis shifting potassium out of cells. However, it will fall rapidly with insulin treatment, thus **potassium should be repleted**, even at "normal" serum levels. Administration of **bicarbonate** has potentially harmful effects, so it should only be given for an arterial blood **pH of 7.0 or less**.

234. The answer is d. *(McPhee, pp 1003-1005.)* Symptoms of **hypothyroidism** include constipation, depression, edema, tongue thickening, cold intolerance, **Queen Anne sign** (missing lateral one-third of eyebrows), muscle cramps, weight gain, goiter, amenorrhea, galactorrhea, pleural effusion, pericardial effusion, cardiomegaly, bradycardia, hypothermia, hyponatremia, anemia, and hypertension. On examination patients have a **prolonged relaxation phase** on testing of deep tendon reflexes. **Amiodarone has high-iodine content and causes hypothyroidism** in 8% of patients. **Myxedema crisis** is a rare severe complication of hypothyroidism; patients present with coma, severe hypotension, hypothermia, hypoventilation, and hypoxemia. The **single best screening test** for primary hypothyroidism is the **serum TSH**.

Cretinism is congenital (infantile) hypothyroidism. **Cushing disease** leads to central obesity, striae, hirsutism, easy bruisability, proximal myopathy, osteoporosis, amenorrhea, hypertension, glucose intolerance, and hypokalemia. Patients with **acromegaly** have tall stature, large hands and feet, prominent mandible, prognathism, coarse facial features, wide tooth spacing, deep voice, macroglossia, and visual field defects. **De Quervain (subacute) thyroiditis** is thought to be viral in origin and presents with a tender, enlarged gland and hyperthyroidism which eventually becomes hypothyroidism.

235. The answer is a. *(Seidel, p 313.)* A pituitary tumor may impinge on the optic chiasm. The temporal field fibers are damaged as they decussate at the optic chiasm, and the result is a **bitemporal hemianopsia**. Lesions of the optic tract cause **homonymous hemianopsias**—a right-sided lesion causes a left homonymous hemianopsia and a lesion on the left, causes a homonymous right-sided visual defect.

236. The answer is d. *(McPhee, pp 798-800.)* This patient has **Chvostek sign**—tapping on cranial nerve VII as it exits the parotid gland will cause spasm or contraction of the facial muscles on the same side of the face that is being tapped—which is indicative of **hypocalcemia.** In this case, it is the result of her parathyroidectomy. Other clinical signs of hypocalcemia include paresthesias, neuromuscular irritability, cramps, **tetany**, **Trousseau phenomenon** (carpal spasm after elevating pressure in a cuff placed over the brachial artery), and a **prolonged QT interval** on electrocardiogram. Hypocalcemia causes rickets in children and osteomalacia in adults. The mnemonic for the clinical presentation of **hypercalcemia** consists of **bones** (fractures, osteitis fibrosa), **stones** (renal calculi), **abdominal groans** (anorexia, constipation, vomiting, peptic ulcers, pancreatitis), and **psychic overtones** (anxiety, depression, and insomnia). Patients with **hypokalemia** present with muscle weakness, muscle cramps, and flaccid paralysis. **Hyperkalemia** may lead to areflexia, flaccid paralysis, and electrocardiographic abnormalities such as peaked T waves, prolongation of the PR interval, widening of the QRS complex, and ventricular tachycardia. The clinical presentation of **hyponatremia** depends on the severity and acuity of the sodium drop-patients may have symptoms ranging from only nausea and malaise to altered mentation and respiratory arrest.

237. The answer is e. *(McPhee, pp 1083-1084.)* Diagnosis of diabetes mellitus dramatically changes a person's lifestyle. Thus, recommendations for screening require **a fasting plasma glucose level of greater than or equal to 126 mg/dL, a random blood glucose of 200 mg/dL or more with symptoms or a 2-hour glucose on an oral glucose tolerance test of greater than or equal to 200 mg/dL on *at least* two occasions. HbA_{1c}** levels reflect the level of glycemia over the preceding 3-month period. Initially used only to follow control of the disease, an international expert committee in 2009 recommended that a level greater than or equal to **6.5%** be diagnostic of diabetes as these values vary less than fasting plasma glucose levels.

238. The answer is d. *(McPhee, pp 1047-1050.)* This patient has chronic adrenocortical insufficiency (**Addison disease**), in the setting of concomitant hypothyroidism, known together as **Schmidt syndrome**. This condition is the result of **polyglandular autoimmune destruction** of the adrenals and the thyroid gland, and may also be accompanied by type 1 diabetes mellitus. Other etiologies of Addison disease include tuberculosis, malignancy, sarcoidosis, trauma, histoplasmosis, hemochromatosis, amyloidosis, sepsis, cytomegalovirus infection, and medications (ketoconazole, rifampin, anticoagulants, and anticonvulsants). Symptoms include weakness, hypotension, anorexia, and weight loss. Laboratory studies may reveal hyponatremia, hyperkalemia, and eosinophilia. On physical examination, patients are hypotensive and **orthostatic**, have scant axillary and pubic hair, and have **hyperpigmentation of the skin** both in exposed and nonexposed areas, most prominently over the posterior neck, elbows, knees, palmar creases and over pressure areas from a belt or brassiere. An **early AM plasma cortisol of less than 3 mcg/dL** makes the diagnosis, but the best way to confirm that a patient has adrenal insufficiency is by administering the **cosyntropin stimulation test**. After obtaining an AM cortisol level, cosyntropin is administered and a repeat serum cortisol level is obtained 1 hour later. The diagnosis is excluded if the serum cortisol rises to at least 20 mcg/dL. **Serum DHEA levels** above 1000 ng/mL exclude the diagnosis, but a low level is not specific enough to diagnose Addison disease. **Fasting blood glucose** may be low as well, but again, may result from other etiologies.

239. The answer is b. *(Fauci, pp 2397-2408.)* **Osteoporosis** is defined as a bone mineral density more than 2.5 standard deviations below maximum level for young healthy gender-matched adults **(T score ≤ 2.5)**. It may be secondary to estrogen deficiency from menopause, medication use (seizure medications, corticosteroids, heparin), hyperthyroidism, anorexia nervosa, malabsorptive disease, hyperparathyroidism, multiple myeloma, immobilization, tobacco use, or alcoholism. Patients have a reduced bone mass with a normal mineral matrix. **Osteomalacia** is a disorder with reduced mineralization of the matrix; patients need to be evaluated for vitamin D deficiency. **Scleromalacia** is an inflammatory disorder often seen in patients with rheumatoid arthritis associated with chemosis and scleral-conjunctival inflammation. Patients with **Paget disease** (increased bone turnover with the formation of disorganized bone) present with pain, enlarging skull bones (increasing hat size and hearing loss), skeletal deformities (bowing of the lower extremities), and increased warmth of the skin overlying the tibias. **Multiple myeloma** affects adults around 65 years old who present with bone pain usually in the back or ribs as well as symptoms associated with anemia or hypercalcemia.

240. The answer is c. *(McPhee, pp 800-802.)* This patient likely has **hypercalcemia** of malignancy which should be treated initially with **intensive hydration using intravenous saline** to force renal excretion of calcium. **Bisphosphonates** (inhibitors of bone resorption) would be the best treatment for hypercalcemia of malignancy; however, these agents take several days to work. Often **calcitonin** is used as bridge therapy until the bisphosphonates are at full strength. Dialysis may be used to treat emergency cases. **Thiazide diuretics** will actually increase serum calcium.

241. The answer is b. *(McPhee, pp 1053-1055.)* **Hirsutism** is growth of coarse, male-pattern hair in a woman. It is a sign of androgen excess, and patients must be evaluated for ovarian or adrenal tumors. The typical workup for hirsutism includes testosterone level, LH, follicle-stimulating hormone (FSH), 17-OH progesterone, and prolactin, as well as possibly DHEAS and androstenedione levels. This patient already in adulthood most likely has a partial **21-hydroxylase deficiency,** which is the most common form of **congenital adrenal hyperplasia**. The highly **elevated 17-OH progesterone concentration** (which will be even higher after stimulation with synthetic ACTH) supports the diagnosis, along with elevated plasma renin activity and androstenedione. **Cushing syndrome** seems unlikely in a patient without cushingoid features (central obesity, buffalo hump, etc.). **Idiopathic hirsutism** applies to patients who have normal adrenal glands and ovaries. Seventy percent of patients with **polycystic ovary disease (PCOD)** present with hirsutism. They have elevated serum testosterone levels and elevated LH values. Patients with PCOD have slightly elevated levels of 17-OH progesterone after ACTH stimulation. Medications such as bodybuilding steroids, minoxidil, cyclosporine, oral contraceptives, and phenytoin can cause hirsutism.

242. The answer is d. *(McPhee, pp 1066-1067.)* **Gynecomastia** is seen in 50% to 60% of adolescent boys and usually **occurs during Tanner stages 2 or 3**. It is usually painful and may be unilateral or bilateral. It gradually appears and resolves spontaneously within 1 to 2 years of onset. Pubertal changes that occur during Tanner stages 2 and 3 include growth spurt, growth of testes and penis, spermarche, acne, axillary perspiration, and appearance of pubic hair. The boy in this case should be reassured and followed monthly. If the gynecomastia does not resolve, it will be necessary to rule out Klinefelter syndrome, adrenal tumors, gonadal tumors, hyperthyroidism, hepatic disorders, and the use of drugs, especially marijuana and bodybuilding steroids.

243. The answer is c. *(McPhee, p 984.)* Patients, like this one, may use **anabolic steroids** to improve athletic performance. The risks associated with use of these agents include mood swings, aggressiveness, paranoid delusions, psychosis, gynecomastia, infertility, testicular atrophy, hepatic tumors, peliosis hepatis, hypertension, and decreased HDL cholesterol levels. Patients with **prolactinomas** (pituitary tumors) generally present with galactorrhea, reduced libido, erectile dysfunction, amenorrhea, infertility, and visual field defects. Chronic **cocaine** use may cause hyperprolactinemia. **Kallmann syndrome** is characterized by cleft palate, anosmia (impaired sense of smell), short fourth metacarpal bones, hypogonadism, and infertility.

244. The answer is c. *(McPhee, pp 1067-1070.)* This patient has **secondary amenorrhea**, the absence of menses for 3 consecutive months after already experiencing menarche. **Pregnancy** is the most common cause in young women and must always be considered in any patient who presents with amenorrhea. Other causes in this age group include stress, aggressive dieting or exercise, organic illness, and anorexia nervosa, as well as prolactin-secreting pituitary tumors.

245. The answer is c. *(McPhee, pp 1058-1060.)* Patients presenting with episodic symptoms of headache, sweating, palpitations, and sustained or paroxysmal hypertension should be evaluated for **pheochromocytoma,** a potentially life-threatening tumor of the sympathetic nervous system usually found in the adrenal glands. Pheochromocytoma may be associated with von Recklinghausen syndrome, neurofibromatosis, and von Hippel-Lindau disease, as well as MEN-2A and MEN-2B syndromes. The diagnosis is made by elevated plasma-fractionated free metanephrines and confirmed by a 24-hour urine for total metanephrines and creatinine, with or without total catecholamines as well. Ten percent of pheochromocytomas are bilateral, and 10% are extra adrenal. Increased levels of **5-HIAA** are associated with **carcinoid syndrome** (facial flushing and diarrhea) from a tumor usually located in the lung or ileum. Patients with **thyroid storm** present with nausea, diarrhea, jaundice, fever, dyspnea, shortness of breath, diaphoresis, delirium, and tachycardia. **Conn syndrome** is due to a unilateral adrenal adenoma that secretes aldosterone and causes moderate hypertension and hypokalemia. **Glucagonomas** are islet cell tumors that cause weight loss, diarrhea, nausea, and peptic ulcers.

246. The answer is d. *(McPhee, pp 431-432.)* Simple goiter, if sufficiently large, may be accompanied by tracheal compression, esophageal compression, dysphagia, odynophagia, mediastinal obstruction, and **superior vena cava syndrome**. Retrosternal goiter may cause mediastinal obstruction and superior vena cava syndrome (swelling of face, neck, and upper extremities with engorged veins in the neck and chest). This patient has **Pemberton sign**, which is a reversible superior vena cava syndrome; when a patient elevates the arms above the head (obstructing the thoracic inlet and preventing venous return), facial plethora and dizziness occur.

247. The answer is e. *(McPhee, pp 1033-1035.)* **Primary hyperparathyroidism** is the most common cause of hypercalcemia in the outpatient setting and it results in elevated excretion of calcium and phosphate by the kidneys. It is seen more frequently in women than in men and is usually due to one parathyroid adenoma (usually in the inferior lobe). Patients often have a history of hypophosphatemia, fatigue, hypertension, depression, peptic ulcer disease, pancreatitis, bone pain, hypercalciuria, and nephrolithiasis from calcium oxalate stones. The most common cause of hypercalcemia in hospitalized patients is **malignancy** (ie, breast, lung, multiple myeloma, pancreas, uterus, and renal cell) due to the secretion of **parathyroid hormone (PTH)–related peptide (PTHrP)**. Patients with **familial hypocalciuric hypercalcemia (FHH)** have hypocalciuria, a positive family history, and no end-organ damage. Other causes of hypercalcemia include sarcoidosis, mycobacteria, milk-alkali syndrome, and medications (ie, thiazide diuretics). **Osteitis fibrosa cystica** (replacement by fibrous tissue) is the cystic bone abnormality seen with hyperparathyroidism.

248. The answer is c. *(Kliegman, p 61.)* There are five Tanner Stages of Development (sexual maturity) for males:

Tanner 1 = young child penis, scrotum, and testes; no pubic hair
Tanner 2 = enlargement of scrotum and testes; penis the same; scrotal skin becomes more red, thinner, and wrinkled; some straight pubic hair at the base of penis
Tanner 3 = enlargement of penis and testes; scrotum descends; dark, curly pubic hair
Tanner 4 = further penile enlargement; increased pigmentation of scrotum; sculpturing of the glans; adult pubic hair but not beyond inguinal fold
Tanner 5 = ample scrotum; penis reaches to bottom of scrotum; hair spreads to medial surface of thighs

249. The answer is a. *(McPhee, pp 1115-1116.)* **Hyperglycemic hyperosmolar state** is seen in patients with non-insulin-dependent diabetes mellitus (NIDDM) and is usually precipitated by an illness. The patient's glucose is markedly elevated with osmotic diuresis and dehydration, but their residual insulin prevents lipolysis and ketogenesis. If patients are unable to keep up with their volume loss, severe hyperosmolality develops that can lead to altered mental status and even coma. **Diabetic ketoacidosis (DKA)** is due to an absolute deficiency of insulin relative to the counterregulatory hormones. The result is gluconeogenesis, ketogenesis, lipolysis, and decreased glucose uptake, causing hyperglycemia and a metabolic acidosis. **Kussmaul respiration** is a respiration pattern of increased tidal volume seen in patients with metabolic acidosis (ie, DKA). **Impaired glucose tolerance** is defined as a 2-hour plasma glucose of 140 to 200 mg/dL after a glucose load of 75 g in a patient whose fasting blood glucose is normal. Glucose intolerance is due to a combination of insulin resistance and impaired insulin secretion. **Glucagonomas** are islet cell tumors that cause hyperglycemia due to tissue insensitivity to insulin. Patients with **barbiturate overdose** generally present with hypoglycemia.

250. The answer is e. *(McPhee, p 1109.)* The location and description of the rash in this diabetic patient most likely describes **necrobiosis lipoidica diabeticorum**—sharply circumscribed plaques on the anterior and lateral surface of the lower legs. **Acanthosis nigricans** is a velvety, hyperpigmented, thickened skin lesion over the dorsum of the neck, axillae, and groin and often precedes the diagnosis of an endocrine (insulin-resistant) disorder. **Eruptive xanthomas**, red-yellow papules often on the buttocks, may result from hypertriglyceridemia associated with hyperglycemia. Patients with DM must be evaluated for both macrovascular and microvascular complications. **Macrovascular complications** include coronary artery disease, cerebrovascular disease, and peripheral vascular disease and **microvascular complications** include retinopathy, nephropathy, and neuropathy.

251. The answer is d. *(Fauci, p 2419.)* This patient is extremely young with a significant family history of hypercholesterolemia. The most common type of familial hyperlipoproteinemia is **type IIA** (elevated LDL). Heterozygous carriers present with a family history of coronary events and often have **tendon xanthomas**. Patients with **type III** dysbetalipoproteinemia (normal LDL with elevated IDL and VLDL) often present with palmar xanthomas and tuberous xanthomas. Hypothyroidism, diabetes mellitus, nephrotic syndrome, and liver disease are secondary causes of hyperlipidemia. Hyperlipidemia occurs in over half of patients with early **nephrotic syndrome**. **Arcus senilis (a gray band in the cornea) seen** before the age of 40 is consistent with hyperlipidemia. Physicians should be able to calculate different cholesterol levels (mg/dL) using the following simple formulas:

1. Total cholesterol = HDL+ VLDL+ LDL
2. VLDL = triglycerides/5
3. LDL = total cholesterol – HDL – (triglycerides/5)

252. The answer is b. *(McPhee, pp 1398-1399.)* **Mucormycosis** is a rare fungal disease limited to persons with preexisting illness and may be seen in poorly controlled diabetic patients. Patients present with fever, nasal congestion, sinus pain, diplopia, and coma. Physical examination may reveal a necrotic nasal turbinate, reduced ocular motion, proptosis, and blindness. CT scan or MRI will reveal the extent of sinus involvement prior to surgery.

253. The answer is a. *(McPhee, pp 1075-1077.)* This patient with a pituitary adenoma most likely has multiple endocrine neoplasia or **MEN-1 (Wermer syndrome)**, an autosomal dominant disorder consisting of tumors of the **P**ancreas, **P**ituitary, and **P**arathyroid gland **(PPP)**. Pituitary adenomas in MEN-1 usually secrete prolactin, growth hormone, or both. **MEN-2A (Sipple syndrome)** consists of **P**heochromocytoma, hyper **P**arathyroidism, and medullary carcinoma of the **T**hyroid **(PPT)**. Patients with **MEN-2B syndrome** present with **P**heochromocytoma, mucosal **N**euromas, and medullary carcinoma of the **T**hyroid **(PNT)**. **Kallman syndrome** is congenital isolated gonadotropin deficiency, presenting with hypogonadism, infertility, anosmia, and unilateral renal agenesis.

254. The answer is b. *(McPhee, p 1122.)* The surreptitious injection of insulin is just as common as insulinoma. **Factitious hypoglycemia** should be suspected when hypoglycemic symptoms appear in health professionals or in relatives of patients with diabetes mellitus and is confirmed by **high insulin levels with low plasma C-peptide levels**. Patients with **insulinoma** have high levels of both C-peptide and insulin.

255. The answer is b. *(Kliegman, p 60.)* There are five Tanner Stages of Development (sexual maturity) for females:

Tanner 1 = no growth of pubic hair; no breasts
Tanner 2 = scarcely pigmented, straight pubic hair along medial border of labia; breast and papilla as small mound with increased size of areola
Tanner 3 = sparse, dark, curly pubic hair on labia; breast and areola enlarged
Tanner 4 = abundant coarse and curly pubic hair; areola and papilla form interior second elevation
Tanner 5 = lateral triangular spreading of adult hair to medial surfaces of thighs; mature nipple projections

256. The answer is d. *(McPhee, p 783.)* Diabetics with peripheral neuropathy are susceptible to developing a **Charcot joint**. The insensitivity of the feet predisposes the patient to multiple silent fractures, causing a deformed joint. The **Somogyi effect** is nocturnal hypoglycemia, which stimulates a surge of counterregulatory hormones to produce a high fasting blood sugar in the morning. The **Dawn phenomenon** is morning hyperglycemia from reduced sensitivity to insulin in the morning hours evoked by spikes of growth hormone released during sleep. **Mature-onset diabetes of the young (MODY)** is a rare autosomal dominant disorder characterized by impaired insulin secretion and the subsequent development of NIDDM in nonobese persons under the age of 25 years. The **Charcot triad** (fever, right upper quadrant pain, and jaundice) is seen in cholangitis.

257. The answer is c. *(McPhee, pp 995-997.)* The man had trauma to his posterior pituitary stalk from the car accident, resulting in **central diabetes insipidus (DI)** due to lack of vasopressin (antidiuretic hormone). Patients develop excessive thirst and pass large volumes of dilute urine. The diagnosis may be made by observing the urine osmolality response to injected vasopressin. **Nephrogenic DI,** in which a defect in the renal tubules will not respond to the stimulation by vasopressin presents similarly to central DI. Patients with the **syndrome of inappropriate antidiuretic hormone secretion (SIADH)** present with hyponatremia.

258. The answer is d. *(McPhee, pp 1518-1519.)* Persons with **Marfan syndrome** are tall, have arm spans that are greater than their height and above-average crown-to-heel height. Joints are hyperextensible, and patients have long, spiderlike, slender fingers **(arachnodactyly)**. **Steinberg sign** or the **thumb sign** is positive when the fingers are clenched over the thumb and the thumb protrudes beyond the ulnar margin of the hand. Patients often have a high-arched palate, kyphoscoliosis with pectus excavatum, subluxation of the lens, and a **murmur of mitral valve prolapse.** Aortic regurgitation and dissection of the aorta may complicate Marfan syndrome. Boys with **Klinefelter syndrome** have a 45XXY karyotype. After puberty they have disproportionately long extremities, gynecomastia and small testes, with azoospermia resulting in infertility. Patients with gonadal dysgenesis or **Turner syndrome** are 45, X; the syndrome is characterized by primary amenorrhea, short stature, webbed neck with low posterior hairline, and multiple congenital abnormalities. Patients with **Ehlers-Danlos syndrome (EDS)** present with hyperelasticity of the skin ("rubber man" syndrome) and hypermobile joints. **Noonan syndrome** is an autosomal dominant disorder characterized by webbed neck, short stature, and congenital heart disease. Patients have normal karyotypes and normal gonads.

259 and 260. The answers are 259-c, 260-a. *(McPhee, pp 862-864.)* Patients are diagnosed with **erectile dysfunction** when they cannot sustain erections to have sexual intercourse. A history of hypertension, hyperlipidemia, diabetes, depression, cardiac disease, pelvic trauma, surgery, or irradiation are all associated with this diagnosis. In addition, up to a quarter of cases are drug-related. Drugs that may cause impotence include antidepressants, anticholinergics, alcohol, methadone, heroin, tobacco, antihypertensives, and sedatives. **Nocturnal penile tumescence** occurs during rapid eye movement (REM) sleep, and if the man gives a history of rigid erections under any circumstances, the most likely etiology of his ED is **psychological** (ie, depression, disinterest, anxiety). In patients with a history of neuropathy, further studies to evaluate impotence are not necessary and are attributed to a **neuropathic** etiology. Patients with peripheral vascular disease should be evaluated with a **penile/brachial index**. An index of less than 0.06 suggests **vascular impotence. Retrograde ejaculation** may result from surgical disruption of the bladder neck or medications. **Premature ejaculation** is usually not rooted in an organic cause, but rather is anxiety-related.

Hematology and Oncology

Questions

261. A 55-year-old man presents with bone pain, especially in the lower back, that is aggravated by movement or weight bearing but tolerable when he is lying down at night. Physical examination is remarkable for pale conjunctivae. Laboratory results show a normocytic anemia and an increased serum globulin level. Peripheral blood smear is significant for rouleaux formation. Osteolytic bone lesions are seen on a radiograph of the spine and pelvis. Bone scan is normal. Which of the following is the most likely diagnosis?

a. Multiple myeloma
b. Paget disease
c. Metastatic bone disease
d. Monoclonal gammopathy of unknown significance (MGUS)
e. Waldenström macroglobulinemia

262. A 56-year-old African American man presents with a 15-lb unintentional weight loss over the last 6 weeks. He states that food "gets stuck" in the middle of his chest. Initially, the patient had difficulty swallowing solids, but the symptoms have since progressed to the point where he has similar problems when swallowing liquids. He also complains of odynophagia. He denies hoarseness and does not have a history of reflux symptoms. He smokes one pack of cigarettes per day and admits to heavily drinking alcohol. Physical examination reveals a left fixed supraclavicular node. Which of the following is the most likely diagnosis?

a. Achalasia
b. Squamous cell carcinoma of the esophagus
c. Adenocarcinoma of the esophagus
d. Esophageal stricture
e. Schatzki ring

263. A 37-year-old man who is in excellent health presents for a routine physical examination. Family history reveals that the patient's mother died of colon cancer at the age of 50 years and a brother, who is 44 years old, was recently diagnosed with colon cancer. The patient also has two maternal aunts with ovarian cancer. Physical examination is normal, and fecal occult blood test (FOBT) is negative. Laboratory data are normal. Which of the following statements best describes this patient?

a. He most likely has the *BRCA2* mutation.
b. He needs an annual colonoscopy beginning at age 36.
c. He should have a prophylactic colectomy.
d. If he develops colon cancer, it would most likely be in the proximal colon.
e. If he develops colon cancer, it would most likely be in the distal colon.

264. A 61-year-old woman presents to the emergency room with dyspnea on exertion and facial swelling for nearly 2 weeks. She has smoked three packs of cigarettes per day for nearly 40 years but does not drink alcohol. Her blood pressure is 120/88 mm Hg, pulse is 90 beats per minute, respirations are 16 breaths per minute, and she is afebrile. Heart and lung examinations are normal. She has dilated veins in the neck and upper chest area. Blood gases are normal. Which of the following is the most likely diagnosis?

a. Tumor lysis syndrome
b. Superior vena cava syndrome
c. Cord compression
d. Hypercalcemia
e. Cardiac tamponade
f. Pancoast syndrome

265. A 19-year-old woman with a lifelong history of easy bruisability presents with menorrhagia. She also reports occasional nosebleeds. She has no family history of bleeding disorders and takes no medications. Physical examination is normal. Laboratory investigation reveals a normal platelet count but a prolonged bleeding time. Which of the following is the most likely diagnosis?

a. Hemophilia A
b. Christmas disease
c. Type III von Willebrand disease
d. Type I von Willebrand disease
e. Bernard-Soulier syndrome

266. A 28-year-old woman with no significant past medical history complains of easy fatigability, tachypnea, and occasional palpitations. On further history, she reports a bizarre craving for ice chips. She has no other symptoms. On physical examination, she has conjunctival pallor and brittle nails, with a 2/6 systolic ejection murmur at the left sternal border, but no other findings. Her hemoglobin level is 7 g/dL and a peripheral smear shows hypochromic, microcytic cells with target cells and an increased number of platelets. What is the most likely etiology of her anemia?

a. Gastrointestinal blood loss
b. Menorrhagia
c. Hemolysis
d. Aplastic anemia
e. Hypersplenism

267. A 43-year-old man presents with a 2-month history of diarrhea and abdominal cramping. He has no nausea or vomiting. He denies melena and hematochezia. He has a 10-lb weight loss. Physical examination reveals edema of the head and neck. His face appears to be flushed. He has bilateral expiratory wheezes and a systolic murmur that increases with inspiration. Abdominal examination is normal. Rectal examination is FOBT negative. Which of the following is the best next step in diagnosis?

a. CT scan of the chest
b. Transthoracic echocardiogram
c. CT scan of the abdomen
d. Twenty-four-hour urine for 5-HIAA
e. Transesophageal echocardiogram

268. A 7-year-old boy with sickle cell disease presents with severe left upper quadrant pain that started suddenly 2 hours before he arrived at the emergency room. He has no previous history of pain in that area. Physical examination reveals a temperature of 37°C (98.6°F) and a normal blood pressure. Heart rate is 108 beats per minute. Heart and lung examinations are normal. There is fullness and tenderness in the left upper quadrant of the abdomen with palpation, but there is no audible rub. There is no hepatomegaly or rebound tenderness, and FOBT is negative. The rest of the physical examination is normal. Hemoglobin is 6.1 g/dL. Which of the following is the most likely diagnosis?

a. Vasoocclusive crisis
b. Splenic infarction
c. Splenic sequestration crisis
d. Left pleural effusion
e. Pulmonary infarction

269. A 37-year-old woman, G0P0, presents with an eczematous scaly eruption on her right nipple. She recently has taken up running and weight lifting and believes that the exercise has irritated her breast. Physical examination reveals a 1.5-cm erythematous and crusted lesion on her right nipple. The nipple is not inverted, and there are no masses or discharge. There are no axillary nodes, and the other breast is normal. Which of the following is the best next step in diagnosis?

a. Biopsy of the lesion
b. Mammogram
c. Topical steroid therapy
d. Topical antifungal therapy
e. Suggest the use of an athletic bra

270. A 42-year-old woman of Italian descent presents for a preemployment physical examination. She has no symptoms, no past medical problems, and takes no medications. Her physical examination is normal except for pale conjunctivae. Fecal occult blood test (FOBT) is negative. Her complete blood count (CBC) is remarkable for a hemoglobin of 11.4 g/dL, a mean corpuscular volume (MCV) of 60 fL, and a reticulocyte count of 0.6%. Her white blood cell count and platelets are normal. Peripheral smear reveals microcytosis, hypochromia, acanthocytes (cells with irregularly spaced projections), and occasional target cells. Which of the following is the most likely diagnosis?

a. Iron-deficiency anemia
b. Sideroblastic anemia
c. Anemia of chronic disease
d. Thalassemia trait
e. Alpha thalassemia major

271. A 23-year-old man with sickle cell disease presents with shortness of breath and pleuritic chest pain. His temperature is 38.5°C (101.3°F), and he is tachypneic and tachycardic. Heart examination is normal. Lung examination is notable for right basilar crackles. The patient's arterial saturation is 88%. He has a leukocytosis, and chest radiograph reveals an infiltrate. Which of the following is the most likely diagnosis?

a. Acute osteomyelitis
b. Acute chest syndrome
c. Myocardial infarction
d. Congestive heart failure
e. Parvovirus B19 infection

272. A 19-year-old woman in her second trimester of pregnancy presents with a deep venous thrombosis (DVT) of her left lower extremity. She has no previous history of DVT and has no family history of thromboembolism. Which of the following is the most likely reason for the patient developing a DVT?

a. Protein C deficiency
b. Protein S deficiency
c. Antithrombin III deficiency
d. Factor V Leiden deficiency
e. Hyperhomocysteinemia

273. A 31-year-old African American man presents to the emergency room and is diagnosed as having a community-acquired pneumonia. After 2 days of antibiotics, the patient becomes jaundiced. His hematocrit is 30% (decreased from 40% on admission), reticulocyte count is 6%, and indirect bilirubin value is 4.5 mg/dL (total bilirubin of 6.0 mg/dL). Peripheral blood smear demonstrates Heinz bodies. The patient recalls a similar problem when he was given antibiotics 5 years ago for an acute sinusitis. His three brothers have a similar reaction to antibiotics. Which of the following is the most likely diagnosis?

a. Sickle cell anemia
b. Sickle cell trait
c. Autoimmune hemolytic anemia
d. Glucose-6-phosphate dehydrogenase deficiency
e. Allergic reaction

274. A 32-year-old woman presents with the recent onset of petechiae of her lower extremities. She denies menorrhagia and gastrointestinal bleeding. She has no family history of a bleeding disorder and has been in excellent health her entire life. She takes no medications and does not drink alcohol. Physical examination is remarkable for petechiae of both legs. There is no hepatosplenomegaly. The rest of the physical examination is normal. Platelet count is 8000/μL. Hemoglobin and white blood cell count are normal. Peripheral smear reveals reduced platelets and an occasional megathrombocyte. Which of the following is the most likely diagnosis?

a. Thrombocytopenic thrombotic purpura (TTP)
b. Hemolytic-uremic syndrome (HUS)
c. Evans syndrome
d. Disseminated intravascular coagulopathy (DIC)
e. Idiopathic thrombocytopenic purpura (ITP)

275. A 52-year-old man presents with a neck mass. He states that after he drinks one to two glasses of wine, the neck mass becomes painful. He also complains of intermittent fever, night sweats, pruritus, and a 10-lb weight loss over the last month. Physical examination reveals a 3-cm mass in the left anterior cervical lymph node chain that is hard and tender to deep palpation. Several other cervical nodes and a left axillary node are palpable. There is no hepatomegaly or splenomegaly. Which of the following is most likely to be found on diagnostic testing?

a. Paratrabecular lymphoid aggregates on bone marrow biopsy
b. Reed-Sternberg cells on lymph node biopsy
c. Auer rod on bone marrow biopsy
d. Cells with numerous cytoplasmic projections on bone marrow biopsy
e. Noncaseating granulomas on lymph node biopsy

276. A 62-year-old man presents for his annual health maintenance visit. The review of systems is positive for occasional fatigue and headache. The patient admits to generalized pruritus following a warm bath or shower. He has plethora and engorgement of the retinal veins. A spleen is palpable on abdominal examination. The patient's hematocrit is 63%, and he has a leukocytosis and thrombocytosis. Peripheral blood smear is normal. The patient does not smoke. Which of the following is the most likely diagnosis?

a. Essential thrombocytosis
b. Myelofibrosis
c. Spurious polycythemia
d. Polycythemia vera
e. Secondary polycythemia

277. A 42-year-old man develops fever and chills within a few hours after a blood transfusion. His temperature is 38.7°C (101.6°F), and his blood pressure is 120/80 mm Hg. He is slightly tachycardic, but his respiratory rate is normal. His CBC is normal except for the anemia for which he was receiving the transfusion. Laboratory data including electrolytes, liver function tests, and urinalysis are normal. Which of the following is the most likely diagnosis?

a. Anaphylaxis to blood transfusion
b. ABO incompatibility
c. Leukoagglutinin reaction to blood transfusion
d. Transfusion-associated circulatory overload
e. Urticarial reaction to blood transfusion

278. A woman with a history of left mastectomy and subsequent radiation therapy for breast cancer 2 years ago presents with a 3-cm mass along the edge of the surgical suture line. She denies fever, chills, night sweats, and weight loss. Physical examination reveals some generalized induration and a tanned appearance of the skin overlying the mastectomy secondary to radiation therapy. There is a nonmobile, nontender mass along the suture line that is not warm or fluctuant. She has no axillary lymphadenopathy. A biopsy specimen of the breast mass is most likely to show which of the following?

a. Fibroadenoma
b. Malignancy
c. Benign cyst
d. Abscess
e. Lipoma

279. A 56-year-old man complains of a 10-lb weight loss over a 2-month period. He has no symptoms except nocturia, hesitancy at starting his urinary stream and mid-back pain that is constant and worse at night. He does not smoke cigarettes, use illicit drugs, or drink alcohol, and he has no past medical history. On physical examination, the patient is afebrile with normal blood pressure. The only abnormal finding on heart, lung, abdominal, lymph node, and musculoskeletal examinations is point tenderness over the thoracic spinous processes. Which of the following is the most likely diagnosis?

a. Musculoskeletal strain
b. Lymphoma
c. Metastatic prostate cancer
d. Metastatic lung cancer
e. Epidural abscess

280. A 28-year-old woman presents with her third episode of left lower extremity deep venous thrombosis. She has a history of two second-trimester miscarriages in the past. Laboratory data reveal an elevated activated partial thromboplastin time (PTT) that is not corrected by dilution with normal plasma and an abnormal dilute Russell viper venom. Which of the following is the most likely diagnosis?

a. Libman-Sacks disease
b. Livedo reticularis
c. Antiphospholipid syndrome
d. Takayasu arteritis
e. Sjögren syndrome

Questions 281 to 285

For each patient with cancer, select the most likely risk factor for the malignancy. Each lettered option may be used once, multiple times, or not at all.

a. *Helicobacter pylori* infection
b. Hepatitis C infection
c. Mutation to *BRCA1*
d. Translocation between chromosome 9 and 22 [t(9;22)]
e. Villous adenomatous polyp
f. Tubular adenomatous polyp
g. Human papillomavirus
h. Tobacco use
i. Schistosomiasis
j. Epstein-Barr virus
k. Herpesvirus type 8 (HHV-8)
l. Human T-cell lymphotrophic/leukemia virus type 1 (HTLV-1)

281. A previously healthy 49-year-old man presents with fever and night sweats. He has splenomegaly. His peripheral white blood cell count is 22,000/μL, and a peripheral smear shows immature leukocytes with an increase in the number of basophils. Leukocyte alkaline phosphatase score is low, and vitamin B_{12} level is elevated.

282. A 29-year-old patient presents with squamous cell carcinoma of the anus. He is sexually promiscuous and is requesting an HIV test.

283. A 57-year-old patient presents with right upper quadrant abdominal pain. Serum alpha-fetoprotein level is higher than 1200 ng/mL. The patient does not drink alcohol and has no history of intravenous drug use or blood transfusions. A hepatic mass is present on CT scan of the abdomen.

284. A 62-year-old woman presents with jaundice, back pain, and weight loss. CT scan of the abdomen demonstrates a mass at the head of the pancreas.

285. A 44-year-old man presents with intermittent epigastric pain and is found to have a gastric lymphoma.

Questions 286 and 287

For each patient with a lung mass, select the most likely malignancy. Each lettered option may be used once, multiple times, or not at all.

a. Adenocarcinoma of the lung
b. Hamartoma
c. Bronchial adenoma
d. Squamous cell carcinoma of the lung
e. Small-cell carcinoma of the lung
f. Bronchioalveolar carcinoma of the lung
g. Mesothelioma

286. A 54-year-old woman presents with a peripheral lung mass. She has no history of tobacco use and has worked as a seamstress all her life. She has no family history of lung cancer.

287. A 39-year-old woman with a tobacco history has a centrally located lung mass and a serum sodium of 121 mEq/L.

Questions 288 to 290

For each cell shown, select the most appropriate abnormality. Each lettered option may be used once, multiple times, or not at all.

a. Howell-Jolly bodies
b. Reed-Sternberg cells
c. Pelger-Hüet cells
d. Heinz bodies
e. Auer rods
f. Hypersegmented polymorphonuclear leukocytes
g. Schistocytes
h. Pappenheimer bodies
i. Döhle bodies
j. Toxic granulations

288. A 53-year-old woman with a history of resection of the ileum presents with glossitis and a hematocrit of 15%. Her peripheral smear is as shown in the following figure.

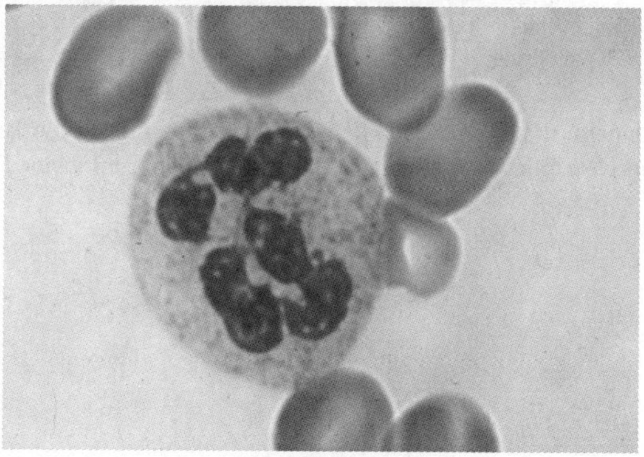

(Reproduced, with permission, from Marshall A. Lichtman, MD.)

289. A 10-year-old boy is admitted to the hospital with acute renal failure after a few days of bloody diarrhea. His peripheral smear is as shown in the following figure.

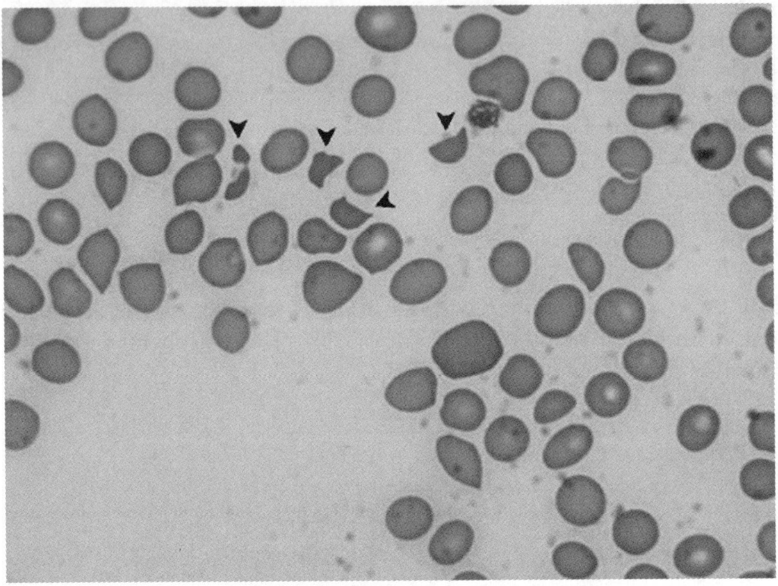

(Reproduced, with permission, from Knoop KJ, Stack LB, Storrow AB, et al. Atlas of Emergency Medicine, *3rd ed. New York, NY: McGraw-Hill; 2009:849. Photo contributor: James P. Elrod, MD, PhD.)*

290. A 22-year-old man presents with a painless mass in his neck. A biopsy shows the cells as in the following figure.

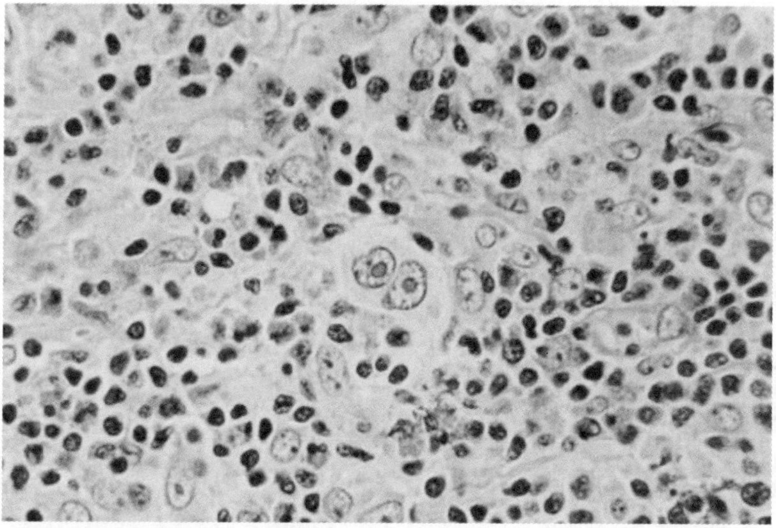

(Reproduced, with permission, from Lichtman MA, Beutler E, Kipps TJ, et al. Williams Hematology, *7th ed. New York, NY: McGraw-Hill; 2006:1464.)*

Questions 291 to 295

For each malignancy, select the most appropriate tumor marker. Each lettered option may be used once, multiple times, or not at all.

a. CA-125
b. LDH
c. PSA
d. CEA
e. AFP
f. hCG
g. 5-HIAA
h. Beta-2 microglobulin

291. Hepatocellular carcinoma

292. Multiple myeloma

293. Colon cancer

294. Ovarian cancer

295. Lymphoma

Hematology and Oncology

Answers

261. The answer is a. *(McPhee, pp 471-473.)* **Multiple myeloma (MM)** is a neoplasm characterized by proliferation of **plasma cells** ("fried-egg-appearing cells") replacing the bone marrow (median age at presentation is 65). The disorder may lead to bone pain often in the back, pathologic fracture, normocytic anemia, susceptibility to infections, renal failure, and hypercalcemia. The bone pain of MM worsens with movement while the pain of metastatic bone disease is typically worse at night. Patients have an increased serum globulin fraction and a **monoclonal IgA or IgG spike (M component) on serum or urine protein electrophoresis**. The monoclonal immunoglobulin causes **rouleaux formation** on blood smear. Urine examination reveals **Bence-Jones (light chain) proteinuria**. **Osteolytic lesions** in the axial skeleton are seen in many bones on plain radiographic studies, but bone scan (technetium Tc 99m) is normal. **MGUS** is monoclonal gammopathy of unknown significance that is more common than MM. However, these patients do not have anemia, renal failure, Bence-Jones proteinuria, lytic bone lesions, or hypercalcemia. Bone marrow aspirate is normal in MGUS. **Paget disease** of bone is increased bone turnover especially in the skull, pelvis and long bones of the upper and lower extremities. In this disease, serum alkaline phosphatase is markedly elevated, calcium is increased and there are osteolytic lesions which are apparent on bone scans. Cancer **metastatic to bone** also lights up on bone scans. **Waldenström macroglobulinemia** is a B-cell malignancy (so is MM) with an **IgM monoclonal protein** and both lymphocytosis and plasmacytosis in the bone marrow. Patients present with bleeding, cytopenia, lymphadenopathy, and hyperviscosity crises.

262. The answer is b. *(McPhee, pp 1465-1469.)* Progressive (solids to liquids) difficulty swallowing **(dysphagia)** accompanied by rapid weight loss and **odynophagia** (painful swallowing) often indicates esophageal carcinoma. Tumor involvement of the recurrent laryngeal nerve would cause hoarseness and the patient's fixed supraclavicular node **(Virchow node)** is consistent with the diagnosis. **Squamous cell carcinoma** is more common in black patients and also has a high incidence in China and Southeast Asia. Risk factors for esophageal squamous cell carcinoma include tobacco and alcohol use, achalasia, and lye ingestion. **Adenocarcinoma** is more common in white patients, commonly arising in the distal third of the esophagus due to Barrett metaplasia from chronic gastroesophageal reflux. Patients with **Schatzki ring** (lower esophageal web) have intermittent dysphagia to solids, and patients with **strictures** typically present with complaints of heartburn. **Achalasia** is loss of peristalsis in the distal two-thirds of the esophagus and impairment of lower esophageal sphincter relaxation; patients often present with progressive dysphagia to solids and liquids as well as respiratory symptoms from regurgitation. Barium esophagogram in achalasia reveals a dilated esophagus with a "bird's beak" tapering distal to the esophageal contraction.

263. The answer is d. *(McPhee, pp 592-593.)* The pedigree of the patient (multiple primary cancers, including ovarian, gastric, renal, endometrial, and small intestinal among others) is most consistent with **hereditary nonpolyposis colon cancer (HNPCC)**. Affected patients develop a few flat polyps that rapidly transform into cancer and at an earlier age than nonfamilial colon cancers—the median age for HNPCC transformation into adenocarcinoma of the colon is 50 years, and **the most common site is the proximal colon**. Inheritance is autosomal dominant, and **members of the family should undergo biennial colonoscopy starting at age 25. Prophylactic colectomy is recommended for patients with familial adenomatous polyposis**, an autosomal dominant disorder characterized by small polyps that develop during the second decade of life and undergo malignant transformation before the age of 40. Breast cancer is not associated with HNPCC (the genetic defect is in DNA mismatch repair genes).

264. The answer is b. *(McPhee, pp 431-432.)* There are several life-threatening complications in cancer patients. This patient is manifesting symptoms consistent with **superior vena cava (SVC) obstruction** which is due to direct extension of lung cancer in 85% of cases and can cause swelling of the neck, face, and upper extremities with dilated veins in the neck and upper chest. Tumors that may cause SVC syndrome include small-cell carcinoma of the lung, squamous cell carcinoma of the lung, lymphoma, and mediastinal tumors like thymomas and germ cell tumors. Tissue diagnosis is preferable prior to starting any treatment. Some malignancies are so responsive to chemotherapy that **tumor lysis syndrome** occurs, resulting in hyperkalemia, hyperphosphatemia, hypocalcemia, hyperuricemia, and renal failure hours after receiving treatment (these tumors require allopurinol prophylaxis prior to chemotherapy to prevent hyperuricemia). Patients with **cord compression** may present with back pain, gait difficulty, weakness, sensory deficits, and incontinence. Patients with **hypercalcemia** from remote effects of malignancy **(paraneoplastic syndrome)** may present with lethargy, weakness, constipation, vomiting, and coma. Cancer patients may develop **cardiac tamponade** from pericardial metastasis; physical examination might demonstrate findings such as hypotension, jugular venous distention, distant heart sounds, and pulsus paradoxus. **Pancoast syndrome** (superior sulcus tumor) is a complication of lung cancer when it extends into the apex. Patients have compression of the C8, T1, and T2 nerves and often complain of arm and shoulder pain.

265. The answer is d. *(McPhee, pp 492-493.)* **von Willebrand disease (vWD)** is the most common inherited bleeding disorder. It is autosomal dominant and caused due to an abnormality in the quantity or quality of **vWF**. The **most common type is type I** (80% of cases), caused by a quantitative decrease in vWF, and patients present with mild symptoms, as in this case. Type IIA and IIB vWD are qualitative disorders; **type III vWD is a rare autosomal recessive disorder** in which vWF is nearly absent—patients with these types have moderate to severe bleeding. Most bleeding from vWD is mucosal (epistaxis, gingival bleeding, menorrhagia) or gastrointestinal, and bleeding is exacerbated by aspirin use. Hemarthroses do not occur in vWD. The treatment for vWD types I and IIA is **desmopressin,** which stimulates the release of vWF from endothelial cells. Spontaneous hemarthroses are characteristic of **hemophilia A or factor VIII deficiency** (classic hemophilia) and **factor IX deficiency (hemophilia B or Christmas disease)**. Hemophilia has an X-linked pattern of inheritance, and the symptoms and prognosis are similar for hemophilia A and B. **Bernard-Soulier syndrome** is a rare platelet disorder in which platelets cannot adhere to the endothelium because they lack receptors for vWF. Patients present with severe bleeding, especially postoperatively. Platelets appear abnormally large on peripheral smear. Measurements of vWF in Bernard-Soulier syndrome are normal.

266. The answer is b. *(McPhee, pp 439-441.)* **Iron deficiency** is the most common etiology of anemia worldwide and patients may present with fatigue, tachycardia, tachypnea, conjunctival pallor, and if severe, nail and mucosal changes. Patients who are iron deficient will sometimes develop pica, a craving for ice or starch. The major storage form of iron is ferritin, and a ferritin level below12 mcg/L indicates iron deficiency. Once patients have been deficient for a while, the peripheral blood smear will show hypochromic, microcytic cells and increased platelets. In women of childbearing age, exceedingly heavy menstruation (menorrhagia) is the most likely cause of iron deficiency, though pregnancy and lactation can strain iron stores as well. In older patients, and in those without menorrhagia, the most important cause to exclude is **blood loss**, especially from the GI tract. **Hemolytic anemias** occur because of inherent problems with the red cell (as in sickle cell or G6PD deficiency) or due to immune disfunction or microangiopathic problems (like TTP or HUS). Patients with hemolysis have a depressed haptoglobin level. **Aplastic anemia** results from bone marrow failure, thus patients present with pancytopenia, fatigue, and bruising on physical examination. **Splenomegaly** resulting from problems such as lymphoproliferative diseases, congestive heart failure, portal hypertension, autoimmune disorders, and infection causes thrombocytopenia due to platelet sequestration.

267. The answer is d. *(McPhee, pp 1473-1474.)* **Carcinoid syndrome** is usually associated with primary carcinoid tumors of the lung or stomach and carcinoid tumors of the small bowel metastatic to the liver. Patients with **carcinoid tumor** who present with the carcinoid syndrome (fewer than 10%) like this patient, experience cutaneous flushing, diarrhea, wheezing, telangiectasias, and paroxysmal hypotension due to the production of **serotonin** by the tumor. Patients often have cardiac lesions, such as tricuspid insufficiency and pulmonic stenosis. The best next step of the choices given in this patient would be a 24-hour urine collection for 5-hydroxyindoleacetic acid (**5-HIAA**), a breakdown product of serotonin that is elevated in carcinoid syndrome.

268. The answer is c. *(Fauci, p 638.)* Patients with hemoglobin SC disease and children with sickle cell disease are at risk for **splenic sequestration** crisis when blood is trapped in the spleen (leading to further splenic enlargement and anemia). **Splenic infarction** is not associated with anemia or sudden splenomegaly; patients often have a **left upper quadrant**

rub on physical examination. Episodes of **vasoocclusive crisis** (pain crises) are not associated with increased hemolysis, anemia, or splenomegaly. Patients with a **left pleural effusion** would have decreased breath sounds at the left lung base, with dullness to percussion and decreased tactile fremitus. **Pulmonary infarction** may result from sickle cell disease and pulmonary emboli, among other things, and can present with hemoptysis and bloody pleural effusions.

269. The answer is a. *(McPhee, p 660.)* The basic lesion of **Paget carcinoma** (1% of all breast cancers) is a usually well-differentiated infiltrative ductal carcinoma or a ductal carcinoma in situ (DCIS). A tumor mass may not be palpable, and there may be few gross nipple changes, leading these lesions to often be overlooked or treated with topical antibacterial or antifungal agents. The diagnosis is established by **biopsy** of the erosion or ulceration. If this lesion is Paget disease of the breast, it will not be best-visualized on mammogram **and it will not respond to the topical therapies** suggested in the answer choices. The **risk factors for breast cancer** include age (80% of cases occur after age 50), family history of breast cancer, previous breast biopsy for benign disease, genetic mutations (*BRCA1* and *BRCA2*), increased breast tissue density on mammogram, early menarche (< 12 years old), nulliparity, late menopause (> 50 years old), and late age at birth of first child (> 30 years old). Breast cancer should always be the primary consideration in any woman who presents with a breast lesion.

270. The answer is d. *(McPhee, pp 442-444.)* The differential diagnosis for **microcytic hypochromic anemia** is **TICLS** (**T**halassemia, **I**ron deficiency, **C**hronic disease, **L**ead toxicity, and **S**ideroblastic anemia). **Thalassemias,** inherited disorders with reduction in the synthesis of alpha- or beta-globin chains, generally produce a greater degree of microcytosis (lower mean corpuscular volume or MCV) for any given level of anemia than does iron deficiency. Alpha thalassemia is found in people from Southeast Asia and China while patients of Mediterranean descent and some Asians develop beta thalassemia. **Acanthocytes** (cells with projections emanating from them) and **target cells** are seen in this disorder, but the latter are also seen in lead poisoning, liver disease, hyposplenism, and hemoglobin C disease. This patient of Mediterranean descent most likely has **thalassemia trait**, meaning she has laboratory abnormalities with no significant clinical disease, **as opposed to thalassemia major which is life-threatening**. The most common cause of a microcytic anemia is **iron deficiency**, but this diagnosis is unlikely in this asymptomatic patient with a negative FOBT. The MCV in anemia of chronic disease is usually normal or slightly reduced, and patients typically have a history of chronic infection or inflammation, cancer, or liver disease. Alcoholics, patients taking antituberculosis medication or chloramphenicol, or those with lead poisoning may develop **sideroblastic anemia** (a failure to incorporate heme into protoporphyrin). Bone marrow staining will demonstrate iron deposits **(ringed sideroblasts)** encircling the nucleus in siderocytes. Coarse **basophilic stippling** of the red blood cells on peripheral smear would be characteristic of **lead poisoning**.

271. The answer is b. *(Fauci, pp 638-639.)* This patient with sickle cell disease most likely has **acute chest syndrome**, which is a life-threatening complication of the disease characterized by fever, dyspnea, cough, leukocytosis, pulmonary infiltrate, and hypoxemia. The usual causes of acute chest syndrome are vasoocclusion, infection, and pulmonary fat embolus from infarcted marrow, and its presentation can mimic pneumonia or pulmonary embolism. This condition is one of the few in sickle cell disease in which transfusion is advocated in order to increase oxygen-carrying capacity of the blood. Sickle cell patients may get **osteomyelitis** (most often from salmonellae or staphylococci) and vasoocclusion may cause **cardiac infarcts**. **Parvovirus B19** causes **aplastic anemia** in patients with sickle cell disease.

272. The answer is d. *(Fauci, p 46.)* Pregnancy itself is a hypercoagulable state, but **factor V Leiden mutation or activated protein C (APC) resistance** is the most common heritable clotting disorder to increase a pregnant woman's risk for development of deep venous thrombosis **(DVT)**. In these women, clots arise much more commonly in the left leg. The defect is a mutation in activated factor V, not in protein C, and is found in 8% of the general population **(exclusively in white populations)**. Forty percent of all patients presenting with DVT have the mutation. All of the primary hypercoagulable states in the question may cause DVT, especially during pregnancy (due to the elevation in estrogen), but these are less common than APC resistance.

273. The answer is d. *(McPhee, pp 449-450.)* The clinical picture strongly suggests **glucose-6-phosphate dehydrogenase (G6PD) deficiency**, an

X-linked recessive condition in which red blood cells are unable to deal with oxidative stresses. Acute hemolysis occurs when affected patients are exposed to an infection or an **oxidizing drug** (dapsone, primaquine, sulfonamides, nitrofurantoin, quinine). Oxidized hemoglobin precipitates into **Heinz bodies** which are ultimately removed by the spleen. The hemolytic episodes are **self-limited,** even if the offending agent is still present, because older red cells with low enzyme activity are removed and replaced by younger red cells with adequate levels of G6PD. Cells that survive a hemolytic episode have adequate amounts of G6PD, so testing is not useful during the acute illness. G6PD deficiency is often called favism in the Mediterranean, as hemolysis can occur after patients eat fava beans.

274. The answer is e. *(McPhee, pp 482-484.)* **Idiopathic thrombocytopenic purpura (ITP)** is an autoimmune disorder in which an IgG autoantibody binds to platelets. Destruction of the platelets takes place in the spleen, where macrophages bind to the antibody-coated platelets. Fifty percent of patients with ITP have no associated disease, but HIV infection, Systemic lupus erythematosus (SLE), or a lymphoproliferative disorder should be considered. ITP is a disease of persons between the ages of 20 and 50 years and occurs in women more than in men. There is **no splenomegaly** in ITP. The diagnosis is one of exclusion, but often megathrombocytes are seen on peripheral smear. Patients with platelet counts below 20,000 or those who are bleeding should be treated with corticosteroids, with or without intravenous immunoglobulin (IVIG). **Evans syndrome** is ITP with coexistent autoimmune hemolytic anemia. **DIC** is a systemic coagulation disorder that can be accompanied by thrombocytopenia. It may be secondary to transfusion, infection, malignancy, trauma, or obstetric complications. **TTP** is unlikely since the patient does not have the pentad of symptoms seen in 40% of patients **(FAT R.N.** = Fever, Autoimmune hemolytic anemia, Thrombocytopenia, Renal disease, Neurologic disease**). HUS** presents with three of the five symptoms seen in TTP **(RAT** = Renal disease, Autoimmune hemolytic anemia, and Thrombocytopenia**)**. Fever and neurologic disease are lacking.

275. The answer is b. *(McPhee, p 471.)* Patients with **Hodgkin lymphoma** often present with **painless regional lymphadenopathy** and the constitutional "**B symptoms**" of fever, drenching night sweats, and weight loss. Occasionally, patients may present with pruritus or pain in an involved lymph node after ingestion of alcohol. There is a bimodal age distribution with one peak in the twenties and a second peak at over age 50. The diagnosis of Hodgkin disease is made by lymph node biopsy with the finding of **Reed-Sternberg cells ("owl eyes")**. The bone marrow in non-Hodgkin lymphoma shows **paratrabecular lymphoid aggregates** and **Auer rods** are **cytoplasmic needle-shaped inclusions found in AML**. Hairy cell leukemia is aptly named for the characteristic **"hairy cells"** (cytoplasmic inclusions make the cells look hairy) which are present on the examination of the bone marrow and **noncaseating granulomas** are found in sarcoidosis.

276. The answer is d. *(McPhee, pp 457-459.)* The patient most likely has **polycythemia vera**, an acquired myeloproliferative disorder characterized by overproduction of all three cell lines, but most prominently there is a **primary erythrocytosis**. The median age at diagnosis is 60 and hematocrits are more than 54% in males and more than 51% in females. Patients present with symptoms related to an increase in blood volume and viscosity, such as headache, dizziness, blurred vision, fatigue, and thrombosis coupled with bleeding episodes. **Pruritus after a warm bath or shower** is due to **histamine release by basophils**. **Splenomegaly** exists in virtually every patient with polycythemia vera. The treatment of choice for polycythemia vera is **phlebotomy**. **Spurious polycythemia** is the result of contracted plasma volume from diuresis, rather than actual increase in red cells mass. **Secondary polycythemia** may be due to smoking, high altitudes, cardiac or pulmonary disease, or erythropoietin-secreting cysts or tumors. Patients with **essential thrombocytosis** have platelet counts of more than 2 million/μL. Patients with **myelofibrosis** have splenomegaly, dry bone marrow taps, and peripheral blood smears showing abnormal and bizarre morphologies and immature forms.

277. The answer is c. *(McPhee, pp 476-479.)* The most common reaction to blood transfusion is the **febrile, nonhemolytic (or leukoagglutinin) reaction**. Patients develop fever and chills several hours after receiving the transfusion because of recipient antibodies to donor leukocyte antigens on white blood cells. **Hemolytic reactions** (manifesting as fever, chills, hemoglobinuria, back pain, flank pain, dyspnea, anxiety, renal failure, DIC, multiorgan failure, and death) are due to erythrocyte (ABO) incompatibility.

Other transfusion reactions, such as **anaphylaxis** with bronchospasm or **urticaria** (recipient antibodies to protein) and **circulatory overload** (pulmonary congestion), are unlikely in this patient.

278. The answer is b. *(McPhee, pp 656-661.)* **Malignant lesions,** as found in this patient, are painless, irregular in contour and shape, hard, nonmobile, and not well demarcated. **Fibroadenomas** are the most common benign neoplasms of the breast. They are well demarcated, rubbery, mobile, and nontender. **Benign cysts** are the most common cause of breast lumps and tend to occur in association with other cysts. They are round, mobile, and soft, with a cystic consistency. They are tender premenstrually, become smaller immediately after menses, and regress after menopause. **Breast abscesses** are localized and are tender, swollen, erythematous, and fluctuant. **Lipomas** are soft, rounded, mobile benign tumors in the subcutaneous tissue.

279. The answer is c. *(Fauci, p 613.)* This patient with BPH symptoms and point tenderness over the vertebrae must be ruled out for **prostate cancer metastatic to his spine.** Metastatic bone tumors are more common than primary bone cancers and travel to bone hematogenously or via local extension. The vast majority of bone metastases come from **prostate, lung, and breast primaries**, but kidney, bladder, and thyroid cancers, as well as sarcomas and lymphomas, also metastasize to the bone. The sites most often affected are the **vertebrae, proximal femur, pelvis, ribs, sternum, proximal humerus, and skull.** Bone pain is usually **localized, constant, unrelieved by rest** (unlike musculoskeletal strain) and **more severe at night**. While **lung cancer** and **lymphoma** can metastasize to the spine as well, this patient's urinary symptoms and lack of other complaints or physical examination findings point to prostate cancer as the most likely cause of his bone pain. A patient with an **epidural abscess** will have infectious symptoms and signs (fever, chills) in addition to point tenderness of the spine **Musculoskeletal strain** in the back usually causes spasm and point tenderness over the paraspinous muscles.

280. The answer is c. *(McPhee, pp 755-756.)* The patient most likely has **antiphospholipid syndrome**. Patients with this antibody are at risk for venous and arterial thrombotic events, probably due to antibody reactivity with platelets or endothelial cell phospholipids. Patients often have a history of recurrent miscarriages, leg ulcers, Raynaud phenomenon, and livedo reticularis. Laboratory data often reveal a positive lupus anticoagulant, thrombocytopenia, a prolonged partial thromboplastin time (PTT; not corrected by adding normal plasma; a clotting factor deficiency would correct with normal plasma), elevated titers of anticardiolipin antibodies, and an **abnormal dilute Russell viper venom. Libman-Sacks disease** is endocarditis in patients with SLE and may be associated with antiphospholipid antibodies. **Livedo reticularis** is characterized by reddish or bluish mottling of the extremities and is usually idiopathic and requires no treatment. Livedo reticularis may be secondary to atheroembolism-induced emboli following an intraarterial procedure. **Takayasu arteritis** (pulseless disease) is a granulomatous arteritis that affects women more than men. Patients are usually in their fourth decade of life. The disease typically affects the aorta and its major branches, including the arteries that supply the upper extremities. Patients have absent pulses in the upper arm and complain of arm claudication. **Sjögren syndrome** affects women predominantly with dryness of the eyes and mouth and is often associated with other connective tissue diseases.

281 to 285. The answers are 281-d, 282-g, 283-b, 284-h, 285-a. *(McPhee, pp 1463-1494.)* Most patients with **chronic myelogenous leukemia (CML)** present in middle age with fatigue, night sweats, splenomegaly, and an elevated white blood count. The majority of these patients have the **Philadelphia chromosome t(9;22)** and the **bcr-abl fusion protein detected on polymerase chain reaction test of the peripheral blood. Squamous cell carcinomas of the anus**, penis, and cervix have been linked to **human papillomavirus (HPV). Hepatitis B and C and hemochromatosis** are the major risk factors for **hepatocellular carcinoma**. Other risk factors include aflatoxin (peanuts) exposure and being from the Far East or Africa (high-incidence areas). **Cigarette smoking** is the most consistently observed risk factor for **pancreatic cancer. Mucosa-associated lymphoid tissue (MALT) tumor of the stomach** has been shown to be secondary to ***H. pylori*. Schistosomiasis** is associated with **squamous cell carcinoma of the bladder**. Patients with the ***BRCA1* gene on chromosome 17** present with breast cancer at a young age with a family history of breast or ovarian cancer. Patients with colonic polyps are at risk for developing colon cancer. **Villous adenomas are more likely to be malignant**, but tubular adenomas are four times more common. **Epstein-Barr virus** is associated with **Burkitt lymphoma and nasopharyngeal cancer**; patients often present with an enlarging neck mass. **HHV-8** is associated with **Kaposi sarcoma**, and **HTLV-1** is associated with **adult T-cell leukemia**.

286 and 287. The answers are 286-a, 287-e. *(McPhee, pp 1452-1459.)* **Adenocarcinoma of the lung** is the most common lung cancer and is increasing in incidence in women. It often occurs in the **absence of a smoking history** (although the role of secondhand smoke is still unknown) and is usually found in the **periphery**. **Small-cell carcinoma of the lung** (20% of all new cases of lung cancer) is usually found **centrally** and is associated with a **history of tobacco use** and the **production of ectopic hormones**, such as antidiuretic hormone (ADH), parathyroid hormone (PTH), and adrenocorticotropic hormone (ACTH). **Squamous cell carcinoma** (another **central** lesion) is associated with PTH production, leading to **hypercalcemia**. Patients with **bronchioalveolar carcinoma** (a variant of adenocarcinoma) may present with an infiltrate on chest radiograph. **Hamartomas** and **bronchial adenomas** are benign lung tumors. Hamartomas are located **peripherally**; bronchial adenomas are located **centrally. Mesothelioma** is associated with **asbestos exposure** but not tobacco use and presents with pleural effusion or thickening.

288 to 290. The answers are 288-f, 289-g, 290-b. *(McPhee, pp 445, 454, 471.)* The patient, who presents after ileal resection with glossitis, has vitamin $\mathbf{B_{12}}$ **deficiency**, thus her peripheral smear reveals **hypersegmented polymorphonuclear cells** (also seen in folic acid deficiency). **Schistocytes** (as well as helmet cells, burr cells, triangular cells, and spherocytes) are seen in **microangiopathic hemolytic anemia**, one of the cardinal findings in TTP and, as in the case of the child with hemorrhagic enteritis, **HUS (hemolytic uremic syndrome)**. The **Reed-Sternberg cell** is the diagnostic "owl-eyes" tumor cell of Hodgkin disease, which often presents as a painless neck mass. **Howell-Jolly bodies** are found in asplenic or hyposplenic patients; **Heinz bodies** are the precipitants of denatured oxidized hemoglobin in G6PD deficiency. The **Pelger-Hüet anomaly** is a benign inherited trait resulting in neutrophils with bilobed nuclei. Prominent cytoplasmic granules called **toxic granulations** and **Döhle bodies,** representing fragments of ribosome-rich endoplasmic reticulum, are seen in immature neutrophils in bacterial infections. **Auer rods** are eosinophilic inclusions seen in acute myelogenous leukemia (AML). **Pappenheimer bodies** are often seen in thalassemia.

291 to 295. The answers are 291-e, 292-h, 293-d, 294-a, 295-b. (*Fauci, p 483.*) Tumor markers should not be used to diagnose cancer, but may be helpful in following patients for whom a diagnosis has already been made. **AFP** is associated with hepatocellular carcinoma. **Beta-2 microglobulin** is the most important prognostic factor for multiple myeloma **and carcinoembryonic antigen (CEA)** is associated with colon and breast cancer. **CA-125** is associated with ovarian cancer. **Lactate dehydrogenase (LDH)** is an important prognostic factor for Hodgkin and other lymphomas. **LDH, alpha fetoprotein (AFP)**, and **human chorionic gonadotropin (hCG)** are associated with testicular cancer. **5-HIAA** is associated with carcinoid syndrome (facial flushing and diarrhea from a tumor usually located in the lung or ileum). **Prostate-specific antigen (PSA)** is associated with prostate cancer. The most commonly used marker for pancreatic cancer is **CA 19-9**.

Rheumatology

Questions

296. A 60-year-old, mildly obese woman presents complaining of bilateral medial right knee pain that occurs with prolonged standing. The pain does not occur with sitting or climbing stairs but seems to be worse with other activities and at the end of the day. The patient does not have morning stiffness but her knees are stiff after sitting for a long time. Examination of the knees reveals no deformity, but there are small effusions. Some mild pain and crepitus are produced with palpation of the medial aspect of the knees. Which of the following is the most likely diagnosis?

a. Rheumatoid arthritis
b. Gouty arthritis
c. Chondromalacia patellae
d. Osteoarthritis
e. Psoriatic arthritis

297. A 72-year-old fair-skinned Caucasian woman with a history of hypertension presents to the emergency room complaining of left hip and groin pain. She remembers that she stumbled on a curb a few days before but did not fall. The pain has become so difficult that she has been unable to bear weight on her left leg. On physical examination her left leg is externally rotated. A hip radiograph confirms a fracture of the left femoral neck. What would you expect to find on further testing?

a. T score on bone densitometry greater than −1.0
b. T score on bone densitometry less than −2.5
c. Normal 25-hydroxyvitamin D levels
d. Low serum calcium
e. Low serum parathyroid hormone

298. A 17-month-old boy has a history of multiple fractures due to "brittle bones." The child is short in stature and has a deformed skull. Physical examination is normal except for the finding of blue scleras. Which of the following is the most likely diagnosis?

a. Osteoporosis
b. Achondroplasia
c. Osteomalacia
d. Osteitis deformans
e. Osteogenesis imperfecta

299. A 34-year-old woman has a 15-year history of Crohn disease. She presents to your office with the acute onset of left knee pain. She recalls a worsening of her gastrointestinal symptoms a few days before the joint symptoms developed. Radiographs of the knee demonstrate soft tissue swelling and small effusions but no bone destruction. Which of the following statements best describes the patient's situation?

a. Her joint inflammation will likely stay limited to her knees as arthritis associated with Crohn disease is usually monoarticular and symmetric.
b. The patient is experiencing the only extraintestinal manifestation of inflammatory bowel disease.
c. Controlling the intestinal symptoms will likely eliminate the knee arthritis.
d. The patient will go on to develop bone erosion and destruction of the knee.
e. The patient requires high-dose nonsteroidal anti-inflammatory drugs (NSAIDs).

300. A 19-year-old man was recently treated for *Chlamydia* urethritis. He now complains of persistent dysuria, watery discharge of his eyes, and swelling of his right knee. On examination he has a low-grade fever, conjunctival injection and warmth of his right knee, with a ballottable patella. Which of the following features will best distinguish this arthritis from gonococcal arthritis?

a. Lack of improvement after 72 hours of antibiotics.
b. Negative synovial fluid culture.
c. The fact that the knee is involved.
d. The fact that the patient is male.
e. The presence of dysuria.

301. A 28-year-old man presents with morning back pain, stiffness with anterior flexion at the waist, and tenderness over the sacroiliac joints. The patient denies any previous history of eye or genitourinary problems. On physical examination, there is diminished chest expansion with breathing and a diastolic rumbling murmur. Which of the following is the most likely diagnosis?

a. Rheumatoid arthritis
b. Sjögren syndrome
c. Ankylosing spondylitis
d. Systemic lupus erythematosus
e. Reiter syndrome

302. A 61-year-old woman with a 10-year history of rheumatoid arthritis presents with painful swelling at the back of the knee that is visible on physical examination only when the patient is standing with the knee extended. Which of the following is the most likely diagnosis?

a. Anserine bursitis
b. Baker cyst
c. Deep venous thrombosis
d. Prepatellar bursitis
e. Infrapatellar bursitis

303. A 28-year-old law student complains of blanching and cyanosis of her fingertips in cold weather and in times of emotional stress. She complains that her fingers become numb and painful during these episodes. She has a 6-month history of dysphagia and arthralgias. She does not smoke or take any medications. On physical examination, the skin of her hands appears to be taut and atrophic, with a flexion deformity from the tight skin. Which of the following is the most likely diagnosis?

a. Rheumatoid arthritis
b. Limited systemic sclerosis
c. Dermatomyositis
d. Pyoderma gangrenosum
e. Sarcoidosis

304. A 9-year-old boy with no past medical history presents with the acute onset of fever, arthralgias, abdominal pain, hematochezia, and hematuria, but no cough or hemoptysis. Physical examination reveals palpable purple discolorations that do not blanch on the patient's lower extremities bilaterally. Which of the following is the most likely diagnosis?

a. Cryoglobulinemia
b. Kawasaki disease
c. Wegener granulomatosis
d. Goodpasture disease
e. Henoch-Schönlein purpura

305. A 49-year-old man presents with painful, recurring episodes of swelling in his left great toe. He takes 25 mg of hydrochlorothiazide daily for blood pressure control but otherwise is in good health. On physical examination, the patient is afebrile, but his great toe is warm, swollen, erythematous, and exquisitely tender to palpation. He has several subcutaneous nodules in his pinna. Which of the following is the most likely cause of his discomfort?

a. Calcium pyrophosphate dihydrate deposition disease
b. Calcium oxalate deposition disease
c. Monosodium urate deposition disease
d. Calcium phosphate deposition disease
e. Osteoarthritis of the great toe

306. A 41-year-old music teacher presents with a 10-month history of prolonged morning stiffness accompanied by swelling of her wrists and the proximal interphalangeal joints of both hands. Now she feels that her knees are also swollen and painful. Physical examination reveals synovial tenderness and swelling of her knees, wrists, and proximal interphalangeal joints. She has subcutaneous nodules in the extensor area of her right forearm. The right knee has a positive bulge sign consistent with an effusion. Which of the following is the best test to confirm your suspected diagnosis?

a. Anti-SCL-70 antibodies
b. Anti-CCP antibodies
c. Anti-double-stranded DNA antibodies
d. Anti-Smith antibodies
e. C-reactive protein

307. A 43-year-old man presents with fever and arthritis. During the past 2 months he has been treated four times for a maxillary sinus infection. He also complains of the recent onset of hematuria. His complete blood count and differential is normal. Chest x-ray reveals nodules with no hilar lymphadenopathy. Which of the following is the most likely diagnosis?

a. Wegener granulomatosis
b. Churg-Strauss syndrome
c. Lofgren syndrome
d. Sjögren syndrome
e. Sarcoidosis

308. A 31-year-old man with no past medical history presents with fever, nausea and vomiting, and arthralgias for 10 days. He complains of inability to move his left foot due to weakness. He also states he has had hematuria for several hours. On physical examination, the patient has a temperature of 38.4°C (101.2°F) and he is hypertensive. He has diffuse abdominal tenderness on palpation but has no rebound tenderness. He has subcutaneous nodules and shallow ulcerations near his medial malleolus on his left leg. Neurologic examination reveals a left footdrop. Which of the following is the most likely diagnosis?

a. Polyarteritis nodosa
b. Behçet syndrome
c. Whipple disease
d. Osteonecrosis
e. Polymyositis

309. A 65-year-old man with end-stage renal disease on hemodialysis and a history of a right knee replacement 3 years ago presents with acute onset of right knee swelling and pain. On examination he has a low-grade fever, but is hemodynamically stable. His cardiac and lung examinations are normal. The right knee is warm to the touch, with a positive bulge sign, and his patella is ballotable. What is the next best step in management of this patient?

a. Obtain a radiograph of the right knee.
b. Obtain an MRI of the right knee.
c. Perform an arthrocentesis of the right knee effusion.
d. Begin empiric broad-spectrum antibiotic therapy.
e. Consult orthopedics for open surgical debridement.

310. A 44-year-old woman presents with diffuse myalgias and excessive fatigue. She has morning stiffness and pain of all her joints, especially her wrists, elbows, shoulders, hips, knees, and neck. She does not sleep well at night. Her symptoms have been progressing for over 4 years. On physical examination, the patient has 13 tender points at the elbows, knees, shoulders, and hips. Which of the following is the most likely diagnosis?

a. Polymyalgia rheumatica
b. Fibromyalgia syndrome
c. Rheumatoid arthritis
d. Scleroderma
e. Polymyositis

Questions 311 and 312

For each patient with joint pain, select the most likely diagnosis. Each lettered option may be used once, multiple times, or not at all.

a. Behçet syndrome
b. Drug-induced lupus
c. Systemic lupus erythematosus
d. Sjögren syndrome
e. Thromboangiitis obliterans

311. A 17-year-old woman complains of intermittent ankle pain and swelling, photosensitivity, and oral ulcers. On physical examination, she has a raised erythematous rash over her nose and cheeks, sparing her nasolabial folds.

312. A 52-year-old woman is unable to wear her contact lenses because of burning and itching of her eyes. On physical examination she has caries at the gum line. Her Schirmer test is abnormal.

Questions 313 to 315

For each patient with rheumatologic complaints, select the most likely diagnosis. Each lettered option may be used once, multiple times, or not at all.

a. Dermatomyositis
b. Polymyositis
c. Polymyalgia rheumatica
d. Felty syndrome
e. Scleroderma

313. A 75-year-old woman presents with malaise and myalgias for the last several months. She is chronically tired and has 1 hour of morning stiffness and pain in the cervical, shoulder, and hip areas. She also has developed headache and jaw pain with chewing. Neurologic examination reveals normal sensation, strength, and reflexes.

314. A 53-year-old woman presents with a 2-month history of difficulty climbing stairs and arising from the seated position. On physical examination, she has a purplish discoloration of the skin over the forehead, eyelids, and cheeks. She has tenderness on palpation of the quadriceps muscles.

315. A patient with a 15-year history of rheumatoid arthritis develops splenomegaly and neutropenia.

Rheumatology

Answers

296. The answer is d. *(McPhee, pp 729-731.)* **Osteoarthritis** is degenerative joint disease that most often affects the **weight-bearing joints** (hips, knees, ankles) in addition to the spine, hands, and any over-used joint, and is associated with obesity or other forms of mechanical stress. It has no systemic manifestations. It is more common in women, and onset is usually after the age of 50. Pain often occurs on exertion and is relieved with rest, after which the joint may become stiff (known as "**gelling**"). In the hands distal interphalangeal joints may be involved, with the production of **Heberden nodes. Bouchard nodes** are often found at the proximal interphalangeal joints. **Crepitus** (the sensation of bone rubbing against bone) is often felt on examination of the involved joint. **Rheumatoid arthritis (RA)** is a systemic disease of women under the age of 40. RA is symmetric and predominantly involves the distal joints—hands, wrists, elbows, feet, ankles, and knees—but may also manifest with nodules or inflammation in the lungs and heart. In the hands, RA **spares the distal interphalangeal joints**, only involving the proximal interphalangeal and metacarpophalangeal joints. Ninety-five percent of **gouty arthritis** occurs in men and inflammation often involves the first metatarsal phalangeal joint (great toe), where it's called **podagra.** *Chondromalacia patellae,* or **chondromalacia,** means softening of the cartilage. Patients present with anterior knee pain and tenderness over the undersurface of the patella. Pain is worse when sitting for long periods of time or when climbing stairs. **Psoriatic arthritis** is an asymmetric oligoarthritis that involves the knees, ankles, shoulders, or digits of the hands and feet and occurs in 50% of patients with psoriasis.

297. The answer is b. *(McPhee, pp 1038-1041.)* This patient who suffered a hip fracture with minimal trauma most assuredly has **osteoporosis**, loss of bone mineral density due to increased bone resorption. This condition occurs postmenopausally in women or due to factors such as genetic disorders, alcohol abuse, or medications like corticosteroids. In this patient who is fair-skinned and likely avoids the sun, the **serum 25-hydroxyvitamin D level is most likely low**. However, **serum calcium, phosphate and**

parathyroid hormone will usually be normal. Bone densitometry **(dual-energy x-ray absorptiometry, or DEXA)** is used to confirm decreased bone mineral density in patients at risk for osteoporosis or in those with pathologic fractures. In postmenopausal white women, a **T score** (comparing a patient's bone mineral density to the sex-matched norm of a young patient) of greater than or equal to 1.0 is normal and a score of less than or equal to **2.5 correlates to severe osteoporosis.**

298. The answer is e. *(Fauci, pp 2463-2465.)* **Osteogenesis imperfecta** is inherited as an autosomal dominant trait and is characterized by decreased bone mass and brittle bones that often lead to multiple fractures. Other characteristics include **blue scleras**, short stature, deformed skull, hearing loss, and dental abnormalities. **Osteoporosis** is loss of bone mineral density due to increased bone resorption and is usually seen in postmenopausal women as well as in patients who have a multitude of diseases (such as hyperthyroidism or Cushing syndrome) or who have used chronic medications, such as steroids. **Osteomalacia** (rickets in children) is a disorder of defective mineralization of the organic matrix of the skeleton. It is due to inadequate intake or metabolism of vitamin D. Patients are susceptible to fractures, weakness, disturbances in growth, and skeletal deformities, but the disorder does not affect the eyes. **Paget disease** of the bone, or **osteitis deformans**, is due to excessive resorption of bone by osteoclasts; patients present after the age of 40 with swelling or deformity of a long bone or enlargement of the skull. **Achondroplasia** results from a decrease in the proliferation of cartilage in the growth plate and causes dwarfism.

299. The answer is c. *(Fauci, pp 1893-1894.)* **Crohn disease** is one of the major types of **inflammatory bowel disease (IBD)**. While it most often presents as bowel inflammation of the terminal ileum or colon, up to one-third of patients will experience extraintestinal manifestations as well, including arthritis, iritis, and erythema nodosum. Up to 20% of patients will develop **asymmetric, polyarticular, migratory arthritis** which usually affects large joints. This joint involvement **worsens with exacerbations of bowel inflammation and is usually eliminated after controlling the gastrointestinal symptoms, without therapy directed at the arthritis itself**. Up to 10% of Crohn patients will have ankylosing spondylitis and two-thirds of these express the HLA-B27 antigen. **HLA-B27** diseases are easy to remember with the mnemonic **PAIR** (**P**soriasis, **A**nkylosing spondylitis, **I**nflammatory bowel disease, and **R**eiter syndrome). These are called the **seronegative spondyloarthropathies**. Other extraintestinal manifestations of IBD include erythema nodosum, uveitis, fatty liver, nephrolithiasis, osteopenia, reactive amyloidosis, and increased risk of thrombosis.

300. The answer is a. *(McPhee, pp 776-777.)* This patient has **reactive arthritis (Reiter syndrome)**, which usually occurs in young men within a month following a gastrointestinal or sexually transmitted infection. The mnemonic to remember the cardinal symptoms of this condition is **"can't see" (conjunctivitis), "can't pee" (urethritis), "can't climb a tree" (oligoarthritis in large weight-bearing joints)**. Reactive arthritis may also manifest with fever and weight loss, as well as mucocutaneous lesions and carditis. **The majority of symptoms will resolve within weeks, but the arthritis may persist**. Synovial fluid will be culture-negative. **Gonococcal (GC)** arthritis may mimic Reiter syndrome. It is found more commonly in woman and in men who have sex with men. Patients present with migratory polyarthralgias of the wrist, elbow, ankle, or knee and less frequently, with purulent monoarthritis and necrotic pustules over the extremities, including the palms and soles. Urethral, throat, and rectal cultures should be performed for diagnosis, as synovial fluid culture is positive in less than half of patients. **GC symptoms will markedly improve within 48 hours** of starting antibiotic treatment.

301. The answer is c. *(McPhee, pp 773-775.)* **Ankylosing spondylitis** is a chronic and progressive inflammatory disease that most commonly affects the spinal, sacroiliac, and hip joints in men beginning in their late teens and twenties. All patients have **symptomatic sacroiliitis,** causing low back pain and stiffness that is worst in the morning. Other symptoms may include **uveitis, peripheral arthritis, aortitis with aortic insufficiency and limited chest expansion** as a result of involvement of costovertebral joints. There is a strong association with **HLA-B27**—it is found in half of black patients and in 90% of white patients. A positive **Schober test** indicates diminished anterior flexion at the waist due to fusion of the spine. **Rheumatoid arthritis** is a systemic disease that presents more often in women with symmetric polyarthritis, almost always involving the hands, and morning stiffness. **Sjogren syndrome** has a female predominance and manifests as sicca symptoms (dry eyes and mouth) in association with rheumatoid arthritis and systemic lupus erythematosus (SLE) among other conditions. **SLE** occurs mostly in young women with symptoms such as malaise, joint complaints, malar rash or discoid changes, alopecia, conjunctivitis, pleurisy, and pericarditis. Patients with **Reiter syndrome** may present with a history of conjunctivitis, urethritis, arthritis, and enthesopathy (Achilles tendinitis).

302. The answer is b. *(Fauci, p 2154.)* This patient has a **Baker cyst**, which occurs in the midline of the popliteal fossa and is often a complication of rheumatoid arthritis or osteoarthritis. The cyst represents a diverticulum of the synovial sac that protrudes through the joint capsule of the knee. The knee is composed of **12** different bursae—usually, the history supports the diagnosis. **Anserine bursitis** occurs with inflammation of the bursa on the medial side of the proximal tibia. There is localized tenderness and swelling over the knee. **Prepatellar bursitis is called "housemaid's knee"** (ie, associated with scrubbing floors) and is characterized by inflammation of the bursa anterior to the patella. Inflammation of **the infrapatellar bursa** is called "**clergyman's** or **carpet-layer's knee.**" **Deep venous thrombosis (DVT)** is due to partial or complete occlusion of a vein by a thrombus and may be asymptomatic or characterized by a unilateral painful, swollen calf or thigh in the setting of immobilization or a hypercoagulable state. Occasionally there is a palpable cord or positive **Homan sign** (pain with dorsiflexion of the foot).

303. The answer is b. *(McPhee, pp 758-759.)* The patient presents with symptoms suggestive of **limited scleroderma (systemic sclerosis). Limited systemic sclerosis (LSSc)** was formerly known as the **CREST** syndrome (**C**alcinosis cutis, **R**aynaud phenomenon, **E**sophageal dysmotility, **S**clerodactyly (tight skin of the fingers), and **T**elangiectasia). **Raynaud phenomenon (blanching of fingertips when exposed to the cold) is usually the initial symptom** and may also be associated with tobacco use, medication use (beta-adrenergic blockers), or diseases such as SLE, rheumatoid arthritis, carpal tunnel syndrome, or thromboangiitis obliterans. In the limited form of scleroderma, the hardening of the skin is limited to the face and hands and patients rarely develop the kidney, cardiac, or interstitial lung disease seen in diffuse scleroderma. This disease, when diffuse, causes pulmonary fibrosis, pericarditis and heart block, fibrosis and atrophy of the

GI tract, and renal crisis. **Dermatomyositis** is a systemic disease characterized by a violaceous rash of the eyelids and periorbital areas **(heliotrope)** and flat, violaceous scaly papules over the knuckles of the PIP and MCP joints **(Gottron sign)**. **Pyoderma gangrenosum** is the rash seen in **ulcerative colitis** involving large, irregular painful ulcers that drain a purulent, hemorrhagic exudate. **Sarcoidosis** is a systemic disease with skin manifestations, bilateral hilar adenopathy, and pulmonary disease. Patients with sarcoidosis may present with **erythema nodosum,** which typically takes the form of multiple firm, red, painful plaques that are bilateral and most frequently distributed on the legs. Musculoskeletal findings in sarcoidosis include arthritis and tenosynovitis.

304. The answer is e. *(McPhee, p 771.)* The multisystem disease described in this patient is most likely **Henoch-Schönlein purpura (HSP)**, which is a small-vessel vasculitis that affects mostly children, with a **male** predominance. The purpura (nonblanching purple lesions) and all of the other symptoms described are a result of the vasculitis. Histopathology of the vasculitic lesions reveals the deposition of IgA in the walls of the small vessels (postcapillary venules). The mnemonic for HSP is **AGAR**—**A**bdominal symptoms (nausea, pain, melena), **G**lomerulonephritis, **A**rthralgia (knees and ankles most commonly), and **R**ash (palpable purpura, usually on the lower extremities). The prognosis for HSP is excellent. **Cryoglobulinemia** is associated with hepatitis B or C virus and causes necrotizing skin lesions in dependent areas, fever, arthralgias, abdominal pain, and glomerulonephritis. **Kawasaki disease (KD)**, or mucocutaneous lymph node syndrome, is idiopathic and uncommon in children over the age of 8 years. It is characterized by fever, a desquamating, edematous, blotchy-appearing, mucocutaneous erythema, cervical lymphadenitis, and aneurysms of the coronary arteries. **Wegener disease** and **Goodpasture syndrome** usually have glomerulonephritis and pulmonary involvement.

305. The answer is c. *(McPhee, pp 732-735.)* Tophaceous **gout** is characterized by the finding in synovial fluid of **monosodium urate crystals** that are needle-shaped and strongly negatively birefringent (bright yellow when parallel to the axis). Gouty attacks may be precipitated by trauma, medications that inhibit tubular secretion of uric acid (aspirin, hydrochlorothiazide), surgery, stress, alcohol, or a high-protein diet. The **metatarsalphalangeal (MTP) joint of the great toe is most often affected ("podagra")**, and after years of attacks, patients may have an accumulation of tophi in and around the olecranon, prepatellar bursae, and earlobes. In chronic gout, radiographs may show "**rat bite**" erosions. **Pseudogout** is due to **calcium pyrophosphate dihydrate (CPPD)** deposition disease; the crystals here are rhomboid-shaped and weakly positive birefringent (blue when parallel to the axis). **Calcium oxalate** deposition disease is usually seen in patients with end-stage renal disease; **calcium phosphate** deposition disease causes **calcific tendonitis** or **Milwaukee shoulder**.

306. The answer is b. *(McPhee, pp 747-751.)* The patient most likely has **rheumatoid arthritis,** a chronic systemic inflammatory disease, since she meets four of the seven criteria as classified by the American College of Rheumatology:

1. Symmetric polyarthritis for over 3 months (almost always involves the hands)
2. Morning stiffness lasting more than 1 hour
3. Rheumatoid nodules (found in 20% of patients over bony prominences)
4. Arthritis of more than three joint areas (spares the DIP joints)
5. Involvement of the joints of the hands and wrists; patients may have **swan-neck deformity** (hyperextension of the proximal interphalangeal joints with compensatory flexion of the distal joint), **boutonnière deformity** (extension of the distal interphalangeal joint), or **ulnar deviation** of the digits
6. A positive rheumatoid factor (RF)
7. Erosions or decalcification on radiographs (seen after 6 months of symptoms)

Anti-CCP antibodies are the most specific blood test for rheumatoid arthritis. **Rheumatoid factor** is present in up to 80% of patients with established symptoms, but may also occur in other autoimmune diseases, hepatitis C, syphilis, and tuberculosis. The **ESR and C-reactive protein (CRP)** are elevated proportional to disease activity but are very nonspecific and are elevated in almost any inflammatory state. **Antibodies to double-stranded DNA and anti-Smith antibodies** are specific for systemic lupus erythematosus. The **anti-SCL-70** antibody is found in one-third of patients with scleroderma.

307. The answer is a. *(McPhee, pp 768-769.)* **Wegener granulomatosis is a potentially fatal systemic vasculitis** that involves the upper airways (manifesting as **sinusitis, otitis media, or upper respiratory tract symptoms) with necrotizing granulomas of the lungs, glomerulonephritis in three-quarters of patients and a migratory oligoarthritis.** The diagnosis is made by the clinical picture coupled with a positive antineutrophil cytoplasmic antibody with a cytoplasmic staining pattern **(C-ANCA)**, which has a high specificity for this disease. Confirmation of diagnosis is made by tissue biopsy showing necrotizing granulomas. The typical history for **Churg-Strauss syndrome** (allergic angiitis and granulomatosis) is asthma followed by systemic vasculitis with peripheral eosinophilia (mnemonic is **RAVE: R**hinitis, **A**sthma, **V**asculitis, and **E**osinophilia). **Lofgren syndrome** is a benign form of sarcoidosis that causes bilateral hilar adenopathy, periarthritis of the ankles, and erythema nodosum of the anterior tibial regions of the lower extremities. **Sjögren syndrome** is a slowly progressive autoimmune disease that primarily affects middle-aged women; it affects the lacrimal and salivary glands, resulting in xerostomia and dry eyes. It may occur alone (primary) or in association with other autoimmune diseases such as rheumatoid arthritis or SLE. **Sarcoidosis** is a systemic disease involving noncaseating granulomas in the lung, hilar or diffuse lymphadenopathy, and often other findings such as erythema nodosum or parotid gland enlargement.

308. The answer is a. *(McPhee, pp 764-766.)* The most probable diagnosis is **polyarteritis nodosa (PAN)**, a life-threatening vasculitis of the medium-sized vessels. PAN often presents insidiously with systemic symptoms like malaise, fever, and abdominal pain coupled with vasculitic neuropathy, known as **mononeuritis multiplex, manifesting itself as wristdrop or footdrop**. Skin findings of PAN include **subcutaneous nodules and ulcers** occurring in the lower extremity **near the malleoli. Hepatitis B** has been shown to be present in 50% of patients with PAN. **Behçet syndrome** presents as recurrent painful aphthous ulcers of the mouth and genitals with erythema nodosum-like lesions and uveitis. **Whipple disease** causes a synovitis of the hands, feet, and knees. Often, the patient exhibits fever, lymphadenopathy, and signs of malabsorption, such as diarrhea. Whipple disease is caused by the infectious agent *Tropheryma whippelii*. **Osteonecrosis** is usually found in the hips or knees of patients with conditions such as sickle cell disease or long-term steroid use, but does not have systemic symptoms. **Polymyositis** presents as gradual muscle weakness involving proximal muscle groups of the extremities and the neck and occasionally causes dysphagia.

309. The answer is c. (*McPhee, pp 777-778.*) This patient has **septic (bacterial) arthritis** of his knee, typically presenting as acute inflammation of a large weight-bearing joint, usually the knee. Patients at risk for this problem are usually immunocompromised, have damaged or prosthetic joints, or have a source of bacteremia. This patient's knee replacement, combined with his end-stage renal disease and likely infected dialysis catheter site make this the leading diagnosis, and he should be hospitalized. A **radiograph or MRI of the right knee** will not diagnose the etiology of the effusion present—**it is imperative to tap potentially septic joint effusions**. They often are large, with white blood counts more than 50,000/μL, 90% of which are usually PMNs. While Gram stain of the synovial fluid may be negative in a minority of cases, bacterial culture is positive in up to 90% of patients. The most common etiologic agent is *Staphylococcus aureus*, though methicillin-resistant *S. aureus* (MRSA) and gram-negative bacteria may cause septic arthritis as well. **Antibiotic therapy** is given for 6 weeks and should be tailored to the culture results. Orthopedics should be consulted for arthroscopic lavage and debridement with drain placement, with **open surgical debridement** if standard management fails.

310. The answer is b. (*McPhee, pp 741-742.*) The history of chronic pain and fatigue with a physical examination revealing tender points make **fibromyalgia** syndrome the most likely diagnosis. This is a disorder predominantly of females between the ages of 20 and 50; patients complain of insomnia, easy fatigability, and widespread musculoskeletal pain and stiffness. Fibromyalgia is a diagnosis of exclusion: there are up to **18** symmetrical bilateral tender points, without objective evidence of inflammation, occurring in the same locations on all patients. Laboratory data are normal in primary fibromyalgia syndrome. Effective treatment involves exercise programs and improving sleep. **Polymyalgia rheumatica** causes pain and stiffness in the shoulder and hip girdles in patients over 50 and may be accompanied by temporal arteritis. **Rheumatoid arthritis** is a systemic inflammatory disease that affects symmetrical joints and causes morning stiffness, along with possible pericarditis or pleuritis. **Scleroderma** causes thickening of the skin often with Raynaud phenomenon, esophageal dysmotility, and pulmonary fibrosis. **Polymyositis** causes progressive muscle weakness of the proximal muscle groups.

311 and 312. The answers are 311-c, 312-d. *(McPhee, pp 752-755, 762-763.)* The 17-year-old woman has 4 of the 11 criteria (see following discussion) for **systemic lupus erythematosus**. Drugs may also cause lupus, such as dilantin, procainamide, quinidine, hydralazine, and isoniazid. Patients with **drug-induced lupus** are usually older, have fever, malaise, arthritis, serositis, and rash, but renal involvement is rare. **Sjögren syndrome** almost exclusively affects women and the most common symptoms are **keratoconjunctivitis sicca** (dry eyes) and **xerostomia** (dry mouth), which may cause dental caries, especially at the gum line. The **Schirmer test** can be used to measure the quantity of tears secreted. **Behçet syndrome** is a multisystem disorder that involves the eye and causes painful oral and genital ulcerations. The nondeforming arthritis of BehÁet syndrome affects the knees and ankles. **Thromboangiitis obliterans,** or **Buerger disease,** is an inflammatory peripheral vascular disease of the upper and lower extremities that usually affects men under the age of 40 who smoke. Patients may complain of extremity claudication or Raynaud phenomenon. The treatment of Buerger disease is to quit smoking cigarettes.

The American College of Rheumatology criteria for SLE (need 4 of the 11: **BRAIN SOAP M.D.**) are the following:

Blood or hematologic (hemolytic anemia, thrombocytopenia, or lymphopenia)
Renal (proteinuria or cellular casts)
ANA (abnormal antinuclear antibody titer)
Immunologic (anti-dsDNA Ab or anti-Smith Ab and/or antiphospholipid Ab)
Neurologic (seizures or psychosis)
Serositis (pericarditis, pleuritis)
Oral ulcers
Arthritis that is nonerosive and involves more than two joints
Photosensitivity
Malar rash
Discoid rash

313 to 315. The answers are 313-c, 314-a, 315-d. *(McPhee, pp 748, 759-761, 766-767.)* **Polymyalgia rheumatica** affects older patients. They present with weight loss, profound fatigue, and pain and stiffness of the neck, shoulders, thighs, and hips, preventing them from rising from a chair or brushing their hair. Patients have no objective weakness on physical examination. **Temporal (giant cell) arteritis** may be seen in one-third of patients with polymyalgia rheumatica and must always be ruled out as it may lead to blindness. Classic presenting symptoms include headache, jaw claudication, and diplopia or amaurosis fugax. **Dermatomyositis** is an autoimmune disease that causes proximal muscle weakness along with a violaceous **(heliotrope)** rash over the eyelids, erythema of the face, neck, shoulders, upper chest, and back **("shawl sign")** and scaly patches over the MCP and PIP joints **(Gottron papules)**; **polymyositis** spares the skin. Patients with severe rheumatoid arthritis who develop splenomegaly and neutropenia are said to have **Felty syndrome**. **Scleroderma** involves tightening of the skin of the face and extremities, often accompanied by more severe sequelae such as interstitial lung disease.

Musculoskeletal System

Questions

316. A 52-year-old nurse has a history of low back pain for 2 months. She states that the pain started after she lifted a heavy patient at work. It is a nagging pain that worsens with bed rest. She has tried nonsteroidal anti-inflammatory agents (NSAIDs) without any relief and has continued to work. She has a past medical history significant for breast cancer 8 years ago and, except for a recent 10-lb weight loss, has been well since her lumpectomy. She has tenderness over the lumbar vertebral bodies but her neurologic examination and straight-leg raising test are normal. The rest of her physical examination is unremarkable. Which of the following is the most likely diagnosis?

a. Lumbosacral strain
b. Metastatic breast cancer
c. Disk herniation of L5-S1
d. Spondylolysis
e. Spondylolisthesis

317. A 33-year-old graduate student complains of low back pain after carrying heavy suitcases on a recent vacation in Europe. Because of his pain, he went to a neurologist in London who recommended bed rest and NSAIDs. After 10 days, the back pain resolved, but the patient comes to see you because of new weakness of his right anterior tibialis. The rest of the physical examination is normal. Which of the following is the most likely diagnosis?

a. Nerve root impingement
b. Tibial stress fracture
c. Anterior compartment syndrome
d. Gastrocnemius muscle tear
e. Baker cyst

318. A 45-year-old swimmer presents with a sore right shoulder for nearly 2 months. He was taking NSAIDs throughout this period with minimal relief. Over the last several days, he has developed pain with elevation of his arm above the horizontal. On examination he has some stiffness of passive motion in external rotation and with abduction and a negative drop arm sign. The pain is relieved after you inject 2 mL of lidocaine into the subacromial space. Which of the following is the most likely diagnosis?

a. Fracture of the surgical neck of the humerus
b. Bicipital tendinitis due to snapping
c. Cervical radiculopathy due to a herniated disk
d. Complete rotator cuff tear
e. Frozen shoulder due to a partial rotator cuff injury

319. A 12-year-old boy presents with a 3-week history of pain of his anterior tibia, just below his patella. He plays baseball and soccer, but does not recall any history of trauma. On physical examination, he has swelling and tenderness to palpation over the tibial tubercle. Which of the following is the most likely diagnosis?

a. Osgood-Schlatter disease
b. Legg-Calvé-Perthes disease
c. Muscular dystrophy
d. Rickets
e. Juvenile rheumatoid arthritis

320. A 20-year-old college student develops left shoulder pain after jumping into a lake from a swinging rope. She presents to the emergency department holding her arm adducted beside her body and avoiding any shoulder movement. On examination, the rounded contour of the shoulder is lost and the head of the humerus is felt under the coracoid process. Which of the following is the most likely diagnosis?

a. Inferior glenohumeral dislocation
b. Rupture of the long head of the biceps
c. Posterior glenohumeral dislocation
d. Anterior glenohumeral dislocation
e. Subacromial bursitis

321. A 47-year-old man fell on his outstretched right hand while rollerblading. Several days later, he develops right wrist pain below his thumb that is constant and progressive. Pain is primarily in the area of the anatomical snuffbox and is worse with wrist flexion, extension, and ulnar deviation. On examination, the anatomical snuffbox is tender to palpation with mild swelling. The Finkelstein test is negative. Which of the following is the most likely diagnosis?

a. Cervical radiculopathy
b. Scaphoid fracture
c. Compartment syndrome
d. de Quervain disease
e. Boxer's fracture

322. A 31-year-old man has left ankle pain after stepping off a curb yesterday. He treated the injury with ice overnight, but today he cannot walk due to the pain. On examination of the ankle in the emergency department, you notice that it is swollen and ecchymotic. There is tenderness to palpation in the anterior aspect of the ankle and over the lateral malleolus. Passive inversion of the ankle is painful. The patient is unable to bear weight on his left foot. Which of the following is the next best step in management?

a. X-ray series of the ankle
b. MRI of the ankle
c. CT scan of the ankle
d. Treatment with oral anti-inflammatory agents
e. Application of a compression dressing

323. A 61-year-old woman has recurrent back pain in her lumbar area that radiates to her right buttock and laterally down her leg to her knee. Both sitting and walking aggravate the pain. She does not report bladder or bowel dysfunction. On physical examination, the patient has normal sensation and reflexes of the right lower limb. Straight-leg raising and cross-leg raising tests are positive for reproduction of right lower limb symptoms. The patient has no spinal deformities. Which of the following is the most likely diagnosis?

a. Sciatica
b. Osteomyelitis
c. Cauda equina syndrome
d. Kyphosis
e. Epidural abscess

324. A 12-year-old boy is brought to your office 2 days after a fracture of the humerus in its distal third. The patient complains that he is unable to extend the wrist. On examination he has a wristdrop but his distal pulses in his arm are intact. Which of the following structures was most likely damaged?

a. Median nerve
b. Ulnar nerve
c. Radial nerve
d. Axillary nerve
e. Artery supplying the brachial plexus

325. A 70-year-old man complains of aching lower back pain that radiates to his buttocks and upper thighs over the past few months. He does not recall any trauma and has no past medical history except for allergic rhinitis. He notes that the pain worsens with walking, especially downhill, and gets better with sitting or leaning forward. On physical examination, bilateral straight-leg raise test is negative and his deep tendon reflexes are normal in his lower extremities. He has slight proximal thigh weakness with flexion at the hip but his upper extremity strength is 5/5 in all muscle groups bilaterally. His dorsalis pedis and posterior tibial pulses are 2+ in both legs. What is the most likely diagnosis?

a. Sciatica
b. Lumbar disk herniation
c. Claudication
d. Polymyalgia rheumatica
e. Lumbar spinal stenosis

326. An 18-year-old gymnast heard a popping sound in her left knee while practicing for the Olympic Games. Her knee immediately became swollen and painful. On physical examination, it is obvious that the left knee has an effusion. Which of the following tests is best to confirm an anterior cruciate ligament tear?

a. Lachman test
b. McMurray test
c. Apley grind test
d. Posterior drawer test
e. Ballottement

327. A 15-year-old adolescent presents with complaints of pain in the left distal thigh, close to his knee. The pain has been present for approximately 3 weeks and is increasing in severity and he has recently noticed swelling in the area as well. There is no history of trauma or previous hip or leg problems. A plain film of the area reveals a moth-eaten appearance of the distal femur with a spiculated periosteal reaction. Which of the following is the most likely diagnosis?

a. Osteoid osteoma
b. Paget disease
c. Osteosarcoma
d. Chondrosarcoma
e. Muscle strain

328. A 17-year-old football player with his foot planted is tackled from the side, causing a forced valgus bending of the knee. On physical examination, there is tenderness over the medial femoral condyle. McMurray test is negative for any palpable clicks but there is valgus laxity with the knee fully extended. Which of the following is the most likely diagnosis?

a. Tear of the lateral meniscus
b. Rupture of the lateral collateral ligament
c. Rupture of the medial collateral ligament
d. Dislocation of the patella
e. Subluxation of the patella

329. A 30-year-old woman, who works as a court reporter, presents with a 3-week history of hand tingling and numbness that often awakens her from sleep. The symptoms resolve after she shakes her hands for a few minutes. On physical examination, there is no sensory or motor deficit of her hands but there is reproducibility of the tingling when tapping on the volar side of her wrist. Which of the following is the most likely diagnosis?

a. Thoracic outlet syndrome
b. Carpal tunnel syndrome
c. Dupuytren contracture
d. Trigger finger
e. Ganglion cyst

330. A 41-year-old construction worker complains of the sudden onset of severe back pain after lifting some heavy equipment. He describes the pain as being in his right lower back and radiating down the posterior aspect of his right buttock to above the knee area. He has no bladder or bowel dysfunction. The pain has improved with bed rest. On physical examination, the patient has tenderness in his lumbar paraspinous area with palpation. The straight-leg maneuver with the right leg increases the back pain at 80°. The straight-leg maneuver with the left leg causes posterior thigh pain. Sensation, strength, and reflexes are normal. Which of the following is the most likely diagnosis?

a. Nerve root compression
b. Paravertebral abscess
c. Lumbosacral strain
d. Osteoporosis compression fracture
e. Paget disease

331. A 73-year-old man presents complaining of right lateral hip pain that worsens when he lies on his right side or when he is standing. He has no other complaints. On physical examination, there is tenderness with palpation of the lateral aspect of the hip, but range-of-motion testing of the hip is normal. Which of the following is the most likely diagnosis?

a. Ischial bursitis
b. Osteoarthritis of the hip
c. Avascular necrosis of the hip
d. Trochanteric bursitis
e. Fracture of the proximal femur

332. A 13-year-old adolescent presents with left knee pain. He does not play sports and does not recall any trauma. On physical examination, he is obese, but taller than normal for his age. When he walks to the examination table, you note an antalgic gait. Upon examination, his hip strength is 4/5 and he has reduced ability to actively rotate the hip internally. Which of the following is the most likely diagnosis?

a. Sprengel deformity
b. Juvenile rheumatoid arthritis
c. Slipped capital femoral epiphysis
d. Arnold-Chiari malformation
e. Cerebral palsy

333. A 34-year-old female attorney presents to your office complaining of right heel pain. As the weather has recently improved, she has been running her usual daily 5 miles outside on the pavement and recently she has been involved in a trial which requires her to stand in court a lot during the day. She states that her pain is worst when she steps out of bed barefoot in the morning and after she has been sitting at her desk for a long time, though it seems to be better as she continues to walk around in heels during the day. She has no systemic symptoms or other joint involvement. On examination, she has tenderness upon palpation of the inferior heel near the medial tuberosity of the calcaneus. What is the most appropriate next step in management?

a. Application of ice and stretching exercises
b. Plain radiograph of the right heel
c. Bone scan
d. Ultrasonography of the right heel
e. MRI of the right heel

334. A 42-year-old man presents with a crush injury to his left lower extremity. He complains of severe leg pain that seems out of proportion to his injury. He also complains of paresthesias of the injured extremity. Leg examination is significant for pallor and coldness. The dorsalis pedis and posterior tibialis pulses are not palpable. Which of the following is the most likely diagnosis?

a. Arterial insufficiency
b. Pelvic fracture
c. Aortic insufficiency
d. Aortic dissection
e. Compartment syndrome

335. A 20-year-old woman presents complaining of proximal forearm pain exacerbated by extension of the wrist against resistance with the elbow extended. She denies trauma but is an avid racquetball player. Which of the following is the most likely diagnosis?

a. Lateral epicondylar tendinitis
b. Medial epicondylar tendinitis
c. Olecranon bursitis
d. Biceps tendinitis
e. Long thoracic nerve early paralysis

336. A 41-year-old man was recently in a motor vehicle accident in which he was the driver. He states that he was wearing his seat belt at the time of the accident. A day after the accident, he developed neck pain that has now continued for 10 days. He notices crunching on extension and lateral bending of the neck. Physical examination reveals no neurologic deficits. His neck has no areas of tenderness and there are no areas of spasm. He has normal lateral bend, extension, and flexion of the neck. Which of the following is the most likely diagnosis?

a. Ankylosing spondylitis
b. Osteoarthritis
c. Reiter syndrome
d. Cervical strain
e. Polymyalgia rheumatica

Questions 337 to 339

For each patient with a foot problem, select the most likely diagnosis. Each lettered option may be used once, multiple times, or not at all.

a. Hammertoe
b. March fracture
c. Genu valgum
d. Genu varum
e. Bunion
f. Genu recurvatum
g. Gout
h. Genu impressum
i. Pes planus
j. Morton neuroma

337. A patient with hallux valgus develops lateral displacement of the extensor and flexor hallucis longus tendons.

338. A long-distance runner develops foot pain with exercise.

339. A patient develops painful swelling of the first metatarsophalangeal joint.

Questions 340 and 341

For each patient with a joint complaint, select the most likely diagnosis. Each lettered option may be used once, multiple times, or not at all.

a. Complex regional pain syndrome
b. Ankylosing spondylitis
c. Reiter syndrome
d. Hypertrophic osteoarthropathy
e. Charcot joint

340. A 67-year-old man with lung cancer presents with metacarpophalangeal joint pain. On physical examination, there is pain on moving his fingers and a spongy sensation when palpating the proximal aspects of the fingernails.

341. A 58-year-old woman with a long-standing history of diabetes, complicated by neuropathy, retinopathy, and nephropathy comes for an initial visit. On physical examination of her feet, sensation is absent, and on the right one she has an enlarged, boggy, painless mid-foot.

Questions 342 and 343

For each patient described, select the most likely root that is affected. Each lettered option may be used once, multiple times, or not at all.

a. S1 nerve root
b. L5 nerve root
c. L4 nerve root
d. L2 nerve root
e. L3 nerve root

342. A 37-year-old man presents complaining of difficulty walking. On physical examination, he is unable to walk on his heels.

343. A 71-year-old woman has difficulty squatting or rising out of a chair.

Questions 344 and 345

For each possible diagnosis choose the most appropriate maneuver, sign, or test. Each lettered option may be used once, multiple times, or not at all.

a. McMurray test
b. Bulge sign
c. Apley grind test
d. Phalen test
e. Hawkins test

344. Carpal tunnel syndrome

345. Rotator cuff tear

Musculoskeletal System

Answers

316. The answer is b. *(Fauci, pp 107-115.)* **Low back pain** is a very common complaint. The differential diagnosis includes soft tissue problems (muscles and ligaments), disk problems (prolapse), facet problems (degenerative joint disease), spinal canal disease (spinal stenosis), and vertebral body diseases (osteoporosis causing a compression fracture, infection, metastatic disease, spondylolisthesis). Although radiologic studies are needed in this patient to make a definitive diagnosis, the leading diagnosis with her history of breast cancer and weight loss is **metastatic disease** to the vertebral bodies in the lumbosacral area, with possible pathologic fracture. **Pain that is constant and made worse by lying down or at night** may be a red flag of malignancy or infection. Patients with **disk herniation** at L5-S1 may present with S1 nerve root compression (the herniated disk affects the nerve root below the lesion), causing pain radiating down the buttock to below the knee. The patient is unable to stand on his or her toes and has an absent Achilles reflex (S1). In **disk herniation at L4, L5, and S1 levels,** the **straight-leg raising test** causes pain below the knee in a dermatomal pattern when the leg is raised with the knee straight with the patient in a supine position. **Spondylolysis** is a defect of a lumbar vertebra (lack of ossification of the articular processes) and rarely causes symptoms. **Spondylolisthesis** occurs when the vertebra slips forward from its position and is generally a consequence of spondylolysis or degenerative joint disease (DJD) without spondylolysis. It, too, is usually asymptomatic, but may also cause low back pain and nerve root injury. A **back strain** is an injury to a ligament or muscle; it may mimic disk disease, or cause tenderness over the paraspinous muscles, but the neurologic examination and straight-leg raising test generally remain normal and the pain is relieved by rest.

317. The answer is a. *(Fauci, pp 110-111.)* **Lumbar disk herniation** may occur rapidly after lifting heavy objects awkwardly or with poor technique but usually resolves with a short period of rest ("unloading the spine") and NSAIDs. If a patient develops **radicular pain** (radiating down the leg below the knee) or **significant neurologic deficit** after the initial pain has resolved, the diagnosis is most likely nerve impingement due to a herniation of the disk. Intervertebral disk surgery is indicated for progressive motor weakness from nerve root injury, signs of spinal cord compression like bowel or bladder dysfunction and severe nerve root pain despite conservative treatment. **Tibial stress fractures (shin splints)** may occur due to weight-bearing exercises or training errors. These injuries cause anterior tibial pain after exercise, but not weakness. **Anterior compartment syndrome** occurring after weight-bearing exercise may cause a neuropraxia of the peroneal nerve, leading to foot-drop. A **gastrocnemius muscle tear** usually occurs suddenly after rapid dorsiflexion of the ankle and causes severe midcalf pain. In a few days, the calf characteristically develops a bluish discoloration. A popliteal cyst (**Baker cyst**) causes calf pain, swelling, and knee effusion. It is often a complication of osteoarthritis or rheumatoid arthritis and represents a diverticulum of the synovial sac that protrudes through the posterior joint capsule of the knee.

318. The answer is e. *(McPhee, p 744.)* **Passive range of motion (ROM) tests** are performed by the examiner if **active ROM tests** are unable to be performed by the patient. The loss of passive range of motion indicates a stiffening shoulder **(frozen shoulder or adhesive capsulitis)**. The most likely etiology in this patient would be **impingement of the rotator cuff**, causing inflammation, degeneration, and possibly a partial tear. The **rotator cuff**, which is formed by the **SITS** tendons of the Supraspinatus, Infraspinatus, Teres minor, and Subscapularis muscles, stabilizes the glenohumeral joint and prevents upward movement of the head of the humerus. Injuries may occur from overhead activities including freestyle and butterfly-style swimming. In a **complete rotator cuff** tear, the **drop arm sign** may be **positive** (abduct the arm to 180° and ask the patient to bring it down slowly—at 90° the arm will drop quickly due to weakness). An injection of lidocaine often relieves the inflammation in the subacromial space in patients with rotator cuff tendinitis and alleviates the symptoms. **Fracture of the surgical head of the humerus** is usually seen in the elderly after a fall. Swelling, deformity, and ecchymosis are visible. **Cervical radiculopathy** typically results in decreased sensation, strength, and reflexes all matching one root level of the upper extremity. **Bicipital tendonitis** may be seen with overuse and trauma, but pain is typically felt over the anterior aspect of the shoulder, and palpation of the biceps tendon in the bicipital groove elicits tenderness. Pain produced on supination of the forearm against resistance **(Yergason sign)** confirms bicipital tendinitis. Lidocaine injection into the synovial sheath of the long head of the biceps relieves pain.

319. The answer is a. *(Kliegman, pp 2798-2799.)* **Osgood-Schlatter disease** is more common in males, occurs in adolescence, and is usually self-limited. It is due to patellar tendon stress, which causes **pain, and often swelling, in the region of the tibial tuberosity**. The tubercle is painful on palpation and when the patient extends the knee against resistance. Therapy involves restriction of activities and an exercise program aimed at increasing flexibility, though the disorder will resolve on its own within 2 years. **Legg-Calvé-Perthes disease** (osteochondrosis) is an uncommon disorder that affects boys more than girls between the ages of 2 and 12. The hallmark is temporary loss of blood supply to the proximal femoral epiphysis leading to avascular necrosis. Consequently, children with Legg-Calvé-Perthes disease are of short stature and present with a limp that may become painful with activity. **Rickets** is attributed to **vitamin D deficiency** and is manifested by bowing of the long bones, enlargement of the epiphyses of the long bones, delayed closure of the fontanels, and enlargement of the costochondral junctions of the ribs (rachitic rosary). **Juvenile rheumatoid arthritis** is an inflammatory disorder that begins in childhood and may produce extra-articular symptoms, including iridocyclitis, fever, rash, anemia, and pericarditis. **Muscular dystrophy** is characterized by progressive weakness and muscle atrophy.

320. The answer is d. *(Kliegman, p 2854.)* **Glenohumeral dislocations** may be anterior, posterior, or inferior, depending on the position of the head of the humerus in relation to the glenoid. By far, the **most common dislocation is anterior** and is due to forceful external rotation or extension when the arm is abducted to 90°. There is typically flattening of the deltoid inferior to the acromion process and palpable anterior displacement of the head of the humerus, causing a **squared-off appearance** of the shoulder. The patient is usually in severe pain and holds the arm in slight abduction and external rotation; when asked, he cannot touch the opposite shoulder with his involved arm. **Posterior dislocations** are typically seen following a seizure or fall on an outstretched arm, and the patient holds the arm in adduction and internal rotation. **Inferior dislocations** are very rare and are caused by force applied to an arm raised overhead. In this case, the arm is fully abducted with the elbow behind the head and the humeral head palpable on the lateral chest wall. Possible complications of shoulder dislocation include damage to the axillary artery, axillary nerve (deltoid paralysis), and brachial plexus, with inferior dislocations almost always associated with a fracture. First-time dislocation requires short-term immobilization and therapeutic exercise, with surgical repair reserved for repeated dislocation or for athletes in high-collision sports as 80% of patients will have a recurrence. **Rupture of the long head of the biceps** causes a bulge in the lower half of the arm and pain on elbow flexion. Patients with **subacromial bursitis** report pain with adduction and internal rotation of the shoulder, and on examination, direct pressure over the subacromial bursa just under the acromion process causes pain.

321. The answer is b. *(Seidel, p 751.)* **Scaphoid fractures** occur as a result of a fall on an outstretched hand and manifest as **pain and swelling at the base of the thumb**. These fractures heal poorly and may lead to avascular necrosis due to a poor blood supply in this area. Radiographs done early may be negative, but later radiographs may show evidence of healing (callus fracture). A **boxer's fracture** causes flattening or loss of the fifth knuckle prominence due to displacement of the metacarpal toward the palm. It is usually the result of striking an object with a clenched fist. **Cervical (C6-C8) radiculopathy** causes pain, numbness, and tingling from the neck to the hand. **de Quervain tenosynovitis**, or inflammation of the tendon sheath of the extensor pollicis brevis and abductor pollicis longus, causes swelling and tenderness of the anatomic snuffbox. This disorder is usually found in middle-aged women who perform repetitive activity. The **Finkelstein test** is positive (patient makes a fist around his or her own thumb; pain is produced with adduction toward the ulnar side) in de Quervain disease. **Compartment syndrome** is a surgical emergency and is due to a tight cast or swelling, causing compression of the blood vessels and nerves in the forearm.

322. The answer is a. *(McPhee, pp 746-747.)* Ligament injuries of the ankle are common and occur when the foot twists as it lands on the ground. The **lateral ligament** is most commonly injured, often with inversion, and the **medial ligament** is typically injured with eversion. The lateral ligament is composed of three parts: the **anterior talofibular ligament** (the one most often injured), the calcaneofibular ligament, and the posterior talofibular ligament. The injured ligament is usually tender to palpation, ecchymotic, and swollen. The **Ottawa ankle rules** have almost a 100% sensitivity and 50% specificity in helping to identify patients in whom an x-ray would likely reveal a fracture: those with bone tenderness along the tip of the lateral or medial malleolus or along the posterior edge of the tibia or fibula and those unable to bear weight for at least four steps immediately following the injury or in the emergency department. As this patient meets these criteria, an x-ray series should be obtained before management with anti-inflammatory agents and "**RICE**"—**R**est, **I**ce, **C**ompression, and **E**levation.

323. The answer is a. *(McPhee, p 738.)* The most common cause of **sciatica** is a herniated disk, usually occurring at the L4-L5 or L5-S1 levels, but it may also occur from causes as seemingly benign as compression from a wallet. The sciatic nerve is located between the ischial tuberosity and the greater trochanter, and inflammation of this nerve causes pain radiating down the buttock and leg to below the knee. On examination, the **straight-leg raising test is usually positive** in sciatic nerve irritation (reproduction of the radicular pain is produced with elevation of less than 60° and worsened with dorsiflexion of foot or **Lasègue sign**). A pulling or tight sensation in the hamstring is not a positive straight-leg raising test. In patients who may be malingering, it may be helpful to perform the straight-leg raise with the patient sitting up, elevating the lower leg to 180° at the knee, while dorsiflexing the foot. The **cross-leg raising test** (elevation of the unaffected leg causes pain in the affected leg) may also be positive. **Osteomyelitis** and **epidural abscesses** are usually accompanied by systemic symptoms (ie, fever) and are found in patients who are immunocompromised. The typical presentation for **cauda equina syndrome** is progressive weakness and numbness of the lower extremities bilaterally with urinary retention. There is also perineal and perianal sensory loss **(saddle anesthesia)** and a lax anal sphincter causing bowel incontinence. The cauda equina syndrome is a true surgical emergency. **Kyphosis** (hunchback) is a smooth and rounded backward convexity of the thoracic region that occurs with aging.

324. The answer is c. *(McPhee, p 927.)* The **radial nerve** lies next to the shaft of the humerus in the spiral groove. It may be injured as a result of humeral fractures, especially those involving the distal third of the humerus, or as a result of deep sleep during intoxication (**"Saturday night**

palsy"). The **radial nerve (C6-C8)** supplies the extensor muscles of the wrist; damage to it results in **wristdrop**, a condition in which the patient is unable to extend the wrist. **Clawhand** is due to paralyzed interosseous and lumbrical muscles from an **ulnar nerve (C8-T1) injury**. The **median nerve (C6-T1)** supplies most of the flexors in the forearm (motor branches) and supplies sensory branches to the radial part of the hand; an injury will cause **carpal tunnel syndrome** and thenar atrophy. The **axillary nerve** carries fibers from **C5-C6** and may be injured in anterior shoulder dislocations, causing paralysis of the deltoid, teres minor or the long head of the triceps. Lack of arterial supply to the **brachial plexus** can cause unilateral weakness and burning in an upper extremity.

325. The answer is e. *(McPhee, pp 740-741.)* **Lumbar spinal stenosis** usually occurs in people over age 60 and results from spinal osteophytes, hypertrophy of the ligamentum flavum, or bulging of intervertebral disks. Patients usually complain of gradual onset of aching and numbness starting in the lower back and radiating into the thigh and sometimes as far as below the knee. The pain is often bilateral, exacerbated by prolonged standing or walking **(pseudoclaudication)**, and relieved by lumbar flexion or sitting (the **stoop sign**). On physical examination over half of patients will have slight proximal muscle weakness, but few will have a positive straight-leg raise test or diminished deep tendon reflexes. The diagnosis of spinal stenosis is best confirmed with a spinal MRI. Normal distal pulses rule out **claudication** and lack of shoulder and neck weakness distinguishes this presentation from **polymyalgia rheumatica**. **Lumbar disk herniation** and **sciatica** cause neuropathic pain radiating from the buttocks down the leg to below the knee. On examination, the straight-leg raise will be positive and patients will occasionally manifest a lower extremity motor deficit.

326. The answer is a. *(Seidel, pp 732-733.)* The anterior and posterior cruciate ligaments are intra-articular ligaments and contribute to the stability of the knee. The most likely diagnosis in this gymnast is tear of the **anterior cruciate ligament (ACL)**. Both the **Lachman test** (the patient is placed in the supine position with the knee flexed at 15° while the examiner stabilizes the distal thigh with one hand and grasps the patient's leg distal to the tibiofemoral joint with the other hand; the test is positive if the examiner is able to move the tibia anteriorly) and the **anterior drawer test**

(the foot is immobilized while the hip and knee are flexed to 90°, then the tibia is moved anterior relative to the femur; a positive test occurs with forward displacement of the tibia of more than 0.5 cm) are positive in this kind of injury. **The Lachman test is more sensitive than the drawer test.** Aspirated joint fluid is usually bloody in ACL injuries. An MRI is helpful in diagnosing this injury. A **posterior cruciate ligament (PCL)** tear would have a positive **posterior drawer test** whereby posterior displacement of the tibia is elicited on physical examination. Medial meniscus tears are more common than lateral meniscus tears and are usually due to twisting injuries. Unlike the immediate swelling seen with tears of vascular structures such as the ACL, the relatively cartilaginous meniscus causes more gradual swelling and patients often complain of the knee catching, locking, and clicking. **Ballotability** of the patella just confirms the presence of an effusion. **Meniscal tears** can be detected using the **Apley grind test** (clicking or locking when grinding the tibia into the femur with the knee flexed at 90°) and the **McMurray test** (with the patient supine, flex the knee and hold the foot in one hand; to look for a **torn medical meniscus** rotate the leg outward and slowly extend the knee while palpating the posteromedial margin of the joint for a palpable click as the femur passes over the torn meniscus. To detect a **torn lateral meniscus**, palpate the posterolateral margin of the knee joint with the leg in full internal rotation as the knee is extended.

327. The answer is c. *(Fauci, p 612.)* The most common malignant tumors of bone include osteosarcoma (45%), chondrosarcoma (25%), and Ewing sarcoma (15%). This patient presenting with swelling and pain in the distal femur and radiographic changes likely has an **osteosarcoma**. These malignant extremity tumors usually occur in children and adolescents, but may also occur in older adults with a history of Paget disease or radiation therapy. The most likely sites of involvement include the distal femur, proximal tibia, and proximal humerus. Plain films reveal a **moth-eaten destruction** of bone with a **"sunburst appearance"** correlating to a spiculated periosteal reaction. Long-term survival rates range from 60% to 80%. **Chondrosarcomas have a predilection for shoulder and pelvic girdle** and are seen in older patients (40-50 years old). A history of pain that increases in severity, worsens at night, and is relieved by aspirin suggests the diagnosis of **osteoid osteoma**. This benign tumor is more common in males than females, and patients present between 20 and 30 years of age.

The proximal femur is the most common site for this tumor. Other benign tumors of bone include giant cell tumor (osteoclastoma), osteochondroma, chondroblastoma, and osteoblastoma. A **muscle strain** would be common in an active adolescent, but the plain film results point to something else. **Paget disease** usually is diagnosed after the age of 40 and manifests as bone pain, kyphosis, bowed tibias, an enlarging skull, and a markedly elevated serum alkaline phosphatase.

328. The answer is c. *(Seidel, p 733.)* The lateral and medial collateral ligaments stabilize the knee laterally. Forced valgus (lateral pushing toward medial) bending of the knee from a lateral force may rupture the **medial collateral ligament (MCL)**, also called the tibial collateral ligament. Patients present with pain over the medial aspect of the knee and pulling against the medial distal tibia while stabilizing the knee laterally will reveal valgus laxity when compared to the other, noninjured knee (known as the **valgus stress test**). Injuries to the MCL may in turn tear the medial meniscus, since the MCL is attached to the medial meniscus. Patients **with medial or lateral meniscal tears** may complain of locking of the knee in flexion with activity while walking and on examination, the McMurray test would be positive. Injuries of the **lateral (fibular) collateral ligament** cause tenderness over the lateral knee with palpation, but these injuries are not common. **Dislocation or subluxation of the patella** is due to a great force. Locking is common, and the patella is usually displaced laterally. Subluxation reduces by itself, while dislocation requires reduction.

329. The answer is b. *(McPhee, p 742.)* **Carpal tunnel syndrome (CTS)** is the most likely diagnosis. It is due to median nerve compression by the transverse carpal ligament. Risk factors for this disorder include repetitive use of the hands, especially bending at the wrists, and underlying conditions such as diabetes mellitus, pregnancy, hypothyroidism, rheumatoid arthritis, repetitive activity, and acromegaly. Patients may complain of pain and tingling in the distribution of the median nerve: the thenar eminence, and the first three digits. The diagnosis is confirmed in this patient by **Tinel sign** (paresthesias or pain reproduced with percussion of the volar surface of the wrist) and **Phalen sign** (symptoms are reproduced by holding the wrist in palmar flexion for 1 minute) may also be positive. **Thoracic outlet syndrome** usually causes medial arm pain and paresthesia when using the arms. The presence of a cervical rib is a risk factor for this disorder.

Dupuytren contracture is a fibrotic process of the palmar fascia that causes fixed flexion of the ring finger and is often found in alcoholics and patients with chronic diseases. A **ganglion cyst** is a painless, firm cystic mass arising from any joint or tendon sheath that often moves with flexion and extension of the tendon. A **trigger finger** occurs when an enlarged flexor tendon sheath passes through the pulleys of the digits, causing locking or catching.

330. The answer is c. *(McPhee, pp 738-740.)* Since the patient has pain not radiating below the knee, paraspinous tenderness, and no neurologic compromise, the most likely diagnosis is **lumbosacral back strain**. Strain is common in people in their forties. It is exacerbated by activity and improves with rest. A **straight-leg maneuver** is positive for **nerve root compression from disk herniation** when radicular pain is produced down the leg, to **below the knee**, at less than 70° of elevation. **Crossover pain** (straight-leg maneuver of nonpainful leg worsens pain of involved leg) is also a strong indicator of nerve root compression, but only if pain is produced below the knee. Pain in the hamstrings is *not* a positive straight-leg raise. **Paravertebral abscess** usually presents with fever and tenderness with percussion of the affected area of the spine. Risk factors for **osteoporosis** include female gender, menopause, lack of activity, slim body habitus, older age, inadequate calcium intake, medications such as corticosteroids, and racial–ethnic background (Asian and northern European descent). This loss of bone mineralization of the spine predisposes affected patients to **compression fractures** which present with significant pain and tenderness to palpation over the affected area of the spine. **Paget disease** (osteitis deformans) is a slowly progressing disease of bone that may be asymptomatic or may cause bone pain, deformities (such as a large skull or leg bowing), hearing loss, and fractures. It begins in middle-aged men and is thought to be due to an inborn error of metabolism causing the formation of poorly organized bone.

331. The answer is d. *(Fauci, p 2155.)* **Trochanteric bursitis** is a common cause of hip pain in the elderly but may also be seen in bicyclists and runners. Pain is exacerbated by standing and by external rotation. Lying on the affected side compresses the inflamed bursa and pain is reproducible with palpation over the greater trochanter, as in this patient. **Ischial bursitis (weaver's bottom,** so named because weavers had to sit for long periods of time, which led to ischial bursitis) causes pain in the buttock made worse with sitting and with hip flexion. Today, it is usually a problem for workers who operate heavy equipment on rough roads. **Hip osteoarthritis** presents with **groin pain** exacerbated by the **FABER maneuver** (also called the **Patrick test**), which is a mnemonic for **F**lexion, **AB**duction, and **E**xternal **R**otation. **Avascular necrosis (AVN)** of the hip may be due to trauma, to medical issues like sickle cell disease, or to medications such as corticosteroids. Patients are usually between the ages of 30 and 60 years and often complain of groin pain made worse with weight bearing. **Fracture of the proximal femur** usually follows trauma. On inspection, the affected lower extremity lies in external rotation and is shorter than the normal side.

332. The answer is c. *(Seidel, p 754.)* Adolescents with **slipped capital femoral epiphysis (SCFE)** are often obese, but tall, males who present with thigh or knee pain. SCFE is a disorder of unknown etiology that causes posterior and medial displacement of the femoral head (more commonly on the left side), leading to a **limp, reduced internal rotation of the hip and leg weakness.** A child with **Sprengel deformity** cannot raise one arm completely due to a small and elevated scapula. **Torticollis** (wry neck due to shortening of the sternocleidomastoid muscle) often accompanies the deformity. Children with **juvenile rheumatoid arthritis (JRA)** present with fever, salmon-colored rash, arthritis, hepatosplenomegaly, nodules, pericarditis, and iridocyclitis (may lead to blindness). There is no diagnostic test for JRA, but the disease resolves by puberty in the majority of children. **Arnold-Chiari malformation** is an abnormality of neural tube closure. **Cerebral palsy (CP)** is a nonprogressive disorder resulting from a perinatal insult; it causes either a spastic paresis of the limbs or extrapyramidal symptoms (chorea, athetosis, ataxia). Patients with CP often have an associated seizure disorder, mental retardation, and speech or sensory deficits.

333. The answer is a. *(Fauci, p 2186.)* This patient's symptoms **(first-step heel pain)** are classic for **plantar fasciitis**, often seen in young, active adults due to repetitive microtrauma, as well as in obese patients, those who stand for a long time or run frequently on hard surfaces and in those with **pes planus** (excessive pronation of the foot) or **pes cavus** (high arch). The plantar fascia tightens the longitudinal arch and helps with the push-off phase of walking. The diagnosis can be made on history and with reproducibility of tenderness with palpation of the inferior heel at its attachment to the medial tuberosity of the calcaneus. **No further radiologic studies** are usually necessary and plain radiographs may show heel spurs that may not be related to symptoms. Treatment involves discontinuing activities that incite the pain, application of **ice, massage, and stretching of the plantar fascia** with maneuvers such as lowering the heel off a step. **Orthotics** for arch support and a short course of **NSAIDs** may help as well. Glucocorticoid injections may help, but increase the risk of tendon rupture and fasciotomy is reserved for those patients who fail to experience resolution of symptoms with conservative therapy within 6 months to a year.

334. The answer is e. *(Kliegman, p 2860.)* The patient most likely has **compartment syndrome** from elevated pressure in a confined space compromising nerve, soft tissue, and muscle perfusion. Etiologies include burn injuries, crush injuries, and fractures. Compartment syndrome is often referred to as the disorder of **six P's** (**P**ain, **P**allor, **P**aralysis, **P**aresthesias, **P**oikilothermia, and **P**ulselessness). Immediate fasciotomy and restoration of tissue perfusion is the treatment for compartment syndrome.

335. The answer is a. *(McPhee, p 745.)* **Tennis elbow**, or **lateral epicondylar tendinitis**, is most commonly characterized by tenderness of the common extensor muscles at their origin (the lateral epicondyle of the humerus). Passive flexion of the fingers and wrist and having the patient extend the wrist against resistance causes pain. **Golfer's elbow**, or **medial epicondylar tendinitis**, is a similar disorder of the common flexor muscle group at its origin, the medial epicondyle of the humerus. **Olecranon bursitis** is an inflammation of the bursa over the olecranon process caused by acute or chronic trauma **(student's elbow)** or secondary to gout, rheumatoid arthritis, or infection. Clinically, there is swelling or pain on palpation of the posterior elbow. Direct pressure of the biceps tendon in the bicipital groove indicates **biceps tendinitis.** Paralysis of the serratus anterior muscle (innervated by the **long thoracic nerve**) causes the scapula to protrude posteriorly from the posterior thoracic wall when the patient is asked to push against a wall **(winged scapula)**.

336. The answer is d. *(McPhee, p 736.)* The most likely diagnosis in this patient is **whiplash**, or **cervical musculoligamental sprain or strain**. Whiplash-associated disorders begin after a symptom-free period following a hyperextension or hyperflexion injury, usually in an MVA. It is vital to perform a complete neurologic examination to exclude other causes of neck pain. **Ankylosing spondylitis** is a chronic and progressive inflammatory disease that most commonly affects spinal, sacroiliac, and hip joints. **Osteoarthritis** most often affects the weight-bearing joints and the cervical or other areas of the spine, but usually is more chronic than this patient's presentation. **Reiter syndrome** usually causes arthritis of the hips, and there is often a history of urethritis, conjunctivitis, and foot involvement. **Polymyalgia rheumatica** causes weakness and pain in the shoulder and hip girdles.

337 to 339. The answers are 337-e, 338-b, 339-g. *(Seidel, pp 724-725.)* Improper footwear results in lateral deviations of the great toe, extensor, and flexor hallucis longus tendons **(bunions)**. **Stress fractures** result in bone resorption followed by insufficient remodeling due to continued activity, such as running. Stress fractures occur in the tibia as well as the metatarsal; examination typically reveals point tenderness and swelling. A stress fracture of a metatarsal is called a **march fracture.** Painful swelling and erythema of the first metatarsophalangeal joint is the typical presentation of **gout**, and is called **podagra**. **Hammertoe** often affects the second toe. The metatarsophalangeal joint is dorsiflexed, and the proximal interphalangeal joint displays plantar flexion. In **genu varum (bowleg)**, the lateral femoral condyles are widely separated when the feet are placed together in the extended position. In **genu recurvatum,** the knee hyperextends, and in **genu impressum,** there is flattening and bending of the knee to one side with displacement of the patella. **Pes planus** is a flattened longitudinal arch of the foot, often called flat foot. **Morton neuroma** causes pain in the forefoot that radiates to one or two toes with tenderness between the two metatarsals. The pain may be further aggravated by squeezing the metatarsals together.

340 and 341. The answers are 340-d, 341-e. *(McPhee, pp 743, 748-749.)* **Hypertrophic osteoarthropathy** is nail clubbing accompanied by a symmetrical polyarthritis involving the large joints and occasionally the metacarpophalangeal joints. This condition may be seen secondary to malignancy, endocarditis, vasculitis, and other pulmonary and cardiac diseases. **Charcot joint** is a complication of peripheral neuropathy seen in diabetic patients. Repetitive minor trauma to the foot causes deformities, which may lead to skin breakdown, erythema, edema, and callus formation. The pathogenesis of **complex regional pain syndrome** (formerly **reflex sympathetic dystrophy**) is unknown. The presentation may be seen after peripheral limb injury; early symptoms include diffuse pain in the limb and edema, often also with changes of color and temperature in the limb. This disorder may lead to contractures. **Ankylosing spondylitis (AS)** is a chronic and progressive inflammatory disease, seen mostly in men in their thirties, that most commonly affects the spinal, sacroiliac, and hip joints. It may go undiagnosed for many years, and bilateral hip pain due to sacroiliac involvement may be clinically undetectable. It is strongly associated with HLA-B27 test. Examination of the spine usually reveals limitation in movement; patients in advanced stages may have a characteristic bent-over posture. Patients with AS may present with an acute nongranulomatous uveitis and limited chest expansion due to involvement of the costovertebral joints. The **Schober test** is positive in AS (with the patient erect, marks are made 5 cm below and 10 cm above the lumbosacral junction between the posterior superior iliac spines; the patient bends, marks are measured, and if the distance between the two marks increases by less than 4 cm there is spinal immobility).

342 and 343. The answers are 342-b, 343-c. *(Seidel, p 748.)* Ninety percent of radiculopathies involve the L5 or S1 nerve roots.

L5 motor: assessed by asking the patient to walk on the heels
sensory: medial forefoot and lateral aspect of the leg

S1 motor: assessed by asking the patient to walk on the toes
sensory: lateral foot
reflex: Achilles reflex

L4 motor: assessed by asking the patient to squat and rise (knee flexion and extension)
sensory: medial aspect of the leg
reflex: patella

L2/3 motor: assessed by hip flexion and for L3, hip adduction

344 and 345. The answers are 344-d, 345-e. *(Seidel, pp 727-733.)* In patients with possible carpal tunnel syndrome, **Phalen test** (holding both wrists in palmar flexion for 1 minute) will reproduce numbness and pain in the distribution of the median nerve. Shoulder pain on the **Hawkins**

test (the patient forward flexes the shoulder to 90° and flexes the elbow to 90° while internally rotating the arm to its limit) is associated with rotator cuff inflammation or tear. The **Apley grind test** and the **McMurray test** are used to detect a torn meniscus. A positive test occurs when there is pain, clicking, or locking of the knee with rotation. The **bulge sign** (sometimes called the **balloon sign**) detects a knee effusion. A positive bulge test occurs when a bulge of fluid returns to the medial aspect of the knee with lateral tapping.

Neurology

Questions

346. A 31-year-old man complains of daily throbbing headaches for the last 2 weeks. He has approximately eight episodes per day, each lasting 20 minutes. The headaches are localized to the left periorbital area and are accompanied by tearing of the left eye, left ptosis, rhinorrhea, and left facial redness. The patient remembers having a similar problem 2 years ago that lasted for 3 weeks. He did not seek medical help at that time. The patient thinks that the headaches are often precipitated by drinking a glass of wine. Which of the following is the most likely diagnosis?

a. Migraine headache
b. Cluster headache
c. Tension headache
d. Trigeminal neuralgia
e. Sinusitis

347. A 28-year-old woman presents with the chief complaint of diplopia for several weeks. She admits to occasional vertigo and ataxia. Six months ago, she had urinary incontinence for 1 month. Examination of the eyes reveals nystagmus, and funduscopic examination reveals swelling of the optic nerve. The patient has increased muscle tone of the lower extremities and is hyperreflexic. She has bilateral extensor plantar reflexes and loss of position sense. Which of the following is the most likely diagnosis?

a. Multiple sclerosis
b. Friedreich ataxia
c. Acute transverse myelitis
d. Brown-Séquard syndrome
e. Syringomyelia

348. A 49-year-old woman is brought to the emergency room after suddenly losing consciousness. Her husband states that the patient was in good health until 2 hours ago, when she suddenly complained of a severe headache. After one episode of vomiting, the patient lost consciousness. The husband states that there were no seizure-like movements and no incontinence. The patient does not take any medications, smoke, drink, or use illicit drugs. On physical examination, the patient has a regular heart rate of 100 beats per minute, respiratory rate of 16 breaths per minute, and blood pressure of 120/80 mm Hg, and is afebrile. Heart and lung examinations are normal but she has neck stiffness. On neurologic examination, the patient responds only to painful stimuli and her deep tendon reflexes are bilaterally equal. She has bilateral flexor plantar responses. Which of the following is the best initial diagnostic test?

a. Lumbar puncture
b. MRI of the brain
c. MR angiography
d. CT scan of the brain
e. Cerebral arteriography

349. A 39-year-old man presents with progressive weakness of his arms and legs. He noticed difficulty in performing tasks such as buttoning his shirt several months ago, and his symptoms have continued to worsen. On physical examination, cranial nerve and sensory findings are normal. Severe atrophy and fasciculations are seen in the legs, arms, and tongue. The patient has a spastic muscle tone, hyperactive reflexes, and bilateral extensor plantar reflexes. Which of the following is the most likely diagnosis?

a. Guillain-Barré syndrome
b. Multiple sclerosis
c. Amyotrophic lateral sclerosis
d. Todd paralysis
e. Poliomyelitis

350. When testing a patient's extraocular muscle movements, you detect that the right eye cannot adduct past the midline. However, when you move a fingertip toward the patient's nose, convergence does occur. Additionally, the patient has horizontal nystagmus in the left eye on lateral gaze. Which of the following is the most likely diagnosis?

a. Paralysis of cranial nerve VI
b. Paralysis of cranial nerve III
c. Internuclear ophthalmoplegia
d. Retrobulbar optic neuritis
e. Paralysis of cranial nerve IV

351. A 30-year-old obese woman presents with a 2-month history of a nonthrobbing headache that is constant and dull in nature. The patient also complains of blurred vision and occasional diplopia. Funduscopic examination reveals blurring of the optic discs bilaterally and no other neurologic deficit. CT scan of the brain reveals no masses and cerebrospinal fluid analysis is normal. Which of the following is the first step in management?

a. Repeat lumbar puncture
b. Oral acetazolamide therapy
c. Vitamin A therapy
d. Oral contraceptive therapy
e. Placement of a lumboperitoneal shunt

352. A 44-year-old man presents with facial asymmetry. On physical examination, touching the cornea of either eye with a cotton swab results in blinking of only the left eye. The patient states that he feels the cotton swab touch in both eyes. Which of the following is the most likely diagnosis?

a. Left trigeminal palsy
b. Right trigeminal palsy
c. Right facial nerve palsy
d. Left facial nerve palsy
e. Left oculomotor nerve palsy

353. A 52-year-old unresponsive pedestrian is brought to the emergency room after being struck by a speeding automobile. He is intubated and stabilized by paramedics. On physical examination, the oculocephalic maneuver reveals the eyes to move disconjugately when the head is moved rapidly from side to side. Which of the following is the most likely cause of these findings?

a. The brainstem is intact.
b. The brainstem is partially intact.
c. The brainstem is not intact.
d. The patient has locked-in syndrome.
e. The patient is in a vegetative state.

354. A 51-year-old alcoholic presents to the emergency room with horizontal nystagmus, ataxic gait, and confusion. Which of the following is the most likely diagnosis?

a. Wernicke syndrome
b. Niacin deficiency
c. Korsakoff syndrome
d. Klüver-Bucy syndrome
e. Delirium tremens

355. An 18-year-old presents with bilateral leg weakness that has progressed over the last several days. He noticed some numbness and tingling of the toes and feet that has now progressed to his thigh and pelvic areas. He has no bladder or bowel incontinence. He denies use of tobacco, alcohol, or drugs and takes no medications. Past medical history is unremarkable except for an upper respiratory tract infection 2 weeks ago. On physical examination, the vital signs are normal. Neurologic examination reveals an inability to move the muscles of facial expression on the left side of the face. There is bilateral symmetric weakness and deficit to pinprick and vibration of the lower extremities. Deep tendon reflexes are absent in the lower extremities. Which of the following is the most likely diagnosis?

a. Myasthenia gravis
b. Multiple sclerosis
c. Poliomyelitis
d. Charcot-Marie-Tooth disease
e. Guillain-Barré syndrome

356. A 76-year-old woman has deviation of her tongue to the left after a recent stroke. Which of the following is the most likely cause for these findings?

a. Right hypoglossal nerve paralysis
b. Left hypoglossal nerve paralysis
c. Right glossopharyngeal nerve paralysis
d. Left glossopharyngeal nerve paralysis
e. Right vagus nerve paralysis

357. A 37-year-old woman underwent a total abdominal hysterectomy for fibroids under general anesthesia. In the days following her surgery, she complains of numbness and tingling in her ring finger and little finger of her left hand. On examination she has some diminished sensation in these fingers. She is also noted to have flexion of these digits at rest with inability to extend them and decreased grip strength. Which of the following is the most likely diagnosis?

a. Radial neuropathy
b. Ulnar neuropathy
c. Erb-Duchenne palsy
d. Cervical radiculopathy
e. Carpal tunnel syndrome

358. A 46-year-old man has a 1-month history of headache. He has no past medical history of headache and no family history of headache. He does not use illicit drugs, drink alcohol, or smoke cigarettes. Physical examination reveals alexia, agraphia, acalculia, right-left confusion, and finger agnosia as well as an abnormally painful response to touch. An MRI of the brain with gadolinium is most likely to show which of the following?

a. Frontal lobe lesion
b. Parietal lobe lesion
c. Temporal lobe lesion
d. Occipital lobe lesion
e. Cerebellar lesion

359. A 66-year-old obese woman has the chief complaint of pain and numbness over the lateral aspect of the right thigh. She has no back pain or difficulty ambulating and her symptoms are relieved by sitting. Physical examination is normal except for impaired cutaneous sensation over the affected lateral aspect of the right thigh. There is a negative straight-leg raise maneuver; motor strength and deep tendon reflexes are normal. Romberg test is negative. Which of the following is the most likely diagnosis?

a. Peroneal nerve palsy
b. Vitamin B_{12} deficiency
c. Meralgia paresthetica
d. Sciatica
e. Femoral neuropathy

360. A 14-year-old adolescent presents with a history of intermittent facial grimacing, twitching, and eye blinking since childhood. The movements are repetitive and often move from one part of the face to another. On physical examination, cranial nerve, sensory, and cerebellar examinations are normal. Motor examination reveals frequent and quick repetitive eye blinking, nasal twitching, and facial grimacing accompanied by an occasional snort or grunt. Which of the following is the most likely diagnosis?

a. Tardive dyskinesia
b. Gilles de la Tourette syndrome
c. Asterixis
d. Sydenham chorea
e. Huntington chorea

361. A 26-year-old woman presents with the chief complaint of weakness that worsens throughout the day. She especially notices weakness and feeling tired when chewing food. The patient states that she feels strong on arising in the morning but the weakness develops over the course of the day. She also complains of her eyelids drooping and occasional diplopia. Neurologic examination reveals ptosis after 1 minute of sustained upward gaze. Which of the following is the most likely diagnosis?

a. Lambert-Eaton syndrome
b. Botulism
c. Myasthenia gravis
d. Multiple sclerosis
e. Friedreich ataxia

362. Examination of a patient's visual fields reveals complete blindness in the left eye but the right eye is unaffected. Ophthalmoscopic examination is normal. Which of the following lesions is most likely causing this abnormality?

a. A lesion between the optic chiasm and the lateral geniculate body
b. A lesion between the retina and the optic chiasm
c. A lesion between the lateral geniculate body and the visual cortex
d. A lesion at the medial longitudinal fasciculus
e. Bilateral lesions of the occipital lobes

363. A 32-year-old previously healthy man is brought to the emergency room after having a seizure. He has no family history of seizure and denies alcohol use, illicit drug use, and trauma. A family member states that recently the patient has been complaining of a headache and has been acting bizarre, which is a change in his personality. Physical examination reveals a temperature of 38.3°C (100.9°F). Blood pressure and heart rate are normal. During examination, the patient has a partial complex seizure. CT scan of the head reveals hemorrhagic necrosis of the temporal lobes. Which of the following is the most likely diagnosis?

a. Lyme disease
b. Cysticercosis
c. Waterhouse-Friderichsen syndrome
d. Herpes encephalitis
e. Rabies

364. A 29-year-old woman was an unbelted passenger in a motor vehicle accident. On arrival at the hospital, the paramedics inform you that her calculated Glasgow Coma Scale (GCS) score is 5. Which of the following is included in the physical examination assessment as part of the calculation of the GCS score?

a. Thought content
b. Cold calorics
c. Eye opening
d. Stereognosia
e. Graphesthesia

365. A 67-year-old woman presents to your office complaining of "losing her taste buds." She cooks with table salt and adds it to meals but has difficulty tasting the salt. On physical examination, her tongue is normal in size, consistency, and color. The patient fails to sense stimulation of the tongue with sugar or salt. Bitter and sour taste sensations are intact. Which of the following cranial nerves is most likely responsible for the lack of sensation?

a. Glossopharyngeal nerve
b. Vagus nerve
c. Facial nerve
d. Maxillary branch of the trigeminal nerve
e. Mandibular branch of the trigeminal nerve

366. A 66-year-old nursing home resident was recently started on haloperidol for behavioral problems. One week later, the patient develops a temperature of 40.3°C (104.5°F) and is transferred to the hospital. The patient is awake but not responsive. His heart rate is 110 beats per minute, his respiratory rate is 24 breaths per minute, and he is diaphoretic. Neurologic examination reveals a rigid muscle tone and catatonia. Which of the following is the most likely diagnosis?

a. Tardive dyskinesia
b. Neuroleptic malignant syndrome
c. Acute schizophrenia
d. Dystonic reaction
e. Drug-induced parkinsonism

Questions 367 to 370

For each patient with neurologic deficits, select the most likely diagnosis. Each lettered option may be used once, multiple times, or not at all.

a. Basilar artery stroke
b. Middle cerebral stroke
c. Anterior cerebral stroke
d. Transient ischemic attack
e. Posterior cerebral stroke
f. Lacunar infarct
g. Wallenberg syndrome

367. A 52-year-old man presents with locked-in syndrome. On neurologic examination, the patient is quadriplegic with sensory loss and cranial nerve involvement. He is able to respond to questions using his eyes.

368. A 71-year-old woman presents with aphasia and severe right-sided hemiparesis greater in the arm than the leg. Her eyes deviate to the left.

369. A 57-year-old man presents with an episode of right face, arm, and leg weakness that resolved on arrival at the emergency room.

370. A 61-year-old woman with poorly controlled diabetes and hypertension presents with slurred speech and clumsiness of her left hand.

Questions 371 to 374

For each patient with neurologic deficits, select the most likely diagnosis. Each lettered option may be used once, multiple times, or not at all.

a. Upper motor neuron disease
b. Lower motor neuron disease
c. Myelopathy
d. Radiculopathy
e. Broca aphasia
f. Wernicke aphasia

371. A 61-year-old man presents with flaccid paralysis, atrophy, fasciculations, and hyporeflexia.

372. A 48-year-old man presents with spastic paralysis, 4+ deep tendon reflexes, and an extensor plantar reflex.

373. A 41-year-old man presents with spastic legs, bilateral extensor plantar reflexes, hyperreflexia, and loss of sensation (position sense and vibration) of the lower extremities.

374. A 70-year-old woman presents with poorly articulated phrases but understands commands.

Questions 375 and 376

For each patient with headache, select the most likely etiology of the symptoms presented. Each lettered option may be used once, multiple times, or not at all.

a. Complicated migraine
b. Basilar artery migraine
c. Classic migraine
d. Common migraine
e. Sinus headache
f. Temporal arteritis

375. A 24-year-old woman has a 2-year history of recurrent right-sided headaches that are throbbing in nature and are preceded by 30 minutes of scintillating scotomas.

376. A 23-year-old woman complains of periodic, throbbing, right-sided headaches accompanied by nausea and vomiting. On physical examination during the time of headache, the patient demonstrates a right oculomotor nerve palsy. MRI is normal.

Questions 377 to 380

For each patient with a gait disturbance, select the most likely kind of gait disturbance. Each lettered option may be used once, multiple times, or not at all.

a. Antalgic gait
b. Parkinsonian gait
c. Spastic hemiparetic gait
d. Steppage gait
e. Scissor gait

377. A 60-year-old man ambulates with his upper torso stooped forward. His feet shuffle and he has lost his arm swing.

378. A 55-year-old woman walks by lifting one foot farther off the ground than the other.

379. A 62-year-old man is limping due to a painful hip.

380. A 49-year-old woman walks by moving her right leg forward by abduction and circumduction.

Questions 381 to 384

For each patient with head trauma, select the most likely diagnosis. Each lettered option may be used once, multiple times, or not at all.

a. Cerebellar tonsillar herniation
b. Uncal herniation
c. Basilar skull fracture
d. Subdural hematoma
e. Epidural hematoma
f. Cerebral concussion
g. Contusion

381. A 49-year-old man presents after a fall from a platform that is 15 ft high. On physical examination, the patient has raccoon eyes, blood in the soft tissue overlying the left mastoid bone and has cerebrospinal fluid (CSF) rhinorrhea.

382. A woman survives a motor vehicle accident and is alert, oriented, and neurologically intact on arrival at the emergency room. Within 1 hour she becomes less arousable, and she expires while being transported to the radiology department for imaging studies.

383. A 9-year-old boy falls off a skateboard and strikes his head. He momentarily loses consciousness but subsequently has no neurologic deficit and appears fine. He complains of a slight headache but no dizziness or personality changes.

384. A 55-year-old man is the victim of a mugging in which he was hit on the head repeatedly with a baseball bat. On arrival at the emergency room, his right pupil is dilated and nonreactive. The patient rapidly progresses to coma and expires.

Questions 385 to 387

For each patient with an abnormal level of consciousness, select the most appropriate description of the level of consciousness. Each lettered option may be used once, multiple times, or not at all.

a. Confusion
b. Lethargy
c. Delirium
d. Stupor
e. Decorticate
f. Decerebrate

385. A 67-year-old man, who has recently been resuscitated after a motor vehicle accident, is arousable for short periods of time to visual, verbal, or painful stimuli. He responds by moving slowly or by moaning.

386. A 73-year-old woman is admitted to the cardiac unit for elective placement of a pacemaker. While in the hospital, she becomes confused and experiences hallucinations. She has a diminished attention span, is anxious, and reacts inappropriately to stimuli.

387. A patient with urosepsis presents drowsy and falls asleep several times during physical examination. Once aroused, the patient is cooperative and responds to questions and commands appropriately.

Neurology

Answers

346. The answer is b. *(McPhee, pp 872-876.)* **Cluster headaches** are often referred to as "**suicide headaches**" because of the severity of the symptoms. These recurring headaches are often accompanied by facial flushing, nasal stuffiness, eye tearing, and a partial Horner syndrome (there is no anhidrosis). They are more common in men (the usual age range is 20-50) and are exacerbated by alcohol use or stress. **Inhalation of 100% oxygen is often effective treatment. Migraine headaches** do not recur so many times during the day or have such a short duration, and are accompanied by nausea or photophobia rather than the associated symptoms listed for this patient. **Tension headaches** are bilateral, nonthrobbing, and symmetric, usually located in the frontal or occipital areas of the skull. They are thought to be related to muscle contraction and are often described as being viselike. The **headache of sinusitis** is not abrupt in onset or cessation, and patients often have tenderness with percussion of the sinuses. **Trigeminal neuralgia (tic douloureux)** is a paroxysmal severe facial pain over the distribution of the trigeminal nerve. Women are affected more than men, and patients are usually over the age of 40. The pain of trigeminal neuralgia can be triggered by simply touching the skin near the nostril.

347. The answer is a. *(McPhee, pp 912-914.)* The patient most likely has **multiple sclerosis (MS)**, a demyelinating disease characterized by symptoms such as visual impairment, an afferent pupillary defect **(Marcus Gunn pupil)**, diplopia, nystagmus, limb weakness, spasticity, hyperreflexia, extensor plantar reflexes, vertigo, ataxia, dysarthria, scanning speech, emotional lability, and bladder dysfunction. Patients like this one with optic neuritis are at risk for developing blindness. MS may be relapsing and remitting or progressive. As it may be devastating to a patient, the diagnosis should only be given if the patient has more than one symptomatic episode with two or more regions of central white matter affected at different times on MRI of the brain. **Friedreich ataxia** is an autosomal recessive disease in which young patients present with pes cavus foot deformity, spasticity, areflexia, ataxia, and cardiomyopathy. Patients with **acute transverse myelitis**

initially present with back pain followed by weakness and loss of sensation below the level of the pain. Often, there may be bladder and bowel incontinence. Transverse myelitis may be seen after vaccination or infections. **Brown-Séquard syndrome (cord hemisection)** is characterized by contralateral loss of pain and temperature and ipsilateral spasticity, weakness, hyperreflexia, extensor plantar reflex, and loss of proprioception (vibration and position sense). Patients with **syringomyelia** have bilateral paralysis, muscle atrophy, and fasciculations, along with pain and temperature sensory loss in a shawl-like or cape-like distribution.

348. The answer is d. *(McPhee, pp 893-894.)* There are three types of stroke: subarachnoid hemorrhage, cerebral infarction, and intracerebral hemorrhage. This patient presented after complaining of a severe headache with nuchal rigidity and no focal deficit on neurologic examination. The loss of consciousness requires bihemispheral dysfunction, and this along with the abrupt history is most consistent with a **subarachnoid hemorrhage (SAH)**. Common causes of SAH include ruptured aneurysm (ie, berry) and arteriovenous malformation (AVM). A **CT scan (or CT angiogram)** should be performed as soon as possible to confirm the hemorrhage and find its source as it is faster and more sensitive for detecting a bleed in the first 24 hours than an **MRI**. If the CT is normal and the diagnosis is still highly suspected, a lumbar puncture should be done to look for **xanthochromia** (blood in the CSF). **Cerebral arteriography is preferable to MR angiography** and is only performed once the patient is stable enough to possibly go for surgical repair. **Intracerebral hemorrhage (ICH)** rarely produces coma (it must be significantly large to do so), and patients do not complain of headache (as it does not involve the meninges). Patients with ICH have focal deficits that appear abruptly and slowly progress over hours. An **embolic stroke** can involve any cerebral artery but must be bilateral to cause loss of consciousness. Patients often have a history of atrial fibrillation or cardiac problems.

349. The answer is c. *(McPhee, pp 920-921.)* This patient presenting with a combination of upper and lower motor neuron signs most likely has **amyotrophic lateral sclerosis (ALS)**, a degenerative disease that is the result of lower (anterior horn cells) and upper (corticospinal tracts) motor neuron loss. Patients present with asymmetric muscle weakness, atrophy, fasciculations, spasticity, hyperactive reflexes, and extensor plantar reflexes. Later, they may also complain of dysphagia and difficulty holding up their heads. MS may be continuous or relapsing and remitting episodes of symptoms such as diplopia, nystagmus, limb weakness, spasticity, hyperreflexia, extensor plantar reflexes, vertigo, ataxia, dysarthria, scanning speech, emotional lability, and bladder dysfunction. **Guillain-Barré** is an ascending paralysis that may ultimately cause respiratory compromise. **Todd paralysis** is a transient paralysis following a seizure. **Poliomyelitis** is a lower motor neuron disease.

350. The answer is c. *(Fauci, pp 194-195.)* **Internuclear ophthalmoplegia (INO)** is caused by a lesion in the medial longitudinal fasciculus (MLF) and may be due to glioma in children, multiple sclerosis in young adults, or vascular infarction in the geriatric age group. INO commonly causes paresis of adduction of the ipsilateral eye (patients cannot look medially) and horizontal nystagmus in the contralateral abducting eye, but convergence is intact. **Paralysis of cranial nerve III** would cause ptosis and impairment of medial gaze, as well as function of the superior rectus, inferior rectus and inferior oblique muscles. **Paralysis of cranial nerve IV** would interfere with a person's ability to internally rotate and depress the eye to look toward the nose. **Cranial nerve VI** innervates the lateral rectus, thus paralysis would impair lateral gaze. **Optic neuritis** would cause pain and loss of vision in the affected eye.

351. The answer is b. *(McPhee, p 903.)* Patients with **pseudotumor cerebri (benign intracranial hypertension)** are often obese women in their childbearing years who present with headache and papilledema. Possible causes include **hypervitaminosis A** and the use of **oral contraceptives** or antibiotics (tetracycline). Lumbar puncture will reveal an elevated opening pressure but normal cerebrospinal fluid (CSF) and CT scan will not show any masses in the brain. Treatment includes weight reduction, and while **repeated lumbar puncture** to reduce intracranial pressure is beneficial, a more noninvasive approach with **oral acetazolamide** to reduce CSF formation is preferred. Discontinuing possible inciting medications is warranted as well. A complication of pseudotumor cerebri is blindness; patients without improvement with conservative treatment may require **emergency optic nerve sheath decompression**.

352. The answer is c. *(Seidel, p 778.)* The **corneal reflex** is normal when touching the cornea (**trigeminal nerve provides sensation**) causes bilateral eye closure (**facial nerve provides motor**). This reflex will not occur on the side of a facial nerve paralysis.

353. The answer is c. *(Fauci, pp 1717-1718.)* The test for the **oculocephalic**, or **doll's eyes, reflex** is performed by rapidly rotating the head from side to side. If the **brainstem** is intact in a comatose patient, the eyes will move conjugately in the direction opposite to the head rotation. If the brainstem is not intact, the eyes will move disconjugately or not at all. The **oculovestibular reflex**, or **cold caloric testing caloric**, is performed by introducing ice water into the external auditory canal. The comatose patient with an intact brainstem will respond with deviation of the eyes to the side of the irrigation and nystagmus oppositely. If the brainstem is not intact, the reflex will be absent or the eyes will move disconjugately. "**COWS**" is a helpful mnemonic to remember the direction of nystagmus: "**C**old water (causes nystagmus to) **O**pposite (side); **W**arm water (nystagmus to) **S**ame (side as water)." **Locked-in syndrome** typically results from a pontine hemorrhage or infarct. Patients have intact cognitive function but are quadriplegic and cannot show facial expression, move, speak, or breathe. Patients in a **vegetative state** have no cognitive function or awareness of their environment but maintain their respiratory and cardiac function and may have eye movements and spontaneous movements such as yawning.

354. The answer is a. *(McPhee, p 915.)* The triad of nystagmus or paralysis of eye muscles, ataxia, and confusion is associated with **Wernicke encephalopathy. Korsakoff syndrome** consists of confabulation, confusion, and inability to form new memories or remember past events. These disorders are often found in thiamine (vitamin B_1)–deficient malnourished alcoholics and are secondary to lesions in the mammillary bodies. **Niacin deficiency** (pellagra or vitamin B_3 deficiency) causes the triad of D's (dementia, dermatitis, and diarrhea). **Klüver-Bucy syndrome** is due to lesions in the amygdala; patients present with hypersexuality, compulsive attention to detail, docile behavior, and an inability to recognize objects visually (agnosia). **Delirium tremens** is seen 48 to 96 hours following abstinence from alcohol; patients present with insomnia, confusion, tremors, delusions, visual hallucinations, and hyperactivity of the autonomic nervous system (ie, sweating, tachycardia, fever, and dilated pupils).

355. The answer is e. *(McPhee, pp 925-926.)* **Guillain-Barré syndrome, or acute idiopathic polyneuropathy**, is a progressive, symmetrical, autoimmune demyelinating disorder that affects the motor function of the legs first and proceeds proximally to involve weakness of the arms, trunk, and intercostal, neck, and facial muscles. More severely, this condition may cause autonomic dysfunction and respiratory compromise. Patients often have an antecedent viral infection (respiratory or gastrointestinal) or a history of a recent immunization. **Myasthenia gravis** manifests as weakness that worsens as the day progresses and is better with rest. Symptoms include dysphagia, eyelid drooping, diplopia, and motor weakness with chewing or using extremities. **MS** usually presents between age 20 and 40 with muscle symptoms that include imbalance, neuropathic symptoms, muscle spasms, and extremity weakness. **Poliomyelitis** is a viral meningoencephalitis that destroys the anterior horn cells and causes an asymmetric flaccid weakness with fasciculations and hyporeflexia (lower motor neuron). **Charcot-Marie-Tooth disease (CMT)** is an inherited, slowly progressive peripheral sensorimotor neuropathy causing distal muscle atrophy (**"inverted champagne bottle legs**" or "**stork legs**") and sensory loss. Patients with CMT typically have pes cavus or hammertoe foot deformities.

356. The answer is b. *(Seidel, pp 779-780.)* The **hypoglossal nerve** provides **motor function of** the **tongue**. The tongue will **deviate toward the affected side**, thus, this patient has a left hypoglossal nerve palsy. The **glossopharyngeal nerve** affects ability to taste sour and bitter foods and, along with the **vagus nerve**, controls the gag response and ability to swallow.

357. The answer is b. *(McPhee, p 927.)* The patient most likely has **ulnar nerve paralysis** causing numbness and a **claw-hand deformity of the fourth and fifth digits**. Ulnar nerve lesions are most likely to occur at the elbow where the nerve runs behind the medial epicondyle, but can occur at the wrist as well. Causes of ulnar neuropathy include compression (as with immobilization during general anesthesia), diabetes, trauma, venipuncture, and ganglion cysts at the wrist. **Radial nerve palsy** causes **wristdrop. Carpal tunnel syndrome (CTS)** results from compression of the median nerve by the transverse volar ligament of the wrist. Patients complain of pain and paresthesias of the hand and weakness and atrophy of the thenar muscles. **Tinel sign** (tapping the median nerve at the wrist) and **Phalen sign** (forced wrist flexion) intensify the symptoms. Risk factors for CTS include pregnancy, diabetes mellitus, hypothyroidism, rheumatoid arthritis, amyloid infiltration as seen in patients with multiple myeloma, acromegaly, and repetitive trauma. **Erb-Duchenne palsy** (C5-C6) causes weakness of the shoulder and elbow and results in the **waiter's tip position** (arm dangles at the side with palm in a backward position with fingers flexed). Patients with **cervical radiculopathy** (C6 or C7 root) complain of neck pain that radiates to the arm (radicular pain), dermatomal sensory loss, and decreased reflexes.

358. The answer is b. *(McPhee, p 899.)* MRI will most likely reveal a lesion of the **parietal lobe**. Parietal lobe lesions may produce **contralateral hyperpathia** (abnormally painful reaction to a stimulus), spontaneous pain **(thalamic syndrome)**, and **Gerstmann syndrome** (alexia, agraphia, acalculia, right-left confusion, and finger agnosia), as well as difficulty recognizing objects placed in the hand because of inability to recognize their shape, texture, and size.) **Occipital lobe** lesions produce partial visual field defects. **Temporal lobe** lesions produce seizures, lip smacking, olfactory or gustatory hallucinations, and behavioral changes. **Frontal lobe** lesions lead to intellectual decline and personality changes. The most common adult primary tumors are gliomas. **Cerebellar lesions** cause ataxia, incoordination, nystagmus, and sensory problems in the extremities.

359. The answer is c. *(McPhee, pp 927-928.)* The patient describes classic **lateral thigh numbness** with no motor findings, which is attributable to compression of the **lateral femoral cutaneous nerve** arising from the L2 and L3 roots **(meralgia paresthetica)**. This condition is most common in obese or pregnant patients, and entrapment of the nerve at any point, including from hyperextension of the hip, may cause symptoms. Symptoms are usually mild and spontaneously resolve, but patients may require hydrocortisone injections medial to the iliac spine. Patients with **femoral neuropathy** present with weakness and wasting of the quadriceps muscle, sensory impairment, and an absent patellar reflex. **Sciatica** causes pain and numbness in the buttock and lateral thigh radiating down to the knee; if caused by a disk herniation, it will often be associated with a positive straight leg raise test. Entrapment of the **peroneal nerve** causes a footdrop. The **Romberg test** is performed by having the patient stand with feet together, head erect, and eyes open. The patient is examined for steadiness and then asked to close his or her eyes. A positive test occurs when the patient displays increased unsteadiness with the eyes closed but not with the eyes open. A positive Romberg test may be seen in diseases that affect the dorsal columns, such as tabes dorsalis and vitamin **B_{12} deficiency**.

360. The answer is b. *(McPhee pp 911-912.)* **Tourette syndrome** is a disorder, often first diagnosed in childhood, of repetitive motor tics involving the face, head, and shoulders and is often accompanied by vocal tics (ie, grunts, snorts, involuntary swearing, echolalia—repeating the speech of others or coprolalia—obscene speech). **Huntington disease** is an autosomal dominant disorder characterized by abrupt, involuntary, nonrepetitive, jerky movements (chorea), and dementia. Patients with **tardive dyskinesia** have developed purposeless movements, such as mouth smacking and tongue protrusion, after use of a dopamine-blocking neuroleptic drug. **Asterixis** is seen in patients with hepatic encephalopathy or renal failure and is characterized by inability to sustain wrist extension, causing a "flap." **Sydenham chorea** is seen in rheumatic fever and involves darting movements of the tongue and choreiform movements of the upper limbs on one or both sides of the body.

361. The answer is c. *(McPhee, pp 932-933.)* **Myasthenia gravis** is fatigable weakness that primarily affects the respiratory, bulbar, and ocular muscles, as in this patient. The etiology of the disorder is autoimmune, causing destruction of the acetylcholine receptors in the affected muscles. Thymic abnormalities often accompany the disorder, and the **Tensilon test** (injection of edrophonium, which is an acetylcholinesterase inhibitor) often confirms the diagnosis because it transiently results in improvement of symptoms. **Lambert-Eaton myasthenic syndrome (LEMS)** is a progressive generalized weakness that improves with exercise and is associated with small-cell carcinoma of the lung. Ocular and bulbar muscles are spared, but patients often have autonomic dysfunction. **Botulism** causes rapid progressive paralysis of the bulbar (nonreactive dilated pupils) and extraocular muscles and eventually causes skeletal and respiratory muscle weakness. The disorder is caused by ingestion of the exotoxin produced by *Clostridium botulinum,* which blocks acetylcholine release from nerve terminals. Aminoglycosides should be avoided in patients with neuromuscular disturbances, since they prevent the release of acetylcholine from nerve endings. **MS** involves symptoms that include unsteadiness, neuropathy, muscle spasms and extremity weakness. **Friedreich ataxia** is the most common form of inherited ataxia. It presents before age 25 with staggering gait and falling, dysarthria, nystagmus, titubation of the trunk, and in 90% of affected patients there are cardiac abnormalities as well.

362. The answer is b. *(Seidel, p 313.)* When defects are detected in **only one eye**, the lesion must be **anterior to the optic chiasm**. Lesions **at the optic chiasm produce a bitemporal hemianopsia** because this is where the nasal retinal fibers decussate. The **medial longitudinal fasciculus (MLF)** is involved with extraocular muscle contraction; a lesion to the MLF bilaterally **will not allow either eye to look medially**. Lesions of the **optic tract** (between the optic chiasm and lateral geniculate body) cause a **homonymous hemianopsia** while those **between the geniculate body and the visual cortex** produce a **contralateral upper homonymous quadrantanopsia**. **Bilateral lesions of the occipital lobes result in complete loss of vision**, but pupillary reflexes (fibers end in the midbrain) and extraocular muscle movements remain intact.

363. The answer is d. *(McPhee, p 1236.)* Patients with **herpes simplex encephalitis** present with a subacute course consisting of personality changes, fever, headaches, and seizures. **Temporal lobes** are primarily affected, and the disease is fatal without treatment. **Rabies** causes personality changes, headache, dysphagia to even water (hydrophobia), and pharyngeal muscle spasm that makes patients appear to be frothing at the mouth. **Lyme disease** can produce an encephalitis or demyelination that mimics multiple sclerosis, but infection follows a tick bite. **Waterhouse-Friderichsen syndrome** is hemorrhagic infarction of the adrenal glands due to fulminant meningococcemia. **Cysticercosis** is characterized by multiple brain cysts produced by the larval form of the pork tapeworm (*Taenia solium*). Patients coming from endemic areas will present with seizures or other new neurologic deficits.

364. The answer is c. *(Seidel, pp 97-98.)* The **Glasgow Coma Scale (GCS)** is often used to quantify consciousness and assess cerebral cortex and brainstem function by assessing the patient's verbal response, motor response, and eye opening response to stimuli. It may be repeated at intervals to detect improvement or deterioration and is now widely used in coma assessment of patients with hypoxic injury or head trauma. The **minimum score is 3 and the maximum score is 15**. Three behaviors are assessed in the GCS:

Eye Opening Response	Verbal Response	Motor Response
4 = spontaneous	5 = oriented	6 = obeys commands
3 = to verbal stimuli	4 = confused	5 = localizes pain
2 = to pain	3 = inappropriate words	4 = withdraws from pain
1 = none	2 = incoherent	3 = flexion to pain (decorticate posturing)
	1 = none	2 = extension to pain (decerebrate posturing)
		1 = none

365. The answer is c. *(Seidel, p 776.)* The **facial nerve (cranial nerve VII)** mediates taste (**salty** and **sweet**) on the anterior two-thirds of the tongue. The **glossopharyngeal nerve (cranial nerve IX)** mediates taste (**bitter** and **sour**) on the posterior one-third of the tongue.

366. The answer is b. *(McPhee, pp 959-960.)* **Neuroleptic malignant syndrome** is a complication of neuroleptic medications (especially haloperidol) that usually is seen within 30 days of starting a drug, but may occur at any time during medication use. Patients present with **hyperthermia, muscle rigidity, catatonia, labile blood pressure, involuntary movements, confusion, tachycardia, and tachypnea**. **Tardive dyskinesia** is a common complication of neuroleptics; patients present with choreoathetoid movements of the face and mouth (lip smacking). **Dystonic reaction** may also complicate neuroleptic use; patients present with torticollis (neck spasms), rigidity of the back muscles, carpopedal spasm, blepharospasm, or chorea. Symptoms usually resolve with anticholinergic medication. **Drug-induced parkinsonism, including pill-rolling tremor, rigidity, difficulty initiating gait and reduction of face and arm movements**, may be due to dopamine antagonists (eg, reserpine, phenothiazines, or butyrophenones). Although the etiology for all of these neuroleptic complications is unclear, dopamine antagonism probably plays some role in all of these disorders.

367 to 370. The answers are 367-a, 368-b, 369-d, 370-f. *(McPhee, pp 889-891.)* **Transient ischemic attacks** are episodes of stroke symptoms that last less than 24 hours, with return to normal function, while stroke symptoms persist longer than a day and function may be restored or not. **Basilar artery stroke** causes quadriplegia, pinpoint pupils, sensory loss, and cranial nerve involvement; patients may present with coma or locked-in syndrome. **Middle cerebral artery stroke** causes contralateral hemiplegia or hemiparesis greater in the arm than the leg, aphasia, unilateral sensory loss, and homonymous hemianopsia with eyes that deviate to the side of the hemispheric lesion. Patients with **lacunar infarcts** may present with different syndromes, such as dysarthria and mild hemiparesis **(clumsy-hand dysarthria)**. Lacunar infarcts represent small artery occlusions and usually occur in patients with poorly controlled hypertension and diabetes. **Anterior cerebral stroke** causes unilateral leg weakness and sensory loss. **Posterior cerebral artery stroke** causes an occipital stroke and a homonymous hemianopsia. **Wallenberg syndrome**, or lateral medullary syndrome, causes an ipsilateral weakness of the palate and vocal cords, ipsilateral ataxia, ipsilateral Horner syndrome, and ipsilateral loss of facial pain and temperature but contralateral loss of body pain and temperature sensation. There is no limb weakness in Wallenberg syndrome.

371 to 374. The answers are 371-b, 372-a, 373-c, 374-e. *(McPhee, pp 737, 886, 889.)* Upper motor neuron (UMN) disease (above the level of the corticospinal synapses in the gray matter) is characterized by spastic paralysis, hyperreflexia, and the **presence of a Babinski reflex** (upgoing toe on stroking the bottom of the foot)—**everything is up in UMN disease**. Lower motor neuron (LMN) disease (below the level of synapse) is characterized by flaccid paralysis, significant atrophy, fasciculations, hyporeflexia, and a flexor (normal) Babinski reflex—**everything is down in LMN disease**. **Myelopathy** causes severe sensory loss of posterior column sensation (position sense and vibration), spasticity, hyperreflexia, and positive Babinski reflexes. A **radiculopathy** occurs with root compression from a protruded disk that causes sensory loss, weakness, and hyporeflexia in the distribution of the nerve root. **Broca aphasia** (left inferior frontal gyrus) is a nonfluent **expressive** aphasia (***Broca* should remind you of *broken* speech**); **Wernicke aphasia** (left posterior-superior temporal gyri) is a **receptive** aphasia because patients lack auditory comprehension (***Wernicke* should remind you of *wordy* speech that makes no sense**).

Deep tendon reflex (DTR) response is graded on a scale from 0 to 4+:

0 = no response
1+ = sluggish or diminished response
2+ = active or expected response
3+ = more brisk than expected and slightly hyperactive response
4+ = intermittent or transient clonus; hyperactive and brisk response

375 and 376. The answers are 375-c, 376-a. *(McPhee, pp 873-875.)* **Classic migraine** is a unilateral headache that is pulsatile and throbbing in nature and is preceded by a **prodromal aura** consisting of scotomas (black spots), scintillations (light flashes), or hemianopsia. The headache is often accompanied by nausea, vomiting, photophobia, and phonophobia. **Basilar artery migraine** is a variant of classic migraine in which the aura consists of drop attacks, confusion, blindness, and vertigo (all signs of basilar artery ischemia). **Common migraines** lack a prodromal aura. **Complicated migraines** may be preceded by aura and are headaches accompanied by sensory or motor deficits or muscle palsies. The patient described is having a specific kind of complicated migraine called an **ophthalmoplegic migraine**. A mnemonic for migraine is **POUND** (**P**ulsatile, lasts **O**ne day, **U**nilateral, **N**ausea, and interferes with **D**aily activities). Patients with **sinus headache** often have nasal congestion and sinus tenderness to palpation while those with **temporal arteritis** are older (>50 years old) and have headaches along with jaw claudication and tenderness over the temporal artery.

377 to 380. The answers are 377-b, 378-d, 379-a, 380-c. *(Seidel, p 784.)* **Parkinsonian gait** is noted for the forward stoop of the head and shoulders, with arms slightly abducted and forearms partially flexed; there is decreased arm swing as the feet shuffle. **Steppage gait** occurs with footdrop (paralysis of the peroneal nerve); the affected foot is raised higher than normal to prevent dragging of the toe and brought down with a slap. Bilateral footdrop results in a gait resembling that of a **high-stepping horse**. **Antalgic gait** is a limp caused by the patient limiting weight-bearing on a painful leg. **Spastic hemiparetic gait** may be seen in patients after strokes—the leg is stiff with a foot drop and the arm is held flexed and adducted. The lower limb is dragged or moved forward by abduction and circumduction with the arm not swinging from its abnormal position. **Spastic diplegia gait, or scissor gait,** occurs with extrapyramidal disorders.

The patient uses short steps and drags the foot; the legs are extended and stiff and cross on each other.

381 to 384. The answers are 381-c, 382-e, 383-f, 384-b. *(McPhee, p 918.)* Patients with **basilar skull fracture** may present with **Battle sign** (subcutaneous blood in the external auditory meatus due to fracture of the petrous bone) and **raccoon eyes** (subcutaneous blood around the eyes due to fractures through the cranial fossa) and leakage of CSF from the ear or nose. Patients with **epidural hematoma** typically present with headache, confusion, and somnolence several hours after a lucid period. These are arterial hemorrhages from tears of the middle meningeal artery from temporal bone fractures, and death occurs if the bleeding is not controlled. **Epidural hematomas** appear as **convEx (Epidural = EE)** hyperdensities on CT scan. **Subdural hematomas (SDHs)** are venous hemorrhages, slower bleeds than from arteries; patients may present with headache, confusion, and hemiparesis over days. An SDH appears as a **concave** hyperdensity on CT scan. A **concussion** is a temporary impairment of cerebral function without structural cerebral damage. Following a concussion, patients with **postconcussion syndrome** may complain of personality changes, dizziness, and headache. A **contusion** is due to bruising of the brain tissue and may be **coup** (at the site of impact) or **contrecoup** (at the opposite side of the impact). **Uncal herniation** causes compression of cranial nerve III and results in a blown pupil (dilated and nonreactive). **Cerebellar tonsillar herniation** results in compression of the pons and medulla; patients present with severe hypertension, dizziness, ataxia, drowsiness, weakness, spasticity, and, if left untreated, coma and death.

385 to 387. The answers are 385-d, 386-c, 387-b. *(Seidel, p 92.)* **Confused** patients have poor memory and decreased attention span and respond inappropriately to questions. **Lethargic** patients are drowsy and fall asleep easily but, once aroused, respond appropriately. **Delirious** patients are confused and hallucinate. They are anxious and demonstrate motor and sensory excitement. **Stuporous** patients are arousable for short periods of time to visual, verbal, or painful stimuli. They often moan or have slow motor movements in response to stimuli. **Comatose** patients are neither aware nor awake. **DecErebrate** patients **Extend (EE)** to painful stimuli, and **decorticate** patients **flex** to painful stimuli.

Geriatrics

Questions

388. A daughter brings her 81-year-old mother to your office and states that over the last 6 months her mother has become forgetful. The mother has difficulty remembering recent events and often forgets to pay her bills. The patient has been in good health all her life and takes no medications. Vital signs and physical examination are normal. Which of the following should be your first step in diagnosing this patient?

a. Imaging study of the brain
b. Mini-mental status examination (MMSE)
c. Thyroid function tests
d. Lumbar puncture
e. Vitamin levels

389. A 77-year-old nursing home patient is brought to the emergency room because of low-grade fever. She has no vomiting or diarrhea. She has no cough or foul-smelling urine. Her chest radiograph and urinalysis are normal. A 2.5-cm stage 3 pressure ulcer is visible over her sacrum. Antibiotics are started, and the patient is transferred back to the nursing home. Which of the following is the most effective method to prevent further skin lesions?

a. Wet to dry dressings
b. Dry to wet dressings
c. Frequent turning
d. Whirlpool therapy
e. Surgical debridement

390. A 76-year-old woman is admitted to the hospital for a urinary tract infection. The patient takes no medications and does not drink alcohol. During the evening hours the patient suddenly becomes anxious, restless, and combative. The nurses report that the woman is diaphoretic, with a heart rate of 120 beats per minute. They think the patient is hallucinating and has waxing and waning levels of consciousness. Which of the following is the most likely diagnosis?

a. Dementia
b. Mania
c. Delirium
d. Schizophrenia
e. Depression

391. A 74-year-old man presents with complaints of slow vision loss. He reports no eye pain and has no abnormalities of his lids, conjunctivae, or sclerae bilaterally. His funduscopic examination reveals the image in the following figure. The patient reports wavy lines during Amsler grid testing. Which of the following is the most likely diagnosis?

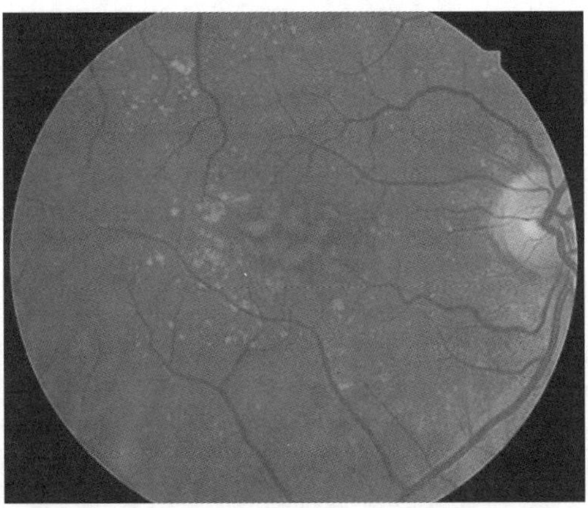

(Reproduced, with permission, from Fauci AS, Braunwald E, Kasper DL, et al. Harrison's Principles of Internal Medicine, *17th ed. New York: McGraw-Hill; 2008:190.)*

a. Glaucoma
b. Macular degeneration
c. Cataracts
d. Pterygium
e. Chemosis

392. A 74-year-old woman presents complaining of a severe right-sided headache for 1 day. She states that the vision in her right eye has diminished, and she complains of pain in the right side of her jaw when she is chewing food. On physical examination, her sinuses are nontender to percussion but her right temple is tender to palpation. Which of the following is the most likely diagnosis?

a. Acute frontal sinusitis
b. Giant cell arteritis
c. Migraine headache
d. Cluster headache
e. Trigeminal neuralgia

393. A 66-year-old woman presents with several weeks of unsteady gait, forgetfulness, and urinary incontinence. She denies headache or any recent trauma. Her past medical history is significant only for meningitis as a child. On physical examination, her blood pressure is 130/85 mm Hg and her heart rate is 82 beats per minute. Her neurologic examination is normal except for a stiff, "magnetic" gait. The patient scores a 22 on the MMSE. After a lumbar puncture, the gait disturbance improves. Which of the following would you find on neuroimaging studies?

a. Cortical atrophy
b. Lacunar infarcts
c. Diffuse white matter disease
d. Enlarged lateral ventricles
e. Nothing abnormal

394. An 81-year-old woman comes to your office for an overdue checkup. She last saw a doctor 3 years ago. She has no complaints other than some forgetfulness that she feels is normal aging. Physical examination reveals mild hypertension, which you plan to control with diet and exercise. MMSE score is 25. Thyroid function tests are normal. Which of the following is the most appropriate next step?

a. A determination of cerebral atrophy by CT scan of the head
b. A determination of arrhythmias by Holter monitor
c. A determination of hearing loss by referral to an audiologist
d. A determination of functionality related to activities of daily living
e. A determination of alcohol use by the CAGE questionnaire

395. A 76-year-old woman presents with the sudden onset of severe sharp left-sided chest pain that radiates in a bandlike fashion only along her left side and back. Vital signs and heart and lung examinations are normal. The patient complains of excruciating pain when the area is lightly touched with a cotton swab. No rash is visible. Electrocardiogram is normal. Which of the following is the most likely diagnosis?

a. Myocardial infarction
b. Gastroesophageal reflux disease
c. Costochondritis
d. Dissecting aortic aneurysm
e. Herpes zoster

396. A 71-year-old woman presents with gradual onset of blurry vision and seeing halos around lights. Her eyes are not painful. On eye examination, the patient has bilaterally diminished vision and you see the problem in the following figure. Which of the following is the most likely diagnosis?

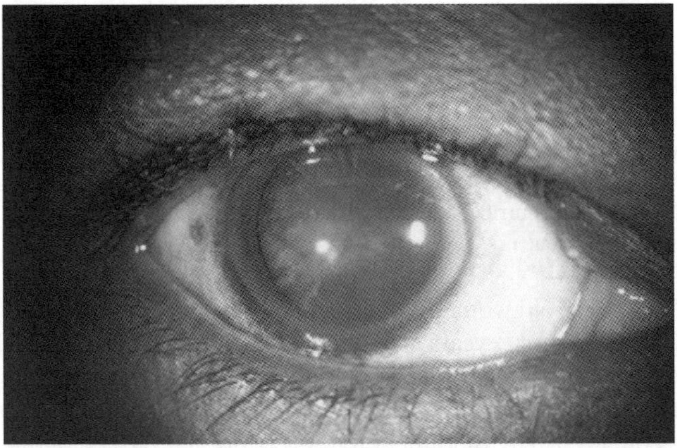

(Reproduced, with permission, from LeBlond RF, Brown DD, DeGowin RL. DeGowin's Diagnostic Examination, *9th ed. New York: McGraw-Hill; 2009: Plate 15.)*

a. Macular degeneration
b. Cataract formation
c. Chronic open-angle glaucoma
d. Chronic angle-closure glaucoma
e. Acute angle-closure glaucoma

397. A 62-year-old man presents with a 2-year history of tremors of the right hand that disappear with voluntary movement. He has no past medical history and takes no medications. Review of systems is positive for anhidrosis and a 5-year history of impotence. On physical examination, the patient is alert and oriented. He has mild postural hypotension on vital signs and a resting tremor of his hands that has a pill-rolling quality. His face is expressionless (mask-like), and his movements are slow. He has difficulty getting out of a chair and is unable to complete the get-up-and-go test in less than 15 seconds. There is a decrease in tone and strength of the extremities. Deep tendon reflexes are diminished. There is no Babinski response. Which of the following is the most likely diagnosis?

a. Benign essential tremor
b. Parkinson disease
c. Shy-Drager syndrome
d. Progressive supranuclear palsy
e. Cerebellar tremor

398. A 67-year-old thin, Caucasian woman presents for evaluation because she feels she is "shrinking." She denies recent trauma and has no weight loss or loss of appetite. She has no fever, chills, or night sweats. She smokes one pack of cigarettes per day. Physical examination reveals a dowager hump and mild kyphotic bowing of the spine with loss of 2 in from her maximum height at age 30. Serum calcium, phosphorus, alkaline phosphatase, and parathyroid hormone levels are normal. Which of the following is the most appropriate next step in diagnosis?

a. Lumbar spine radiographs
b. MRI of the spine
c. CT densitometry of the lumbar spine
d. Dual-energy x-ray absorptiometry
e. Bone scan

399. A 74-year-old woman presents with paresthesias of the feet and an unsteady gait for several months. She takes no medications and does not smoke cigarettes or drink alcohol. The patient has a past medical history only significant for Hashimoto thyroiditis, and on recent labs was noted to have a megaloblastic anemia. On physical examination, she is alert and oriented but cannot recall three objects after 5 minutes. She has glossitis. Which of the following is likely to be found on neurologic physical examination in this patient?

a. Absent patellar and ankle reflexes
b. Flexor plantar reflexes
c. Normal vibration and position sense in the feet
d. Negative Romberg test
e. Diminished muscle strength of the lower extremities

400. A 68-year-old asymptomatic man is found on routine testing to have a peripheral white blood count of 79,000/μL with 20% neutrophils, 75% lymphocytes, and 5% monocytes. His hemoglobin is 14.2 g/dL and his platelet count is 210,000/μL. Peripheral smear reveals well-differentiated lymphocytes and the presence of smudge cells. Physical examination reveals no lymphadenopathy and no hepatosplenomegaly. Which of the following statements is most likely to be true regarding disease in this patient?

a. His disease is a clonal proliferation of B cells.
b. His disease is a clonal proliferation of T cells.
c. He is likely to have hypogammaglobulinemia.
d. He is not expected to survive more than 5 years.
e. His disease will most likely transform into an acute leukemia.

401. A 76-year-old man currently treated for diabetes, hypertension, osteoarthritis of his knees, and benign prostatic hypertrophy is brought by his daughter to clinic because of repeated falls at home. On examination you note that his gait is slow and he is somewhat unsteady upon standing. Which of the following is likely the most reversible cause of his fall risk?

a. Macular degeneration
b. Postural hypotension
c. Cognitive decline
d. Degenerative joint disease
e. Impairment in gait and transfer

402. A 67-year-old man, with a past medical history significant only for moderate bilateral hearing loss, presents with the chief complaint of leg pain, causing him to limp. He also notes that his hat size has increased inexplicably. On physical examination, the patient has bowing of the lower extremities, and the right lower extremity is longer than the left lower extremity. Both legs are warm to the touch anteriorly. The rest of the physical examination is normal. Laboratory data reveal an isolated elevated serum alkaline phosphatase level. Which of the following is the most likely diagnosis?

a. Cerebral vascular accident
b. Paget disease
c. Parkinson disease
d. Metastatic bone disease
e. Vitamin D deficiency

403. A 74-year-old woman presents with an inability to walk after a fall at her home yesterday. On physical examination, the left leg is shorter than the right leg. The injured extremity is in abduction and is slightly externally rotated. Which of the following is the most likely diagnosis?

a. Tibial fracture
b. Fibular fracture
c. Bursitis of the hip
d. Fracture of the femoral neck
e. Quadriceps muscle rupture

404. A 76-year-old man, who has been healthy all of his life, presents to the emergency room after a syncopal episode. He was strolling through the supermarket and had just turned to look at some tomatoes when he suddenly lost consciousness. He denies chest pain, dizziness, or palpitations. He has no previous history of syncope and takes no medications. He was not incontinent of bladder or bowel and had no tonic-clonic movements. When he awoke in the ambulance, he was oriented and asymptomatic. Vital signs and physical examination are completely normal. The patient has no orthostatic changes. The electrocardiogram is normal. Which of the following is the most likely diagnosis?

a. Vasovagal syncope
b. Cardiac syncope
c. Carotid sinus hypersensitivity
d. Cerebral transient ischemia attack
e. Subclavian steal syndrome

405. A 78-year-old woman who has lived with her truck-driver son for a year because of cognitive decline comes in for follow-up. Her past medical history is significant for an arm fracture from a fall 6 months ago. Upon examining her, you note that her hair is uncombed and she smells of urine with skin breakdown over her buttocks. She also has linear bruises over her abdomen horizontally, and when you ask her about them she responds that her son does not want her to get hurt while he is away, so he restrains her in a chair. Which of the following is the most appropriate next step?

a. Order a PT/PTT to investigate the easy bruising.
b. Tell her to rotate her position every few hours to avoid skin breakdown.
c. Order a urinalysis to rule out a urinary tract infection.
d. Contact adult protective services.
e. Advise her to take a multivitamin to prevent skin breakdown.

406. An 80-year-old woman presents from the nursing home where she has lived for 1 month following a stroke to the emergency room with cough, pleuritic chest pain, and shortness of breath. Her cough is productive of purulent sputum. She tells you that this is the first time she has had anything like this. On examination, she is febrile, tachycardic, and tachypneic. Lung auscultation reveals increased fremitus, egophony, dullness, and crackles at the right base. Which of the following is the most likely diagnosis?

a. Health-care-associated pneumonia
b. Community-acquired pneumonia
c. Pulmonary embolus
d. Bronchiectasis
e. Asthma

407. A 72-year-old man was recently admitted to a nursing home after having had a hip fracture. For the last 2 weeks, the patient has eaten very little and has no interest in the social activities of the nursing home. He sleeps most of the day and refuses to get out of bed. He lacks energy and seems uninterested in participating in daily rehabilitation. Most of the time, he states that he wishes to be left alone. When he speaks, he remarks about being a burden to his family. On physical examination he has no tremor or bradykinesia and his MMSE score is 29. Which of the following is the most likely diagnosis?

a. Schizophrenia
b. Depression
c. Dementia
d. Delirium
e. Parkinson disease

408. An 87-year-old man has been living alone. He has no chore worker or caregiver. His neighbor is concerned because the patient is often disheveled and forgetful. He has been late paying his rent and appears to have difficulty ambulating. Which of the following is the most likely intervention for this patient?

a. Assisted living situation
b. Nursing home placement
c. Arrange for a part-time chore worker
d. Arrange for a day program
e. Arrange for a boarding home situation

409. An 81-year-old man is admitted to the hospital with a 1-month history of generalized weakness, lethargy, and a 10-lb weight loss. He states that recently his dietary intake has decreased secondary to poor dentition. Physical examination reveals an emaciated man with bitemporal wasting but otherwise normal HEENT examination. He has no goiter, peripheral edema, or rash. Serum albumin level is normal. Which of the following is the most likely diagnosis?

a. Kwashiorkor
b. Hypothyroidism
c. Zinc deficiency
d. Riboflavin deficiency
e. Protein-energy malnutrition

Questions 410 to 412

For each patient with incontinence, select the most likely explanation for the symptoms. Each lettered option may be used once, multiple times, or not at all.

a. Urge incontinence
b. Stress incontinence
c. Overflow incontinence
d. Functional incontinence
e. Urinary tract infection

410. A 71-year-old woman with a recent history of stroke is newly incontinent of large amounts of urine. She reports no fever or dysuria. She ambulates slowly with her walker and takes no medications. Her postvoid residual urine volume is 35 mL.

411. A 54-year-old mother of five children complains of chronically wetting her undergarments whenever she coughs, laughs, or sneezes.

412. A 66-year-old man with a 15-year history of diabetes mellitus and benign prostatic hyperplasia (BPH) presents with dribbling of his urine. He has a sensation of abdominal fullness and inadequate emptying. Palpation of the lower abdomen reveals a smooth, round, tense mass. Prostate examination reveals an enlarged (50 g) symmetric, nonnodular gland. The patient's postvoid residual urine volume is 800 mL.

Geriatrics

Answers

388. The answer is b. *(Seidel, pp 91-92.)* The best first test to evaluate changes in mental status in elderly patients is the **Folstein mini-mental status examination (MMSE)**. A score of 23 or less out of a possible 30 is consistent with dementia. The differential diagnosis for dementia includes Alzheimer disease (the most common etiology), but other causes must be considered, such as multi-infarct dementia (stepwise decline), normal pressure hydrocephalus (NPH), hypothyroidism, vitamin B_{12} deficiency, folic acid deficiency, depression (pseudodementia), neurosyphilis, HIV, and subdural hematoma. The other answers provided would be appropriate in the work-up of a cognitive deficit confirmed by the MMSE.

389. The answer is c. *(Seidel, p 202.)* **Pressure sores, or decubitus ulcers** can be best prevented by **frequent turning**. The other answer choices are appropriate treatments for already existent ulcers.

The grading system for pressure ulcers is as follows:

Stage 1 = skin is red but not broken
Stage 2 = damage through the epidermis and dermis
Stage 3 = damage through to the subcutaneous tissue
Stage 4 = muscle and possible bone involvement

390. The answer is c. *(Fauci, pp 158-162.)* While **dementia** is a progressive deterioration in cognition, including memory and language, **delirium** is a transient confusional state characterized by waxing and waning levels of consciousness, hallucinations, anxiety, restlessness, combative behavior, paranoia, disorganized thinking, short attention span, autonomic disturbances (tachycardia and diaphoresis), and decreased short-term memory. Elderly patients, like this one, may become delirious because of infections and symptoms often worsen in the evening hours **(sundowning)**. Causes for delirium include (a helpful mnemonic is **I WATCH DEATH**):

Infections (UTI, pneumonia, meningitis, etc.)
Withdrawal (alcohol, sedatives)
Acute metabolic causes (acidosis, electrolyte disturbances, liver or kidney failure)
Trauma (heat stroke, burns, postoperative)
CNS pathology (abscess, tumor, hemorrhage, stroke, etc.)
Hypoxia (from hypotension, PE, CHF)
Deficiencies (vitamin B_{12}, niacin, thiamine)
Endocrine abnormalities (hyper- or hypoglycemia, hyper- or hypothyroidism, etc.)
Acute vascular problems (hypertensive encephalopathy)
Toxins/drugs (drugs of abuse, medications, ingestions)
Heavy metals (lead, mercury)

Mania involves periods of abnormally elevated mood which may involve behaviors such as insomnia, increased speed of speech, hypersexuality, and poor judgment. **Depressed** patients experience a sad mood and low energy level, loss of interest in activities they previously enjoyed and often feelings of guilt, worthlessness, or even suicide. **Schizophrenia** is characterized by delusions, hallucinations, and physical agitation.

391. The answer is b. *(McPhee, pp 162-163.)* **Macular degeneration** is the leading cause of blindness in older persons. Patients complain of a progressive, painless loss of central vision. Funduscopic examination as seen in the image, often reveals small, yellow-white **drusen deposits** around the macula and posterior pole of the eye, subretinal neovascularization, and degenerative changes (depigmentation and atrophy) of the retinal epithelium. **Amsler grid testing** is a method of evaluating the function of the entire macula. The patient looks at a square grid pattern; if he or she sees irregularities in the grid in the form of wavy or fuzzy lines, this indicates macular involvement. **Glaucoma** may occur without visual symptoms, and patients at risk for the disease should be screened carefully. Patients at risk include the elderly, African Americans, those with a family history of glaucoma, and those with a history of hypertension, diabetes mellitus, or myopia. Signs of glaucoma include asymmetry of the cup/disc ratios (even if normal), **cup/disc ratio greater than 0.5**, and flame hemorrhages at the edge of the disc. The disc of glaucoma is pale, not hyperemic. **Cataracts** are opacities of the lens; patients often complain of glare and the inability to see well in reduced light (contrast sensitivity). Eye examination reveals a reduced red reflex. A **pterygium** is an abnormal triangular fold of membrane extending from the conjunctiva to the cornea that results from irritants such as sand, dust, or ultraviolet light. **Chemosis** is conjunctival edema.

392. The answer is b. *(McPhee, pp 766-767.)* This patient has **giant cell arteritis,** or **temporal arteritis,** which usually appears after the age of 55 and is more common in women than in men. Patients typically present with severe headache, malaise, fever, and tenderness over the involved temporal artery. Patients may have ocular symptoms due to ischemic optic neuropathy (**blindness** is an irreversible complication) and complain of jaw pain when chewing (**jaw claudication**). **Polymyalgia rheumatica** (limb girdle stiffness and pain, weight loss, malaise) may be seen in up to 30% of patients with temporal arteritis. Patients suspected of having temporal arteritis require immediate corticosteroids; diagnosis is confirmed by temporal artery biopsy. **Trigeminal neuralgia** (tic douloureux) causes severe unilateral facial pain but is not associated with vision changes or claudication. **Cluster headaches** occur mostly in men and are characterized by periorbital or temporal pain lasting up to 2 hours and accompanied by lacrimation and ptosis. Patients complain of several attacks a day for several weeks, followed by a period of remission. This patient's symptoms are not consistent with **migraine** and she has no fever or sinus tenderness indicative of **sinusitis**.

393. The answer is d. *(Fauci, p 2546.)* The patient has **normal pressure hydrocephalus (NPH)**, which is characterized by a triad of **incontinence, ataxia, and dementia (patients are "wet, wobbly, and weird")** in a patient with a past history of meningitis or subarachnoid hemorrhage. CT scan will show **large lateral ventricles** with no cortical atrophy. None of the other answer choices lead to this constellation of symptoms and signs.

394. The answer is d. *(McPhee, pp 61-63.)* Physicians must determine the degree of functional capacity of an elderly patient based on both medical and psychosocial evaluations. Determining the **activities of daily living (ADLs)**, the **instrumental activities of daily living (IADLs)**, as well as their socioeconomic circumstances and social support system (who will help the patient in case of illness or in an emergency), are integral early in the functional assessment of an elderly patient as one quarter of patients over age 65 and half over 85 have impairments in these areas. The **ADLs** are **D**ressing, **E**ating, **A**mbulating, **T**oileting, and **H**ygiene **(DEATH)**. The **IADLs** are **S**hopping, **H**ouse-keeping, **A**ccounting, **F**ood preparation, and **T**ransportation **(SHAFT)**. All of the other answer choices would be appropriate later in the workup of specific issues found on history or examination, such as hearing loss (**audiometry**), focal neurologic deficits (**CT scan of the head**), arrhythmias (**Holter monitor**) or evidence of excessive alcohol use (**CAGE questionnaire**).

395. The answer is e. *(McPhee, pp 114-116.)* **Herpes zoster** is due to reactivation of latent varicella (chickenpox) virus; patients like this one typically present with a history of pain, tingling, or itching of the affected area, followed a couple of days later by an eruption of vesicles overlying an erythematous base. Although the disease typically presents unilaterally with involvement of a single dermatome, it can disseminate and produce diffuse eruptions, especially in immunocompromised individuals. While this patient may be at risk for an **MI**, **aortic aneurysm**, and **GERD**, the normal vital signs and ECG, as well as reproducibility of symptoms on touch, make these diagnoses less likely. **Costochondritis** is inflammation of the cartilage that connects ribs to the sternum; it causes tenderness to palpation along the sternal edge, not in the areas described in the question.

396. The answer is b. *(McPhee, pp 157-161.)* This patient has a **cataract**, a cloudy area in the lens of the eye, which develops gradually and leads to decreased or blurry vision. **Macular degeneration** causes progressive central vision loss until blindness occurs. In chronic glaucoma, there is an increased cup/disk ratio (> 0.5) and pallor of the optic disk with progressive loss of vision ultimately to complete blindness. **Chronic open-angle glaucoma** is an insidious form of glaucoma in which the intraocular pressure is elevated due to reduced drainage of aqueous fluid, and is usually bilateral. **Chronic angle-closure glaucoma** involves obstruction of flow of the aqueous fluid into the anterior chamber. **Acute angle-closure glaucoma** (also called **narrow-angle glaucoma**) is an ocular emergency in which the trabeculum suddenly becomes completely occluded by iris tissue. Patients complain of severe eye pain, nausea, and the presence of halos or rainbows around light. The pupil may be fixed and dilated secondary to the abrupt rise in intraocular pressure.

397. The answer is c. *(McPhee, pp 905-906.)* **Parkinson disease (PD)** classically includes a constellation of resting asymmetric tremor, rigidity (cogwheel in nature), postural instability, and bradykinesia. Patients have difficulty getting out of a chair, and gait, which is slow at first, becomes faster with ambulation (festination). This patient has **Shy-Drager syndrome** (also called multiple system atrophy, or MSA), in which **parkinsonism is associated with autonomic dysfunction;** patients may present with anhidrosis, disturbance of sphincter control, impotence, and orthostatic hypotension. Patients typically have signs of LMN involvement ("everything is down or low", meaning flaccid paralysis, diminished reflexes, and flexor Babinski reflex). The **get-up-and-go test** (patient gets out of a chair, walks 10 ft, turns around, and returns to chair in less than 15 seconds) is a good test for assessing gait and will be abnormal in patients with parkinsonism. **Benign essential tremor** (also called senile tremor or familial tremor) is not associated with the other features presented here and is reduced by alcohol use. **Cerebellar tremor** occurs with intention and is absent at rest. Patients usually have other signs of cerebellar disease, such as ataxia. **Progressive supranuclear palsy** is a disorder of bradykinesia and rigidity with dementia, emotional lability, and loss of voluntary control of eye movements.

398. The answer is d. *(McPhee, pp 1038-1042.)* Risk factors for **osteoporosis** include Caucasian, Asian–Pacific Islander, and Native American race; Northwestern European descent; blonde or red hair; freckles; thin body frame; nulliparity; early menopause; family history of osteoporosis; postmenopause; constant dieting; calcium intake less than 500 mg/d; scoliosis; rheumatoid arthritis; poor teeth; previous fractures; cigarette smoking; heavy alcohol use; medications (heparin, steroids, thyroxine); and metabolic disorders (diabetes, hyperthyroidism, hypercortisolism). Of all of the options listed, **dual-energy x-ray absorptiometry (DEXA)** is the best choice to determine the density of any bone and is accurate without significant radiation. It is the best screening test for osteoporosis and allows assessment of response of bone density to therapy. **T scores** compare a patient's bone mineral density to that of the young normal mean and is expressed as a standard deviation score away from this mean. On DEXA scan:

T score ≥ 1.0 is normal
T score -1.0 to -2.5 is osteopenia
T score <-2.5 is osteoporosis

399. The answer is a. *(Fauci, p 2660.)* The neurologic symptoms and megaloblastic anemia point to vitamin B_{12} deficiency due to **pernicious anemia** (lack of intrinsic factor). Though **motor strength is usually preserved**, patients show **loss of posterior column sensation (vibration and position sense), positive Romberg test, mild spasticity, loss of knee and ankle reflexes, and bilateral extensor plantar reflexes (Babinski sign)**. Patients may also present with **glossitis, mild dementia, or psychiatric symptoms.**

400. The answer is a. *(McPhee, pp 467-468.)* The peripheral blood results of a significantly elevated white blood count with **isolated lymphocytosis** are highly suggestive of **chronic lymphocytic leukemia (CLL), a malignant clonal proliferation of B cells**. Ninety percent of cases occur after age 50, with a median age of 70 at diagnosis. Often, smudge cells are seen in the peripheral blood smear. The **life expectancy** of this patient (**stage 0** since he has no lymphadenopathy, hepatosplenomegaly, anemia, or thrombocytopenia) is **greater than 10 years**. **Hypogammaglobulinemia** with subsequent infections from encapsulated organisms is a late manifestation of CLL. **Patients with CLL almost never undergo transformation into acute lymphoblastic leukemia**.

401. The answer is b. *(McPhee, pp 68-69.)* **Age-related physiologic changes** which can lead to falling (and which should be examined thoroughly on a physical examination) include cognitive decline; problems with reflexes (decreased righting reflex, absent ankle reflexes, postural instability); vision deficits resulting from presbyopia (due to decreased lens elasticity), macular degeneration or cataracts; degenerative joint disease impairing gait; urinary urgency from BPH; and balance impairment (slower, forward flexed, unsteady, increased body sway). One of the **most common and reversible causes** of falling is **medication use** (especially diuretics which can worsen **orthostasis** and cognition-altering benzodiazepines and sedative-hypnotics) and often **polypharmacy** (use of multiple medications).

402. The answer is b. *(McPhee, pp 1044-1045.)* **Paget disease of bone (osteitis deformans)** is a disorder in which normal bone is replaced by disorganized trabecular bone. The incidence of this diagnosis reaches 10% by age 80. Patients may be asymptomatic but may present with increased hat size (skull enlargement), hearing loss (involvement of the ossicles of the inner ear), facial pain, headache, backache, leg pain, growth of the lower extremities (one leg may be longer than the other), tibial bowing, and increased blood flow to the involved areas of bone growth. Alkaline phosphatase is usually markedly elevated, and a bone scan will detect lytic lesions in the skull and long bones. A complication of Paget disease is osteosarcoma (< 1%). None of the other answer choices will lead to this combination of symptoms and signs.

403. The answer is d. *(McPhee, p 69.)* When elderly patients fall, if they sustain a fracture, they most often fracture the **hip, wrist, or vertebrae**. **Femoral neck fractures** are common in the elderly and occur more frequently in women than in men, carrying up to a 20% mortality rate at 1 year. **Displaced fractures** cause pain and inability to walk. The involved extremity is often **shorter, slightly externally rotated, and abducted**, as in this patient. Acute ground-level falls do not usually lead to **hip bursitis** or **rupture of the quadriceps muscle**, and neither of these problems lead to the changes seen in this patients left leg.

404. The answer is c. *(Fauci, pp 139-143.)* **Syncope** is a transient loss of consciousness and postural tone which may or may not be preceded by dizziness, diaphoresis, or lightheadedness. It may result from disorders of vascular tone or blood volume (neurocardiogenic syncope, orthostatic hypotension), cardiac valvular disease or arrhythmias, and cerebrovascular causes. This patient most likely has **carotid sinus hypersensitivity**, which can induce syncope by putting pressure on the carotid sinus baroreceptors when turning the head to one side, wearing a tight shirt collar, or shaving over the carotid artery. Patients with this problem are usually men over the age of 50. Patients with **vasovagal**, or **neurocardiogenic**, **syncope** (common fainting) present with bradycardia and hypotension due to activation of the parasympathetic nervous system. **Cardiac syncope** results from a sudden reduction in cardiac output usually caused by an arrhythmia. The **subclavian steal syndrome (transient vertebrobasilar ischemia)** occurs with exercise of the upper extremities. When a subclavian artery is occluded and the patient exercises the upper arms, blood is stolen by the ipsilateral vertebral artery from the contralateral vertebral artery bypassing the subclavian artery (reversal of flow). Patients may have decreased radial pulse amplitude, lower blood pressure in the affected arm, and syncope. While this patient may have had a **TIA**, he likely would have some residual neurologic deficit in such a short time after the event.

405. The answer is d. *(McPhee, p 75.)* This patient appears to be the victim of **elder abuse**, an unfortunately common occurrence in patients 65 and older. **Neglect** is the most common form of abuse, followed by financial and emotional abuse. Lack of appropriate clothing, poor hygiene, unexplained injuries, and change in behavior in the presence of a possibly abusive caregiver should alert a provider to possible abuse. The laws in most states require a provider to report suspected abuse, and all 50 states have **adult protective service agencies** to investigate these claims.

406. The answer is a. *(McPhee, pp 248-249.)* This patient who has developed a lower respiratory tract infection in the nursing home has **health-care-associated pneumonia (HCAP)**. This infection is defined as pneumonia that occurs more than **48 hours after admission to a hospital or other health-care facility.** As a result of her recent stroke, she is at increased risk of aspiration of gastric secretions. The most common organisms causing HCAP are *Pseudomonas aeruginosa*, *Staphylococcus aureus* (including MRSA), *Klebsiella pneumoniae*, *Enterobacter,* and *Escherichia coli*, as well as anaerobic bacteria. Symptoms mimic those of community-acquired pneumonia: productive cough, fever, sweats, and occasionally, rigors, hemoptysis, and pleuritic chest pain. Because of the high mortality risk associated with HCAP, empiric antibiotic therapy should be initiated as soon as possible. While this elderly woman may be at increased risk for a **PE** after having a stroke, the increased fremitus, egophony, and rales would not be present in the event of a PE. **Asthma** would cause wheezing and both this and **bronchiectasis** would likely cause repeated symptomatic episodes, whereas this patient presents with pulmonary symptoms for the first time.

407. The answer is b. *(McPhee, pp 961-970.)* The patient has symptoms (depressed mood, anhedonia, and decreased energy and appetite) that are most consistent with **depression**. This diagnosis often accompanies loss of functional status in the elderly and may mimic or overlap delirium or dementia. In this patient, **delirium** from pain medications for his fracture should also be entertained, but he has no evidence of cognitive dysfunction on the MMSE to point to **dementia**. He also gives no history of altered mentation to suggest **schizophrenia** and has no other findings on physical examination beside a mood disorder, thereby making **Parkinson disease** less likely.

The mnemonic for depression is **SIG E CAPS**.

S = Sleep problems
I = decreased **I**nterest in life (anhedonia)
G = Guilt feelings
E = lowered **E**nergy level
C = decreased **C**oncentration
A = decreased **A**ppetite
P = **P**sychomotor retardation/agitation
S = Suicidal ideation

408. The answer is b. *(McPhee, pp 61-63.)* Patients who are unable to perform **IADLs** may be aided by a chore worker, a daycare program, a boarding home, or an assisted living situation. Once patients are unable to perform **ADLs**, they usually **require a nursing home** level of care or **a full-time caregiver** at home. An elderly patient's decline in function in response to disease usually follows the same pattern. **Hygiene or bathing are lost first,** followed by dressing, toileting, ambulating (transferring), and eating. Recovery usually occurs in the reverse order.

409. The answer is e. *(McPhee, pp 1134-1135.)* **Protein-energy malnutrition (PEM)** or **marasmus** results when the body's requirement for calories and protein is not met by the diet. It is characterized by wasting, loss of lean body mass, weight loss, and loss of subcutaneous fat stores. **Kwashiorkor** or severe deficiency of protein is characterized by edema, skin changes, change in hair pigmentation, and hypoalbuminemia. Although this elderly man should be screened for **hypothyroidism**, patients usually present with weight gain, arthralgias, myalgias cold intolerance, and constipation, among other things. Patients with **zinc deficiency** present with a psoriasiform rash, eczematous scaling, and loss of taste (hypogeusia). Patients with **riboflavin deficiency** present with scrotal dermatosis, photophobia, conjunctival inflammation, glossitis, angular stomatitis, and tongue atrophy.

410 to 412. The answers are 410-d, 411-b, 412-c. *(Seidel, p 578.)* Normal **postvoid residual urine volume (PVR)** is less than 50 mL, and normal bladder capacity is 400 to 600 mL. **Functional incontinence**, as seen in the stroke patient using a walker, is often due to the combination of cognitive impairment and immobility leading a patient to be unable to get to the bathroom in time to void. The urinary tract is intact in functional incontinence. **Stress incontinence** is found in postmenopausal women who have had multiple vaginal deliveries or in people with a history of pelvic surgery, and is characterized by the loss of small amounts of urine during activities that increase abdominal pressure, such as coughing, laughing, sneezing, and exercising. **Overflow incontinence** is caused by (1) an acontractile bladder (diabetes or spinal cord injury), (2) anatomic obstruction (BPH), and (3) detrusor sphincter dyssynergy or neurogenic bladder (multiple sclerosis and spinal cord lesions). Often, a tense, overdistended bladder can be palpated and percussed on abdominal examination. Patients with overflow incontinence often have leakage of small amounts of urine and PVRs of more than 100 mL. Patients with stroke, parkinsonism, dementia, and multiple sclerosis may have **urge incontinence** or **detrusor overactivity**. Urinary incontinence (sometimes of large volume) follows a sudden urge to urinate. The patient senses the need to void at below normal volumes (< 200 mL), and the bladder is unable to tolerate normal bladder capacity. **Urinary tract infections** may result in incontinence as well, but patients are usually symptomatic with symptoms such as dysuria, urgency, hematuria, and fever.

Infectious Diseases

Questions

413. A 25-year-old heterosexual man develops a urethral discharge and dysuria 5 days after having unprotected sexual intercourse with a new partner. Physical examination reveals meatal erythema. There are no penile lesions and no inguinal lymphadenopathy. A purulent urethral discharge is evident. Gram stain of the discharge reveals neutrophils and intracellular gram-negative diplococci, and the patient is treated for *Neisseria gonorrhoeae*. Two weeks after antibiotic therapy (ceftriaxone intramuscular injection), the patient returns with a clear urethral discharge and dysuria. Gram stain reveals many neutrophils but no organisms. Which of the following is the most likely diagnosis?

a. Resistant strain of *N. gonorrhoeae*
b. Lymphogranuloma venereum
c. Chancroid
d. *Chlamydia trachomatis* urethritis
e. Syphilis infection

414. A 41-year-old woman presents with a maculopapular rash on her soles and palms. Both the VDRL (RPR) and FTA-ABS are positive. Two hours after being treated with penicillin, the patient develops fever, chills, myalgias, tachypnea, tachycardia, and leukocytosis. Which of the following is the most likely diagnosis?

a. Neurosyphilis
b. Tertiary syphilis
c. Jarisch-Herxheimer reaction
d. Rocky Mountain spotted fever
e. Endocarditis

415. A 26-year-old woman presents with disseminated gonorrhea. She has a past medical history significant for meningococcal meningitis when she was 19 years old. Which of the following complement deficiencies is the most likely cause of her recurrent infections?

a. C2
b. C3
c. C3, C4
d. C5, C6, C7, C8, C9
e. Clq, Clr, Cls

416. A 19-year-old previously healthy college student presents with a 5-day history of fever, generalized malaise, and sore throat. He denies cough. He does not use illicit drugs and uses condoms every time with his sole sexual partner. He has been vaccinated against hepatitis B. On physical examination the patient appears jaundiced and has a temperature of 38.7°C (101.7°F). The pharynx is erythematous but has no exudate. There is bilateral tender cervical lymphadenopathy. Liver size is 14 cm in the midclavicular line (MCL), and the spleen tip is palpable 2 cm below the left costal margin. The white blood cell count is elevated, and many atypical forms are reported. Which of the following is the most appropriate confirmatory diagnostic test?

a. Blood culture
b. Monospot
c. Hepatitis B surface antigen
d. Hepatitis C antibody
e. Sputum culture

417. A neonate develops meningitis, and you suspect that the responsible organism was acquired during passage through the birth canal. Which of the following organisms is most likely responsible for the neonate's illness?

a. *Staphylococcus aureus*
b. *Pseudomonas*
c. *Rubeola*
d. *Listeria monocytogenes*
e. *Salmonella*

418. A 23-year-old man presents with the acute onset of fever, skin lesions on his extremities that are papular and erythematous with a hemorrhagic and necrotic center, joint pain, and an acute tenosynovitis of the dorsum of his left foot. He has no past medical history and takes no medications. He does not smoke, drink alcohol, or use illicit drugs. On physical examination, the patient has a temperature of 39.1°C (102.4°F). Passive flexion and extension of the left great toe causes severe pain over the dorsum of the midfoot and ankle. Which of the following is the most likely diagnosis?

a. de Quervain tenosynovitis
b. Reiter syndrome
c. Acute gouty attack
d. Disseminated gonococcal infection
e. Still disease

419. A 52-year-old man presents with fever and leukocytosis. He has splinter hemorrhages and a holosystolic murmur that radiates to the axilla. Transesophageal echocardiogram demonstrates several vegetations located on the mitral valve; there is moderate mitral regurgitation. Blood culture bottles continuously reveal no growth of organisms. Which of the following may be the causal agent of the patient's endocarditis?

a. *Staphylococcus aureus*
b. *Campylobacter jejuni*
c. *Haemophilus aphrophilus*
d. *Vibrio parahaemolyticus*
e. *Streptococcus viridans*

420. A 40-year-old gardener presents with painless papules that appeared following a puncture wound from a rose thorn a few weeks earlier. Physical examination reveals a chain of erythematous nodules along the dorsal aspect of the arm. Which of the following is the most likely diagnosis?

a. Coccidioidomycosis
b. Sporotrichosis
c. Blastomycosis
d. Cutaneous larva migrans
e. Histoplasmosis

421. An ill-looking 58-year-old man with a 20-year history of diabetes mellitus presents with severe pain and swelling of his right arm that started 2 days ago after some minor trauma. He has a temperature of 39.8°C (103.6°F). Examination of the arm reveals a 13-cm area of dark red epidermal induration. Large bullae filled with purple fluid are seen in the center of the wound. Some parts of the wound are friable and appear black in color. Crepitus is felt with palpation of the arm. Laboratory data reveal a leukocytosis and an elevated serum creatinine phosphokinase. Which of the following is the most likely diagnosis?

a. Bullous pemphigoid
b. Folliculitis
c. Necrotizing fasciitis
d. Cellulitis
e. Fournier gangrene

422. A 54-year-old man presents with a 2-week history of headache, fever, chills, and night sweats. He complains of myalgias and easy fatigability. He has just returned from a business trip to Africa and the Middle East. Before the trip, the patient received immunizations against poliomyelitis, hepatitis A, hepatitis B, and dengue fever. Throughout the trip, he took chloroquine prophylaxis against malaria. On physical examination, the patient has a temperature of 39.5°C (103.2°F) and is diaphoretic. There is no neck stiffness, photophobia, or lymphadenopathy. Heart and lung examinations are normal. There is mild splenomegaly. Which of the following is the most likely diagnosis in this patient?

a. Malaria
b. Tuberculosis
c. Mononucleosis
d. Trypanosomiasis
e. Toxoplasmosis

423. A 68-year-old man with endocarditis and bacteremia from *Streptococcus bovis* infection may have a high incidence of which of the following malignancies?

a. Prostate cancer
b. Pancreatic cancer
c. Lymphoma
d. Colon cancer
e. Lung cancer

424. A 27-year-old man was recently diagnosed HIV positive. As part of his routine workup for his new diagnosis, his CD4 count was 285/μL and his RPR came back positive at a titer of 1:64. On physical examination he does not have a penile chancre or any findings of the cardiovascular, lung, or neurologic systems. What is the most appropriate next step?

a. Treatment with benzathine penicillin G intramuscularly once
b. Treatment with aqueous penicillin G intravenously
c. Lumbar puncture
d. Blood cultures
e. Repeat nontreponemal serologic tests

425. A 35-year-old woman presents with fever, diarrhea, and right upper quadrant pain. She recently returned from a 2-month business trip in Mexico. Physical examination reveals no jaundice. She has point tenderness over the liver and has a positive fecal occult blood test. Computed tomography (CT) scan of the abdomen reveals several oval lesions in the liver. Which of the following is the most likely etiology of this patient's symptoms?

a. Hepatitis A infection
b. *Echinococcus granulosus*
c. *Enterobius vermicularis*
d. *Entamoeba histolytica*
e. *Campylobacter jejuni*

426. A 46-year-old woman with a recent history of sinusitis presents with a severe headache. She complains of neck stiffness and photophobia. On physical examination she has a temperature of 39.7°C (103.4°F). Blood pressure is normal, and heart rate is 110 beats per minute. She has nuchal rigidity with a normal funduscopic examination and no focal neurologic deficit. Brudzinski and Kernig signs are positive. Which of the following is the most likely diagnosis?

a. Migraine headache
b. Bacterial meningitis
c. Torticollis
d. Cluster headache
e. Cysticercosis

427. A 16-year-old boy is bitten on the leg by a neighbor's dog. The dog is healthy and has proof of a rabies vaccination. The next day, the patient develops a cellulitis at the site of the bite, accompanied by a purulent, foul-smelling discharge. There is unilateral inguinal lymphadenopathy. Which of the following organisms is most likely responsible for the patient's symptoms?

a. Rabies virus
b. *Pasteurella multocida*
c. *Aeromonas hydrophila*
d. *Pseudomonas aeruginosa*
e. *Vibrio parahaemolyticus*

428. A 41-year-old woman develops abdominal cramps and diarrhea 2 hours after eating fried rice. Physical examination is normal except for some mild abdominal tenderness with palpation. Examination of the stool reveals no fecal leukocytes. Which of the following is the most likely etiology for the symptoms?

a. *Shigella*
b. *Salmonella*
c. *Vibrio cholerae*
d. *Bacillus cereus*
e. *Staphylococcus aureus*
f. *Vibrio parahaemolyticus*

429. A 33-year-old woman in her second trimester of her first pregnancy comes to see you in October. She has no prior medical history and no complaints except for rhinitis. So far no one around her has been sick, but she wants to be protected during the upcoming flu season. Her vital signs and the remainder of her physical examination are normal for her stage of pregnancy, other than mildly erythematous nasal mucosa and clear drainage. What is the most appropriate recommendation regarding protection against the flu for this patient?

a. She should receive the influenza intramuscular vaccination at this time.
b. She should receive the influenza vaccine intranasal mist at this time.
c. She should be given prophylaxis with a neuraminidase inhibitor.
d. She should not receive flu vaccination until her rhinitis has resolved.
e. She should not receive flu vaccination because she is pregnant.

430. A 34-year-old woman was recently told by another physician that her blood test was positive for *Helicobacter pylori*. She completed a course of medication but is concerned about this finding. This patient is at risk for which of the following?

a. Squamous cell carcinoma of the esophagus
b. Adenocarcinoma of the esophagus
c. Non-Hodgkin lymphoma of the small intestine
d. Gastroesophageal reflux disease
e. Mucosa-associated tissue lymphomas (MALT)

431. A 22-year-old woman with sickle cell disease presents with a painful pretibial ulcer. Physical examination reveals the presence of purulent material draining from the wound site. The patient has a low-grade fever. Radiographs reveal soft tissue swelling and a periosteal reaction. Which of the following is the most likely pathogen responsible for the symptoms?

a. *Staphylococcus epidermis*
b. *Salmonella*
c. *Shigella*
d. *Streptococcus pyogenes*
e. *Mycobacterium tuberculosis*

432. A 37-year-old postal worker from Atlantic City, New Jersey, presents to the emergency room with the chief complaint of dry cough for several days. He has fever, malaise, dyspnea on exertion, and pleuritic chest pain. He has experienced mild nausea and diffuse abdominal pain. He has been in good health otherwise and has no recent travel history. No contacts have been ill. Physical examination is remarkable for a temperature of 38.5°C (101.4°F) and decreased breath sounds at the lung bases bilaterally. Chest radiograph reveals pleural effusions and a widened mediastinum. Which of the following is the most likely diagnosis?

a. Pneumonic plague
b. Tularemia
c. Hemorrhagic fever
d. Inhalation anthrax
e. Hantavirus pulmonary syndrome

433. A 47-year-old nurse presents to your office complaining of a poorly healing ulcer of her left second digit. The ulcer started a week ago and is painless. The patient has tried using over-the-counter antibacterial and hydrocortisone creams without improvement. She denies trauma to the hand. The patient has a temperature of 38.4°C (101.1°F) and left-sided epitrochlear and axillary adenopathy. She has a 4-cm ulcer on the dorsal side of the left second digit covered by a black eschar and surrounded by an extensive amount of nonpitting edema. Which of the following is the most likely diagnosis?

a. Smallpox infection
b. Cutaneous anthrax
c. Cat-scratch disease
d. Leprosy infection
e. Brown recluse spider bite

434. A 79-year-old woman presents to the emergency room with a 1-week history of fever, myalgias, nausea, vomiting, and diarrhea. Her symptoms started shortly after she ate at a Mexican restaurant with her daughter and son-in-law. She did not eat raw foods, and her family members did not become ill. She has no past medical history and takes no medications. She has a temperature of 39.5°C (103.2°F) and appears extremely ill. She is awake and oriented to person and place but not to time. Heart and lung examinations are normal, and she has no focal neurologic deficits. CT scan of the head is normal. Lumbar puncture reveals pleocytosis, increased protein concentration, and normal glucose. Blood and cerebrospinal fluid cultures identify a gram-positive rod organism. Which of the following is the most likely diagnosis?

a. *Actinomyces* infection
b. *Bacillus cereus* infection
c. Invasive *Listeria* infection
d. Inhalation anthrax infection
e. *Clostridium botulinum* infection

435. A 61-year-old man presents to a Houston emergency room in the summertime with a 3-day history of fever, malaise, sore throat, nausea, and vomiting. While being examined by a medical student, the patient becomes lethargic, then convulses, requiring intravenous benzodiazepam administration. Physical examination is remarkable for a temperature of 38.3°C (101.0°F). There is bilateral papilledema and neck stiffness. Deep tendon reflexes are exaggerated, and spastic paralysis is evident. Which of the following is the most likely diagnosis?

a. Mollaret meningitis
b. Neurosyphilis
c. Herpes simplex virus
d. Cerebrovascular accident
e. Brain abscess
f. West Nile virus
g. Heatstroke

Questions 436 to 438

For each patient with symptoms, select the most likely responsible pathogen. Each lettered option may be used once, multiple times, or not at all.

a. *Giardia lamblia*
b. *Trichinella spiralis*
c. *Chlamydia psittaci*
d. *Acanthamoeba castellanii*
e. *Brucella*
f. *Clostridium tetani*
g. *Taenia solium*

436. A 41-year-old man presents with periorbital edema, myalgias, and eosinophilia 3 weeks after eating some undercooked pork at an outdoor restaurant.

437. A 19-year-old college student develops a keratitis thought to be secondary to use of disposable soft contact lenses.

438. A 28-year-old immigrant from Mexico is brought to the emergency room because of new onset of seizures. CT scan of the head reveals several discrete calcified densities throughout the frontal lobe, brainstem, and cerebellum.

Questions 439 to 441

For each patient listed, choose the **minimum** reaction size of their tuberculin skin test (PPD) that would warrant treatment for latent tuberculosis. Each lettered option may be used once, multiple times, or not at all.

a. ≥ 5 mm
b. ≥ 10 mm
c. ≥ 15 mm
d. ≥ 20 mm
e. ≥ 25 mm

439. An incarcerated 56-year-old man with COPD presents with a chronic cough.

440. A 42-year-old woman who recently emigrated from Guatemala has no history of prior BCG vaccination. She has no cough, fever, or night sweats.

441. A 23-year-old man, newly diagnosed HIV positive, is asymptomatic.

Questions 442 and 443

For each patient with neurologic symptoms, select the most likely diagnosis. Each lettered option may be used once, multiple times, or not at all.

a. Toxoplasmosis
b. Cryptococcal meningitis
c. Progressive multifocal leukoencephalopathy (PML)
d. Human immunodeficiency virus (HIV) dementia

442. A 37-year-old woman with HIV presents with headache, irritability, and confusion. Funduscopic examination reveals bilateral papilledema. India ink smear of the spinal fluid is positive.

443. A 47-year-old woman with HIV presents with new right-sided arm and leg weakness. CT scan of the head reveals multiple ring-enhancing lesions located in both hemispheres and involving the basal ganglia and corticomedullary junction.

Infectious Diseases

Answers

413. The answer is d. *(McPhee, p 1328.)* The patient has been treated for **gonococcal urethritis** which can be diagnosed with Gram stain, culture, or now, more commonly with **nucleic acid amplification tests.** He now needs treatment for concomitant ***C trachomatis*** infection, as **coinfection is common.** A negative nucleic acid amplification test for *Chlamydia* reliably excludes the diagnosis, but since in this case it was not performed, **presumptive therapy is indicated.** Patients require treatment for the gonococcal infection (usually ceftriaxone intramuscularly) and doxycycline, azithromycin, or levofloxacin for eradication of the chlamydial infection. **Gonococcal resistance** to penicillin and tetracycline (but not to ceftriaxone) has developed. Patients with **lymphogranuloma venereum** (*C trachomatis* types L1-L3) present with inguinal buboes. Patients with **chancroid** (*Haemophilus ducreyi*) present with a painful genital ulcer. **Primary syphilis** is characterized by a painless chancre that appears 21 days after exposure and disappears in 3 to 6 weeks.

414. The answer is c. *(McPhee, p 1333.)* The **Jarisch-Herxheimer reaction** is a self-limited, dramatic flu-like reaction that occurs within 2 hours of treatment for early (most commonly secondary) syphilis. It is thought to be due to the massive destruction of spirochetes and the formation of inflammatory mediators **(tumor necrosis factor).** The **Venereal Disease Research Laboratory (VDRL) rapid plasma regain (RPR)** is a nonspecific screening test for syphilis and reverts to negative with treatment. The **fluorescent treponemal antibody absorption (FTA-ABS)** is a sensitive and specific diagnostic test and will remain positive for life. **Neurosyphilis** can occur at any stage and can be asymptomatic or manifest as meningitis, tabes dorsalis (diminished proprioception and vibration sense, Argyll Robertson pupils and hypotonia of musculature), or general confusion. **Tertiary syphilis** is rarely seen in this era of antibiotic therapy and refers to gummas of the skin, bones, and liver as well as aortitis and dementia or psychosis. **Endocarditis** might have the fever and other generalized symptoms described in this case, as well as a new or changing murmur, but these symptoms would not suddenly occur after penicillin treatment. The rash of **Rocky Mountain spotted fever** begins in the palms and soles and spreads centrally; the disease may be confirmed by the **Weil-Felix test**.

415. The answer is d. *(Fauci, pp 2030-2031.)* Patients deficient in terminal complement components **C5, C6, C7, C8,** and **C9** (resulting in the **membrane attack complex**) are susceptible to **gonococcal and meningococcal** infections due to an inability to mount a bactericidal response to these organisms.

416. The answer is b. *(McPhee, pp 1243-1245.)* The patient's symptomatology (fever, sore throat, and malaise) is most consistent with **infectious mononucleosis**, which is transmitted through saliva. Physical examination often reveals **posterior cervical lymphadenopathy, exudative pharyngitis, and splenomegaly** in up to half of patients. **If ampicillin is given** for a mistaken diagnosis of strep pharyngitis, **more than 90% of patients will develop a maculopapular rash.** While the other answer choices might be appropriate as well, a **monospot test or heterophile antibody test** must be ordered to confirm the most likely diagnosis of Epstein-Barr virus (EBV) mononucleosis syndrome. If the heterophile test is negative, the most likely etiology of the mononucleosis is **cytomegalovirus (CMV)**, which usually manifests more commonly with rashes but **without exudative pharyngitis or cervical lymphadenopathy. Atypical lymphocytes** may be seen transiently in EBV, CMV, toxoplasmosis, drug reactions, viral hepatitis, rubella, mumps, and rubeola.

417. The answer is d. *(Kliegman, pp 797-798, 804-807.)* Organisms of the female genital tract may be acquired during passage through the birth canal and may cause meningitis in neonates. The **most common causes** include ***L monocytogenes*, group B β-hemolytic streptococci, and gram-negative rods such as *Escherichia coli*;** however, *Streptococcus pneumoniae, Haemophilus influenzae*, staphylococci, *Klebsiella, Enterobacter, Pseudomonas, Treponema pallidum,* and *M. tuberculosis* may also cause neonatal meningitis. Neonates may develop infections outside the birth canal, namely *Salmonella, S. aureus, Proteus,* and *Pseudomonas,* from contact with contaminated persons or articles after birth. The **TORCHES** organisms (**TO**xoplasmosis, **R**ubella, **C**ytomegalovirus, **HE**rpes simplex, **S**yphilis) and HIV are other intrauterine-acquired infections.

418. The answer is d. *(Fauci, pp 918-919.)* **Disseminated gonococcal infection** is the leading cause of bacterial arthritis in young adults. This disease often starts as an early **tenosynovitis-dermatitis syndrome** (including papules and pustules on the extremities in up to 75% of patients), which is often followed by a **septic arthritis.** The joints most commonly involved include the **knee, wrist, ankle, or elbow.** Gonococci are **only isolated in half of joint fluid cultures**, so blood should also be cultured and consideration should be given to culturing other areas such as the pharynx and urethra as well. **de Quervain tenosynovitis** is a chronic inflammation of the common sheath of the abductor pollicis longus and extensor pollicis brevis tendons due to repetitive use and causes marked pain and tenderness in the region of the anatomic snuffbox in the hand. In **Reiter syndrome**, patients develop an inflammatory arthritis after an episode of urethritis, dysentery, or cervicitis. It is more common in males than in females, and HLA-B27 is present in more than 60% of patients. Other findings in Reiter syndrome include conjunctivitis, circinate balanitis (superficial ulcer on the glans penis), and keratoderma blennorrhagica (papules on the soles of the feet). Patients with **Still disease** present with a salmon-colored rash, symmetrical joint involvement, and hepatosplenomegaly. **Gout** may cause joint inflammation of the ankle and great toe, but would not cause this patient's rash or high fever.

419. The answer is c. *(McPhee, p 1307.)* Specific gram-negative organisms are slow growing (fastidious) and require carbon dioxide for growth. Blood cultures may take 30 days to become positive. These organisms cause less than 5% of cases of endocarditis and are often referred to as the **HACEK** organisms (***H****aemophilus parainfluenzae*, ***H****aemophilus aphrophilus*, ***A****ctinobacillus actinomycetemcomitans*, ***C****ardiobacterium hominis*, ***E****ikenella corrodens*, and ***K****ingella kingae*). Culture-negative endocarditis may also occur in fungal infections or those needing to grow on special media.

420. The answer is b. *(McPhee, pp 1399-1400.)* The occupational history and skin findings are consistent with **sporotrichosis.** The mycotic organism *Sporothrix schenckii* is found in soil. The lesion begins as a painless nodule that eventually becomes fixed and necrotic. After a few weeks, multiple nodules develop along the lymphatic channels, causing a chronic nodular lymphangitis. **Blastomycosis** is endemic in the southeastern United States and may be found in agricultural workers but is characterized by pulmonary symptoms. Skin lesions are usually ulcerated, hyperkeratotic, and verrucous. **Histoplasmosis** is transmitted through bird and bat droppings and is endemic in the Ohio and Mississippi River valleys of the United States. Agricultural workers and others involved in outdoor activities, including cave explorers, are at risk for outbreaks. An acute pulmonary infection typically precedes the skin lesions. **Coccidioidomycosis** is caused by a soil saprophyte endemic to the arid San Joaquin Valley of the United States (Arizona, California, and western Texas). Patients present with respiratory symptoms and skin lesions such as **erythema nodosum.** **Cutaneous larva migrans** is caused by hookworms and is most common in children in the southeastern United States. Patients develop pruritic papules of the hands and feet which develop tracks and then lesions become vesicles or crusts.

421. The answer is c. *(McPhee, p 129.)* **Necrotizing fasciitis** is a painful and rapidly spreading infection of the fascia of muscle that often begins at the site of nonpenetrating minor trauma. It should be suspected in patients who are significantly ill with skin bullae or crepitus (crunching of the skin due to small bubbles of air moving through the tissues due to the presence of gas-producing organisms like *Clostridium perfringens*) and laboratory evidence of rhabdomyolysis or disseminated intravascular coagulation. It is usually due to *S pyogenes,* although infections may be polymicrobial. Toxicity is severe, and patients require immediate surgical exploration to deep fascia and muscle and subsequent debridement. Necrotizing fasciitis that leaks into the peritoneum is called **Fournier gangrene. Bullous pemphigoid** is a benign, self-limited skin disorder found in older adults and characterized by tense blisters in flexural areas. **Cellulitis** is an acute inflammatory condition of the skin that causes erythema, pain, and localized swelling. **Folliculitis** is typically due to *S aureus;* patients present with pustules at the insertion site of hair follicles.

422. The answer is a. *(McPhee, pp 1353-1362.)* ***Plasmodium falciparum***, the predominant species in Africa, is now commonly **resistant to prophylaxis with chloroquine.** Chemoprophylaxis is never entirely reliable, and malaria must always be considered in the differential diagnosis of fever in patients who have traveled to endemic areas, like this patient. **Trypanosomiasis,** caused by the protozoan *Trypanosoma cruzi,* is a parasite found only in the Americas; patients present with **Romaña sign** (unilateral and painless edema of the periocular tissues) and cardiomyopathy **(Chagas**

disease). Patients with **toxoplasmosis** who are immunocompetent are generally asymptomatic and have self-limiting disease, while immunocompromised patients may develop ring-enhancing brain lesions. While this patient's symptoms could be consistent with **TB** or **mononucleosis** (which can be accompanied by fever, fatigue and splenomegaly), his recent travel to an area endemic for malaria make that diagnosis more likely.

423. The answer is d. *(Fauci, p 575.)* For unknown reasons, patients with ***S. bovis*** **bacteremia** have a high incidence of **colon carcinoma** (and perhaps upper gastrointestinal malignancies as well) and require colonoscopy.

424. The answer is c. *(McPhee, pp 1337-1338.)* HIV-positive patients should be screened at least every 6 months with RPR or VDRL to identify latent disease. A **lumbar puncture (LP)** should be performed in HIV patients with **positive nontreponemal antibody titers of greater than or equal to 1:32** and those whose **CD4 counts are less than or equal to 350/μL** as these populations have an increased risk of developing neurosyphilis. In addition, an LP should be performed for all patients with **late latent syphilis or infection of unknown duration**, if **neurologic signs** are present or if they have **failed previous therapy.** Some experts recommend an LP for all HIV positive patients, but it may not be needed in those with primary (presence of a chancre) or secondary syphilis. Patients who are positive for neurosyphilis should be treated with intravenous aqueous penicillin G for 10 to 14 days and also for late latent syphilis with benzathine penicillin G intramuscular weekly for 3 weeks.

425. The answer is d. *(McPhee, p 1366.)* ***Entamoeba histolytica*** is the third most common cause of death by parasites worldwide (after schistosomiasis and malaria). Endemic areas include Mexico, India, Central America, South America, tropical Asia, and Africa. Amebiasis may infect the intestines, causing abdominal pain and diarrhea to more severe hematochezia with dysentery. Physical examination findings may include high fever, abdominal distention, hyperperistalsis, right upper quadrant pain, and hepatomegaly, and stools that are FOBT positive. The most common extraintestinal infection is **amebic liver abscess**, presenting as abdominal pain, fever, right upper quadrant pain, and weight loss. Stool evaluation for organisms is not sensitive, so at least three stool samples should be evaluated. Abdominal ultrasound, CT scan, or MRI typically show the abscesses.

Echinococcus granulosus is a tapeworm infection causing cysts in the lung and liver resulting from exposure to domestic dogs in areas such as Africa, the Middle East, South America, and even the southwestern United States. ***Enterobius vermicularis*** is the pinworm, which usually causes school-age children to experience nocturnal perianal pruritus. **Hepatitis A** is a food-borne viral illness presenting with right upper quadrant pain, malaise, jaundice, and low-grade fever. ***Campylobacter jejuni*** causes a self-limited illness of fever, diarrea that may be bloody, and cramps from undercooked poultry or unpasteurized milk.

426. The answer is b. *(Seidel, pp 791-792.)* This patient demonstrates signs of meningeal irritation: she has **nuchal rigidity** (significant neck stiffness), a positive **Brudzinski sign** (involuntary flexion of the hips and knees when flexing the neck), and a positive **Kernig sign** (flexing the hip and knee when the patient is supine, then straightening out the leg, causes resistance and back pain). Other symptoms and signs of **meningitis** include headache, photophobia, seizures, and altered mental status. Patients with meningitis (< 1%) rarely have papilledema secondary to increased intracranial pressure. Risk factors for meningitis include sinusitis, ear infection, and sick contacts. None of the other answer choices cause the combination of fever, neck stiffness, and specific signs.

427. The answer is b. *(McPhee, pp 1165-1166.)* Dogs are responsible for 80% of animal bites; organisms include ***P multocida* (the single most common isolate),** *Eikenella corrodens,* and *Capnocytophaga canimorsus* (formerly called DF-2). ***Aeromonas hydrophila*** is the organism seen in bite wounds from alligators and other aquatic animals. **Rabies** is an acute viral disease of the central nervous system and is transmitted by infected dogs, cats, skunks, foxes, raccoons, mongooses, wolves, and bats. ***Pseudomonas aeruginosa*** may cause a variety of skin lesions, such as hot tub folliculitis and ecthyma gangrenosum. ***Vibrio parahaemolyticus*** is an organism found in undercooked shellfish; patients present with diarrhea.

428. The answer is d. *(McPhee, pp 1170-1172.)* The incubation period for both ***S aureus*** and ***B cereus*** preformed toxins is 1 to 8 hours after eating. *Bacillus cereus* toxicity is often due to eating reheated fried (**the toxin is heat-stable**) or uncooked rice. *Staphylococcus aureus* toxicity is usually due to eating ham, poultry, potato, or egg salad, mayonnaise, or cream pastries.

All the other organisms require an incubation period of more than 16 hours. ***Vibrio* cholerae** toxicity is due to eating shellfish and causes an inflammatory (presence of fecal leukocytes) diarrhea. ***Vibrio parahaemolyticus*** toxicity is due to eating undercooked mollusks and crustaceans and causes dysentery (production of cytotoxins, bacterial invasion, and destruction of intestinal mucosal cells). ***Salmonella*** toxicity is due to eating beef, poultry, eggs, or dairy products and causes a watery diarrhea. ***Shigella*** causes dysentery and can be present in potato or egg salad, lettuce, or raw vegetables.

429. The answer is a. *(McPhee, pp 1194-1198.)* Pregnant women are considered at increased risk for contracting influenza due to their immunocompromised state. This patient has rhinitis of pregnancy but no other symptoms or fever. As a result, immunization with the **killed influenza virus, via intramuscular injection, is absolutely indicated** in this patient at this time. Ideally pregnant women should wait until after the first trimester, but if it is high flu season, they should be immunized even early on in their pregnancy. **Live attenuated viruses are contraindicated in pregnancy**; therefore, pregnant women should not receive the influenza intranasal spray vaccine. Neuraminidase inhibitors, like zanamivir and oseltamivir, are available for prevention and therapy of influenza A and B, but immunization is preferred as she has not been exposed to anyone with the flu and has no flu symptoms.

430. The answer is e. *(McPhee, pp 1470-1473.)* ***Helicobacter pylori*** is associated with gastritis, duodenal ulcer, gastric ulcer, non-Hodgkin gastric lymphoma, adenocarcinoma of the stomach, and mucosa-associated tissue lymphomas **(MALT)**.

431. The answer is b. *(Fauci, p 961.)* **Osteomyelitis** is usually a polymicrobial infection, but *S. aureus* is the pathogen in more than 50% of all cases. Patients with sickle cell disease are at risk of developing ***Salmonella* osteomyelitis** (> 50% of all cases), most commonly in the humerus, tibia, femur, or lumbar vertebrae. **Pott disease** is spinal tuberculosis; it usually involves the upper thoracic vertebral bodies.

432. The answer is d. *(McPhee, p 1301.)* The postal worker from New Jersey is presenting with symptoms most consistent with **inhalation anthrax.** Sentinel clues include chest pain, shortness of breath, malaise, headache, fever, dry cough, abdominal pain, and nausea. Chest radiograph may show a **widened mediastinum** (mediastinitis) and pleural effusions (thoracentesis will show these to be hemorrhagic). This presentation rapidly leads to sepsis, shock, and respiratory failure. Although anthrax was previously rare except among high-risk groups such as farmers, tannery workers, wool workers, and veterinarians, bioterroristic use has resulted in cases. Patients with **pneumonic plague** present with mucopurulent sputum, chest pain, and hemoptysis. **Tularemia** is a gram-negative coccobacillus that causes pneumonia accompanied by bilateral hilar adenopathy. Patients with **hemorrhagic fever** present with generalized mucous membrane hemorrhage and evidence of pulmonary, renal, neurologic, and hematopoietic dysfunction. **Hantavirus** is a rodent-borne RNA virus more common in the southwestern United States; patients present in a shocklike state with thrombocytopenia and leukocytosis.

433. The answer is b. *(McPhee, p 1300)* Fever, regional adenopathy, and a painless ulcer covered by a black eschar and surrounded by extensive nonpitting edema is a presentation most consistent with **cutaneous anthrax.** Patients with **leprosy** present with pale, anesthetic, and erythematous macular or nodular skin lesions. **Cat-scratch disease** is an acute infection of children and young adults transmitted by cats through a scratch or bite. Patients develop a papule or ulcer at the site of the inoculation and weeks later develop fever, malaise, headache, and regional lymphadenopathy. Patients with **smallpox** present with generalized macular or papular vesicular-pustular eruptions, with the greatest concentration of the rash being on the face and the distal extremities, especially the palms. Although spider bites are rare, the bite of the **brown recluse spider** may cause a severe necrotic reaction and death due to intravascular hemolysis.

434. The answer is c. *(Fauci, pp 895-897.)* The patient is presenting with ***Listeria,*** an intracellular pathogen with a predilection for causing illness in immunocompromised persons, including the elderly, cancer patients, and chronic alcoholics. Transmission is food-borne; implicated foods include coleslaws, soft cheeses such as **Mexican cheeses,** undercooked hot dogs, and deli meats. Patients typically present with bacteremia and meningitis. **Botulism** bacillus is usually found in canned, smoked, or vacuum-packed foods. Patients present with "**the Ds**": **d**ysphagia, **d**ysphonia, visual **d**isturbances, **d**iplopia, ptosis, and fixed and **d**ilated pupils. Patients with

anthrax present with cough, dyspnea, and evidence of mediastinitis and pneumonia. Fried rice consumption is associated with ***B cereus*** infection; patients present with a noninflammatory diarrhea. ***Actinomyces*** species are gram-positive organisms that may branch out into bacillary forms. Infection typically follows trauma, such as a **dental extraction**.

435. The answer is f. *(McPhee, pp 1257-1259.)* Identified in 1999, the **West Nile virus** is an arbovirus (arthropod-borne agent) that causes malaise, lethargy, sore throat, stiff neck, nausea, and vomiting. It progresses to stupor, convulsions, cranial nerve palsies, paralysis of extremities, and exaggerated deep tendon reflexes (signs of upper motor neuron disease). Specific antiviral therapy is not available for West Nile virus infection, and prognosis is almost always guarded. **Neurosyphilis** has a progressive course and patients may present with signs of a chronic meningitis (headache, irritability, unequal reflexes, and irregular pupils) or **tabes dorsalis** (hyporeflexia, hypotonia, and impairment of proprioception and vibration sense). Patients with **heatstroke** typically have core body temperatures above 40.5°C (105°F). **Mollaret meningitis** is a benign recurrent lymphocytic meningitis. **Herpes simplex virus** has been implicated as a major cause of Mollaret meningitis; it is associated with headache, flu-like symptoms, behavioral and speech disturbances, and seizures (often, temporal lobe). Patients with **brain abscesses** and **cerebrovascular accidents** typically present with more focal neurologic findings.

436 to 438. The answers are 436-b, 437-d, 438-g. *(McPhee, pp 1368-1369, 1377-1378, 1383-1384.)* **Trichinosis** is caused by the ingestion of infected pork products. Patients present with abdominal pain, diarrhea, a maculopapular rash, periorbital edema, myositis (especially of the extraocular muscles), eosinophilia, and myocarditis. ***Acanthamoeba castellanii*** can cause a dangerous corneal infection following trauma associated with contact lens usage and contaminated saline solution. **Brucellosis** is transmitted through infected milk or raw meat or inhaled during contact with animals (ie, by slaughterhouse workers, veterinarians, and farmers). Patients present with fever, chills, ophthalmoplegia, joint pain, skin rash, lymphadenopathy, hepatosplenomegaly, cardiac murmur, endocarditis, and meningitis. **Cysticercosis** is associated with the pork tapeworm **(*T solium*)**; patients commonly present with neurologic manifestations, such as seizures and signs of increased intracranial pressure. CT scan of the head often shows the multiple calcified lesions of varying size common in neurocysticercosis. ***Giardia lamblia*** may be asymptomatic or may cause severe diarrhea and malabsorption. Transmission is usually waterborne (ie, camping sites, sewers, reservoirs), since the cysts survive both cold water and routine chlorination. ***Chlamydia psittaci*** is associated with bird exposure; patients present with fever, cough, chest pain, dyspnea, pleural effusion, pleural rub, pericardial effusion, and pneumonia. Patients with ***C tetani*** present with an infected wound, muscle spasms, and increased muscle tone, especially of the masseter muscles **(lockjaw)**.

439 to 441. The answers are 439-b, 440-b. 441-a. *(McPhee, pp 253-254).* The **tuberculin skin test (PPD)** identifies people who have been infected with *M. tuberculosis* (TB) and is performed on those individuals at high risk for contact exposure (eg, inmates or health-care workers) or those who are symptomatic. Purified protein derivative (PPD) is injected intradermally on the forearm and then 48 to 72 hours later, the transverse diameter of induration is measured. It takes between 2 and 10 weeks after tuberculosis infection for a positive response to develop. Asymptomatic individuals with positive test results benefit for treatment of latent infection to reduce their risk of developing active disease.

The threshold for positive results in certain high-risk populations (and at which treatment for latent infection should be initiated) are

≥ 5 mm	Contacts of individuals with active TB
	Immunocompromised individuals (HIV positive, organ transplant patients, etc.)
	Asymptomatic but with evidence of old TB on radiographs
≥ 10 mm	Health-care workers
	Residents of nursing homes or other long-term care facilities
	Inmates of correctional institutions
	Recent immigrants from countries with high TB prevalence
	Patients with certain chronic diseases (eg, diabetes and chronic kidney disease)
	Infants and children exposed to adults at high risk
≥ 15 mm	People with no risk factors for TB

(NOTE: there is no cut-off of ≥ 20 mm or ≥ 25 mm)

442 and 443. The answers are 442-b, 443-a. *(McPhee, pp 1363-1364, 1396.)* Patients with HIV who develop **cryptococcal meningitis** present with headache, irritability, confusion, ataxia, blurred vision, papilledema, and cranial nerve palsies. Fever and neck stiffness are rare. India ink smear of the spinal fluid may demonstrate the encapsulated yeast and confirmation is made with a cerebrospinal fluid cryptococcal antigen test. Lesions of **toxoplasmosis** are usually multiple and ring-enhancing (lymphomas in HIV patients may also appear like this on brain imaging, so this description is not pathognomonic for toxoplasmosis). **PML** is a progressive disorder due to **JC virus.** The disorder is one of demyelination; patients present with visual deficits, mental impairment, and motor deficits. CT scan or MRI may show the hypodense, nonenhancing white matter lesions. Patients with **HIV dementia** present with apathy, hyperreflexia, clumsiness, weakness, ataxia, and loss of memory.

Obstetrics and Gynecology

Questions

444. A 23-year-old woman presents with fever and bilateral lower quadrant abdominal pain for 2 days. She complains of the onset of a mucopurulent vaginal discharge with her menses, which she states is yellowish in color. She has a new sexual partner and uses a nonbarrier method of contraception. Her temperature is 39.5°C (103.2°F). She has only bilateral lower quadrant tenderness with palpation of her abdomen, and pelvic examination reveals cervical and adnexal motion tenderness. Other than an elevated white blood cell count, a complete blood count and chemistry panel including liver enzymes are normal. Which of the following is the most likely diagnosis?

a. Fitz-Hugh–Curtis syndrome
b. Pelvic inflammatory disease
c. Perihepatitis
d. Acute inflammation of Bartholin gland
e. Chancroid

445. A 37-year-old woman in her 32nd week of gestation (G2P1) presents with a seizure. She does not smoke cigarettes, drink alcohol, or use illicit drugs. She has been completely healthy prior to and during her pregnancy but has been poorly compliant in receiving her prenatal care. Physical examination reveals a blood pressure of 150/95 mm Hg. The patient's face and hands appear edematous. Other than the patient being postictal (confused and disoriented after the seizure), the neurologic examination is normal. The urinalysis reveals proteinuria. The rest of the patient's laboratory data are normal. Which of the following is the most likely diagnosis?

a. HELLP syndrome
b. Preeclampsia
c. Eclampsia
d. Essential hypertension
e. Primary seizure disorder

446. A 20-year-old woman presents with the sudden onset of severe lower abdominal pain that radiates to her left shoulder. She has some vaginal bleeding now, but her last menstrual period was 6 weeks ago. She has a history of salpingitis but has never been pregnant. She uses condoms inconsistently, about 50% of the time, with her partner of 18 months. She denies dysuria or frequency. On physical examination, blood pressure is 100/70 mm Hg, heart rate is 100 beats per minute, and temperature is normal. Abdominal examination reveals tenderness and rebound in the left lower quadrant. Pelvic examination reveals a boggy and poorly delineated mass in the left adnexa. The patient's abdominal pain worsens upon slight movement of the cervix. Which of the following is the most likely diagnosis?

a. Pelvic inflammatory disease
b. Pyelonephritis
c. Appendicitis
d. Ectopic pregnancy
e. Ruptured corpus luteum cyst

447. A 53-year-old G2P2 complains of onset of menstrual bleeding 1 year after experiencing cessation of menses with hot flashes and palpitations. She has no weight loss. She has never taken oral contraceptives or hormone therapy. Her last Pap smear, 2 years ago, was normal. Pelvic examination reveals blood at the cervical os but is otherwise normal. Which of the following is the most appropriate next step in management?

a. Follow-up in 6 months
b. Colposcopy
c. Hormone replacement therapy
d. Endometrial sampling
e. Reassurance

448. A 24-year-old G3P2 presents with the chief complaint of some lower abdominal pain accompanied by a small amount of vaginal bleeding. She is 16 weeks' pregnant and has been healthy throughout the pregnancy. She does not smoke cigarettes, drink alcohol, or use illicit drugs. Abdominal examination is normal. Pelvic examination reveals that the internal cervical os is closed. Which of the following is the most likely diagnosis?

a. Complete abortion
b. Incomplete abortion
c. Threatened abortion
d. Inevitable abortion
e. Missed abortion

449. A 42-year-old G2P2 presents with the chief complaint of severe bilateral breast pain that seems to be worse around the time of menses. Physical examination reveals bilateral breast tenderness with palpation. Multiple lumps are palpated in both breasts. Mammogram reveals dense bilateral breast tissue. Which of the following is the most likely diagnosis in this patient?

a. Fibroadenoma
b. Fibrocystic disease
c. Paget disease
d. Mastitis
e. Mammary duct ectasia

450. A 36-year-old woman, pregnant for the fourth time, presents in her third trimester with painless and profuse bright red vaginal bleeding. Pelvic examination is deferred. Transvaginal ultrasonography reveals an abnormally positioned placenta and fetal monitoring reveals no distress. Which of the following is the most likely diagnosis?

a. Placenta accreta
b. Placenta previa
c. Abruptio placentae
d. Bloody show
e. Vasa previa

451. A 52-year-old woman with a past medical history of recurrent deep venous thrombosis states that she has been amenorrheic for 12 months and has recently begun experiencing vaginal dryness and dyspareunia. She also complains of recurrent episodes in which she becomes extremely hot and diaphoretic. During these episodes, she becomes anxious and feels like her heart is racing. Each episode lasts approximately 5 minutes. The episodes are so intense that she must put on the air conditioner or open a window until the episode resolves. Hot weather and stress often precipitate the symptoms. The episodes seem to be worse at night. Physical examination is normal. After talking to several friends, she is interested in starting hormone replacement therapy (HRT). What should you tell her?

a. Her symptoms are atypical and need further evaluation before therapy is instituted.
b. She can start estrogen alone at this time.
c. She needs to take estrogen and progesterone and may start therapy immediately.
d. Her symptoms should resolve soon, so no therapy is needed at this time.
e. She is not a candidate for HRT, but may benefit from other nonhormonal therapy.

452. A 30-year-old woman in week 36 of her first pregnancy presents with a platelet count of 85,000/μL. She has no complaints of easy bruisability or mucosal bleeding but feels fatigued toward the end of her pregnancy. She has no past illnesses and takes no medications. She has no family history of bleeding problems. Her blood pressure is 156/90 mm Hg. Laboratory data reveal a hemoglobin of 6 g/dL, with a normal prothrombin time and partial thromboplastin time. Liver enzymes are elevated and urinalysis reveals microscopic hematuria and proteinuria. Peripheral blood smear reveals schistocytes but normal platelet morphology. Which of the following is the most likely diagnosis?

a. Idiopathic thrombocytopenic purpura (ITP)
b. Pseudothrombocytopenia
c. Gestational thrombocytopenia
d. HELLP syndrome
e. Thrombotic thrombocytopenic purpura (TTP)

453. As you are performing the external portion of a pelvic examination, you palpate a warm, fluctuant mass that is unilateral in the posterolateral portion of the labia majora. The patient states that palpation is painful. The surrounding tissue is inflamed and edematous. Which of the following is the most likely diagnosis?

a. Bartholin cyst
b. Bartholin abscess
c. Rectocele
d. Cystocele
e. Genital herpes

454. A 23-year-old woman presents with vaginal bleeding that is occasionally heavy and has occurred at irregular intervals since beginning menses. She denies fever, weight loss, as well as abdominal or pelvic pain. She is sexually active with one partner and has never been pregnant. The patient's BMI is 34 and she is mildly hirsute. Otherwise, the remainder of her physical, including her pelvic examination, is normal. Which of the following is the most likely diagnosis?

a. Atrophic vaginitis
b. Endometriosis
c. Uterine leiomyoma
d. Endometrial carcinoma
e. Polycystic ovarian syndrome

455. A 29-year-old woman in her first trimester presents with painless profuse vaginal bleeding. Pelvic examination reveals a 24-week-sized uterus. Urinalysis reveals proteinuria. An ultrasound does not show any fetal structures. Which of the following is the most likely diagnosis?

a. Placenta previa
b. Abruptio placenta
c. Hydatidiform mole
d. Normal pregnancy
e. Multiple-gestation pregnancy

456. A 23-year-old woman presents to your office for a prenatal visit. She has not received any previous prenatal care and does not know the date of her last menstrual period. On physical examination, the fundal height is palpated to be at the level of the umbilicus. Which of the following is the estimated number of weeks of gestation?

a. 10
b. 15
c. 20
d. 25
e. 30

Questions 457 to 459

For each patient with a vaginal finding, select the most likely causative organism. Each lettered option may be used once, multiple times, or not at all.

a. *Trichomonas vaginalis*
b. *Neisseria gonorrhoeae*
c. *Gardnerella vaginalis*
d. *Candida albicans*
e. *Chlamydia trachomatis*
f. *Enterobius vermicularis*

457. A 19-year-old woman presents with a malodorous, watery, gray-colored vaginal discharge. The wet-mount preparation is shown. There is a fishy odor to the discharge when mixed with potassium hydroxide (KOH).

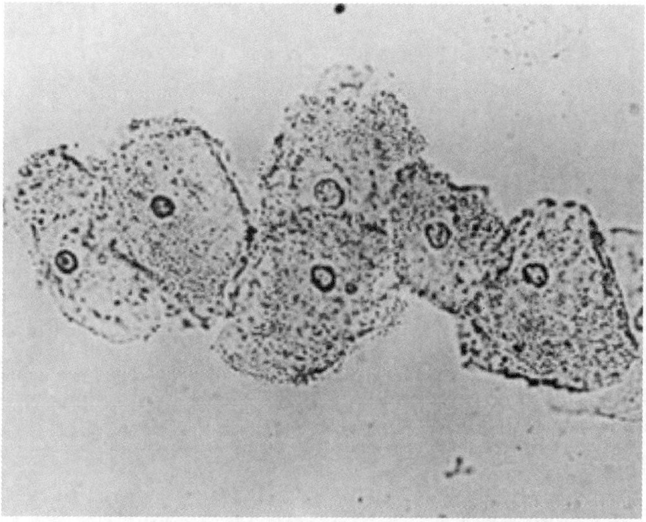

(Reproduced, with permission, from Decherney AH, Nathan L. Current Diagnosis & Treatment: Obstetrics & Gynecology, *10th ed. New York: McGraw-Hill; 2007:600.)*

458. A 35-year-old woman presents with vaginal itching. Examination reveals strawberry petechiae on the cervix and a frothy green-colored discharge. The saline wet-mount is shown.

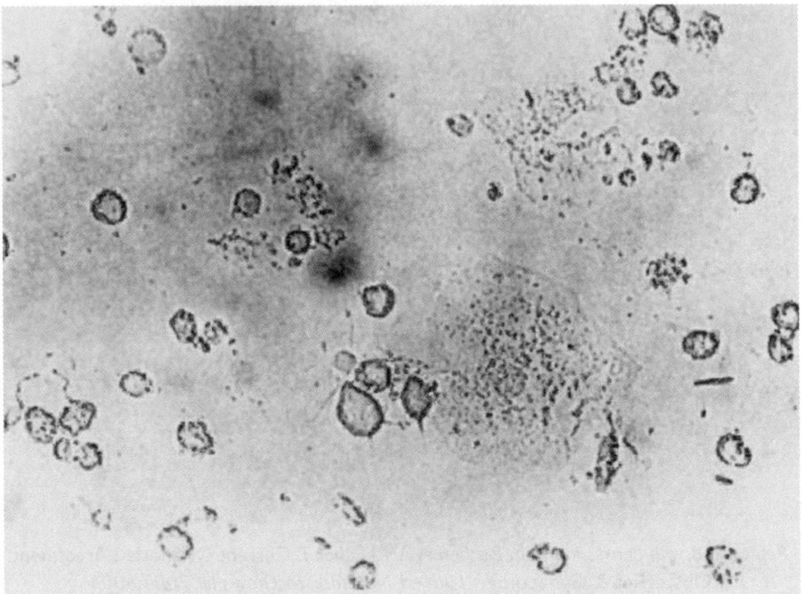

(Reproduced, with permission, from Decherney AH, Nathan L. Current Diagnosis & Treatment: Obstetrics & Gynecology, *10th ed. New York: McGraw-Hill; 2007:600.)*

459. A 31-year-old woman presents with vaginal burning and a white, cheeselike vaginal discharge. Pseudohyphae are visible with a KOH preparation.

Questions 460 to 464

For each patient with a breast finding, select the most likely diagnosis. Each lettered option may be used once, multiple times, or not at all.

a. Breast cancer
b. Paget disease of the breast
c. Inflammatory breast carcinoma
d. Intraductal papilloma
e. Fibroadenoma

460. A 25-year-old woman presents with a palpable breast mass that has well-defined margins and is moveable.

461. A 50-year-old woman presents with a hard, circumscribed, fixed, edematous breast mass. The overlying skin has a peau d'orange (orange peel) appearance.

462. A 52-year-old woman presents with bloody discharge from her right nipple. She has no palpable breast mass.

463. A 36-year-old woman has erythema and a visible erysipeloid margin of her left breast. The involved area is warm and tender to palpation.

464. A 39-year-old woman presents with eczematoid changes of her left nipple, which occasionally itches, burns, oozes, and bleeds.

Obstetrics and Gynecology

Answers

444. The answer is b. *(McPhee, pp 687-689.)* The patient likely has **pelvic inflammatory disease (PID)** (also known as salpingitis or endometritis), which is most often due to **N *gonorrhoeae* or *C trachomatis*.** Patients like this one complain of lower abdominal pain, fever, and yellow mucopurulent vaginal discharge, which is more prominent during menstruation. On physical examination they will have **uterine adnexal or cervical motion tenderness.** Spread of the gonococci (or, in some cases, *Chlamydia*) into the upper abdomen may cause a **perihepatitis**, or **Fitz-Hugh–Curtis syndrome;** in this case, patients will complain of upper abdominal pain and may have an audible **hepatic rub. Acute inflammation of Bartholin gland** (an infected duct) would be visible in the labium majora. **Chancroid** is due to *Haemophilus ducreyi*; patients typically present with a painful ulcer that bleeds easily.

445. The answer is c. *(McPhee, pp 715-718.)* **Preeclampsia** is defined as hypertension and proteinuria (>300 mg/24 h), often accompanied by non-dependent edema of the face and hands. **Risk factors** for preeclampsia include African American race, primagravid state, multiple gestations, extremes of age (<15 or >35), chronic hypertension, and a family history positive for preeclampsia. This patient has **eclampsia**, which is defined as seizures in a patient with preeclampsia. The cure for preeclampsia/eclampsia is delivery. Magnesium sulfate is often used for seizure prophylaxis and management if delivery is not optimal at the time of onset of eclampsia. The **HELLP syndrome** (**H**emolysis, **E**levated **L**iver enzymes, **L**ow **P**latelets) is a variant of preeclampsia, but this patient's lab values are normal. **Essential hypertension** is elevated blood pressure that predates a pregnancy, which this patient does not report in her history. She also has no previous history of a **primary seizure disorder**.

446. The answer is d. *(McPhee, pp 713-714.)* The incidence of **ectopic pregnancy** (outside the uterine cavity) is 1 in 150 pregnancies. Risk factors include anything preventing migration of the fertilized egg to the uterus:

previous history of PID or ectopic pregnancy, use of an intrauterine device (IUD), DES exposure, and prior pelvic surgery. Patients present with abdominal pain that may radiate to the shoulder (indicating irritation of the diaphragm from the hemoperitoneum), vaginal bleeding, cervical motion tenderness (CMT), and the presence of a boggy and poorly delineated **adnexal mass** 1 to 8 weeks after a missed period. The patient may have **other symptoms of pregnancy**, such as nausea, vomiting, and breast tenderness. If the ectopic pregnancy ruptures, the patient may present with signs of shock. The patient's β-hCG will be greater than 2000 mU/mL but ultrasound will reveal an empty uterus. A **ruptured corpus luteum cyst** causes a tender ovary but no palpable mass. **PID** causes fever and bilateral lower quadrant pain and cervical motion tenderness. **Appendicitis** involves fever and right-sided pain while **pyelonephritis** is usually accompanied by urinary symptoms, fever and costovertebral angle tenderness. Pelvic examination is typically normal in appendicitis and pyelonephritis.

447. The answer is d. *(McPhee, p 676.)* The patient has **postmenopausal vaginal bleeding**, which occurs at least 6 months after cessation of menstrual function. Causes for this presentation include endometrial atrophy, polyps, hyperplasia, or cancer. The vulva and vagina should be inspected for ulcers and neoplasms and a Pap smear should be obtained. A **transvaginal ultrasound** can be used to measure endometrial thickness. An **endometrial biopsy or dilatation and curettage (D&C) with hysteroscopy** should be performed for diagnosis and may also be curative. As postmenopausal bleeding could signify endometrial cancer, **reassurance or follow-up** alone would not be sufficient. **Colposcopy** is used to evaluate the cervix after an abnormal pap smear and **hormone replacement therapy** is used primarily to combat the hot flashes and vaginal dryness accompanying menopause.

448. The answer is c. *(McPhee, pp 711-712.)* Threatened abortion, incomplete abortion, complete abortion, and inevitable abortion are all types of spontaneous abortion and present at less than 20 weeks of gestation with vaginal bleeding. Patients like this one, with **threatened abortion**, complain of abdominal pain, and vaginal bleeding. The membranes remain intact and no products of conception are expelled. The internal cervical os is closed and the fetus is viable. In **incomplete abortion** the internal cervical os is open and some products of conception are expelled. In a **complete abortion**, all products of conception are expelled and the internal cervical os is closed. **Inevitable abortion** is when the membranes rupture, the internal cervical os is open, and no products of conception are expelled. Patients complain of abdominal cramps in inevitable abortion. **Missed abortion** is retained fetal tissue with no cardiac activity in a uterus that is not growing. There is no vaginal bleeding, no products of conception are expelled, and the internal cervical os is closed.

449. The answer is b. *(McPhee, pp 649-650.)* Women between the ages of 30 and 55 may develop benign cyst formation of the breasts or **fibrocystic breast disease.** Patients typically state that **cyclic breast pain or multiple asymptomatic or tender masses** worsen premenstrually or as they approach menopause **(decreased progesterone).** Physical examination often reveals bilateral lumpy and tender breasts. Mammography shows dense breast tissue. **Mastitis** is most common in lactating breasts and is usually secondary to *Staphylococcus aureus* infection. The breast is warm, tender, swollen, and erythematous. **Mammary duct ectasia** is a nonmalignant condition that affects menopausal women. The subareolar ducts become blocked with debris, causing pain, inflammation, nipple discharge, and retraction of the nipple. **Fibroadenomas** are benign breast neoplasms found in young women. They are usually round, rubbery, moveable, and nontender. **Paget disease** is rare and affects the nipple, presenting as itching or burning of the nipple with possible ulceration.

450. The answer is b. *(McPhee, p 720.)* **Placenta previa** and **abruptio placenta** are the two most common causes of third-trimester bleeding. This patient has **placenta previa,** which is abnormal implantation of placenta near or at the cervical os, and may be total, partial, marginal, or low-lying. **Risk factors** for placenta previa include advanced maternal age, multiparity, smoking history, and prior cesarean section. Patients present at 30 weeks of gestation with painless vaginal bleeding. There is no fetal distress. Vaginal examination is contraindicated, and ultrasound is required to make the diagnosis. **Abruptio placentae** is premature separation of a normally implanted placenta. Patients present with painful (unremitting abdominal and back pain) vaginal bleeding, and there is fetal distress. **Risk factors** for abruptio placentae include advanced maternal age, multiparity, diabetes, hypertension, tobacco use, alcohol use, and cocaine use. **Placenta accreta** is a placenta that adheres to the myometrium without an intervening decidual layer; it is associated with postpartum hemorrhage. In **vasa previa,** the fetal vessels associated with the cord traverse the lower uterine segment and present in advance of the fetal presenting part, causing rapid bleeding when disrupted during labor. **Bloody show** is a blood-tinged vaginal discharge that occurs when the cervix is dilated and the onset of labor is imminent.

451. The answer is e. *(McPhee, pp 703-704.)* The patient is presenting with symptoms of normal **menopause,** which presents as amenorrhea and may include hot flashes, urinary frequency, dysuria, urinary incontinence, vaginal dryness, vaginal itchiness, and dyspareunia. The average age of onset of menopause in Western societies is 51 years. **Estrogen replacement** (with progesterone if the woman has an intact uterus, to prevent endometrial hyperplasia and cancer) for a maximum of 5 years is the best way to treat vasomotor symptoms; however, there are several contraindications to this therapy. The Women's Health Initiative trial and the Estrogen/Progestin Replacement Study both showed **increased risk of cardiovascular and cerebrovascular events, thromboembolic disease, breast cancer, and gallstones**, thus patients with **previous histories or high risk for these conditions** (as well as first-degree family history of breast cancer) **should not be started on hormone replacement therapy.** For those women who cannot take estrogen replacement, other options include SSRIs (paroxetine, venlafaxine), clonidine and alternative treatments such as soy and black cohosh.

452. The answer is d. *(Fauci, p 1814.)* This peripartum patient presents with the **HELLP** (**H**emolysis, **E**levated **L**iver enzymes, **L**ow **P**latelet count) syndrome, a variant of preeclampsia. Immediate delivery is the treatment for HELLP syndrome. **Gestational thrombocytopenia** develops in the last trimester of pregnancy (in 8% of pregnant women) and is reversible after delivery. It is difficult to differentiate between gestational thrombocytopenia and the autoimmune isolated thrombocytopenia of **ITP**, but ITP will persist after delivery. **Pseudothrombocytopenia** occurs when platelets aggregate in laboratory test tubes, giving falsely decreased platelet counts. Careful inspection of the peripheral smear will show the aggregates. **TTP** is unlikely, since the patient does not have the pentad of symptoms seen in 40% of patients (**FAT R.N.** = **F**ever, **A**utoimmune hemolytic anemia, **T**hrombocytopenia, **R**enal disease, **N**eurologic disease). **HUS** presents with three of the five symptoms seen in TTP (**RAT** = **R**enal disease, **A**utoimmune hemolytic anemia, and **T**hrombocytopenia). TTP and HUS are unlikely in this patient without kidney involvement.

453. The answer is b. *(Seidel, p 597.)* Obstruction of the main duct of **Bartholin gland (located in the posterolateral portion of the labia majora)** results in retention of secretions (cyst) and secondary infection (abscess). **Abscesses** are generally painful to palpation, hot to the touch, and fluctuant. A **rectocele** is a weakness in the fascia of the posterior vaginal wall in which the rectum appears as a bulging mass. A **cystocele** is a protrusion of the bladder into the anterior vaginal wall. Asking the patient to bear down will enhance these protrusions and make them more easily seen. **Herpes** causes often painful grouped vesicles on an erythematous base but is not accompanied by a fluctuant mass.

454. The answer is e. *(McPhee, pp 690-691.)* This patient most likely has **polycystic ovarian syndrome (Stein-Leventhal syndrome)** which affects women of reproductive age and causes chronic anovulation. The etiology of polycystic ovary syndrome is unknown; patients present with obesity, hirsutism, and infertility. Half present with amenorrhea and a third have abnormal uterine bleeding. **Endometriosis** is the most common cause of infertility; patients present with dyspareunia (painful intercourse), abnormal vaginal bleeding, and cyclic pelvic pain. **Uterine leiomyomas** (uterine fibroids) change in size with the menstrual cycle but regress in size during menopause. Often, the fibroid is palpable on pelvic examination. The most common cause of postmenopausal vaginal bleeding is **atrophic vaginitis** (with or without trauma). All postmenopausal women with vaginal bleeding require a **biopsy** to rule out **endometrial carcinoma**.

455. The answer is c. *(McPhee, pp 714-715.)* Gestational trophoblastic disease includes the tumors of **hydatidiform mole**, **invasive mole**, and **choriocarcinoma.** These tumors arise from **fetal tissue**, not maternal tissue. Almost all patients with moles present with **first-trimester vaginal bleeding.** They may also have hyperemesis early on and signs of **preeclampsia** during the second trimester. Typically, patients have increased **β-hCG titers** (greater than expected for gestational age) and rapid enlargement of the uterus (greater than anticipated by dates) with absence of fetal heart sounds and structures. The **cluster of grapes** appearance of the mole makes it easily identifiable on gross examination (with a **snowstorm** appearance on ultrasonography). Rarely, patients with hydatidiform moles may present with **hyperthyroidism** due to the production of thyrotropin by the molar tissue.

Abruptio placentae is premature separation of a normally implanted placenta. **Placenta previa** is abnormal implantation of placenta near or at the cervical os, causing patients to present in the third trimester with painless vaginal bleeding.

456. The answer is c. *(Seidel, p 617.)* At week 12, the uterus is palpable just above the symphysis pubis. By week 16, it reaches halfway between the symphysis and the umbilicus. **At 20 weeks of pregnancy, fundal height is at the level of the umbilicus.** Thereafter, the gestational age in weeks should match the distance in centimeters of the fundus from the symphysis pubis, until just before delivery when the fetus engages into the pelvis. Part of the obstetrics and gynecology history should include a summation of previous pregnancy outcomes, commonly written as **G-TPAL**: Gravida (number of pregnancies, including current one), **T**erm pregnancies, **P**reterm (less than 37 weeks) pregnancies, **A**bortions (spontaneous and elective), and **L**iving children. For example, a woman currently pregnant, with two previous full-term infants and one spontaneous abortion would be G4-T2P0A1L2

457 to 459. The answers are 457-c, 458-a, 459-d. *(McPhee, pp 677-679.)* The normal vaginal flora mostly consists of *Lactobacillus* species in an acidic environment. When the pH of the vagina changes, or the normal flora is replaced by other organisms, the patient develops vaginal discharge and irritation consistent with **vaginitis**. ***Gardnerella vaginalis*** (the organism responsible for **bacterial vaginosis**, the most common cause of vaginitis) causes a profuse, malodorous discharge. Wet-mount preparation will demonstrate **clue cells** (epithelial cells with adherent bacteria that cause their borders to be irregular), and a KOH preparation will release amines, causing the discharge to have a **fishy odor (positive whiff test). Candida** produces a thick, white, cottage-cheese-appearing discharge, and KOH preparation will reveal the characteristic **pseudohyphae.** Ten percent of patients with ***Trichomonas*** will have a **strawberry-appearing** cervix or vaginal mucosa. The vaginal discharge may be green and is often described as frothy. The trichomonal **flagellates** seen in the slide are characteristically motile and **pear-shaped.** Both partners need to be treated for trichomonas to eradicate the infection. A vaginal discharge with leukocytes but no organisms is characteristic of ***Chlamydia. Enterobius vermicularis*** (pin-worms) may cause pruritus of the perineum and perianal area. The diagnosis is made by applying scotch tape to the perineum, then to a slide; microscopic examination will reveal the characteristic double-walled ova of the parasite.

460 to 464. The answers are 460-e, 461-a, 462-d, 463-c, 464-b. *(McPhee, pp 650, 656-660.)* Most **breast cancers** present in the **upper outer quadrant** of the breast; patients may present with a hard, circumscribed mass that is fixed to the skin or deep muscle. Cancer may be nodular with indistinct borders. Patients may also have nipple edema or retraction. A woman under the age of 30 years presenting with a mobile breast mass that has well-defined borders most likely has a **fibroadenoma.** However, breast cancer must still be ruled out since clinical examination and even mammography are not sufficient to exclude the diagnosis. **Intraductal papilloma** is a benign tumor; patients often present with a bloody discharge from the nipple in the absence of a breast mass. Patients who present with an erythematous and warm breast (which eventually becomes indurated and firm) may have **inflammatory breast carcinoma.** Patients with **Paget disease** (a well-differentiated infiltrating ductal carcinoma or ductal carcinoma in situ) classically present with eczematoid changes in the nipple (ie, itching, oozing, and bleeding), all of which occur over a relatively long period of time. Mammography may be negative, and biopsy is required to make the diagnosis.

Pediatrics and Neonatology

Questions

465. An 18-month-old boy is brought to the pediatrician because of progressively worsening episodes of cyanosis. The child has moments when he turns blue and becomes dyspneic. During these episodes the child becomes irritable and remains in a squatting position. Physical examination reveals a small and thin child with clubbing of the fingers and toes. Lungs are normal. Heart auscultation reveals a right ventricular (RV) lift and a grade 3/4 harsh systolic-ejection murmur at the upper left sternal border. Which of the following is the most likely diagnosis?

a. Transposition of the great vessels (TOGV)
b. Tetralogy of Fallot (TOF)
c. Truncus arteriosus
d. Tricuspid atresia
e. Total anomalous pulmonary venous return

466. A 3-year-old boy is brought to the emergency room with lethargy, irritability, and ataxia. The child often complains of diffuse abdominal pain and is constipated. On physical examination, the tongue size is normal but a black line is visible along the gingiva. He is anemic on complete blood count and his peripheral smear is shown in the following figure. Which of the following is the most likely diagnosis?

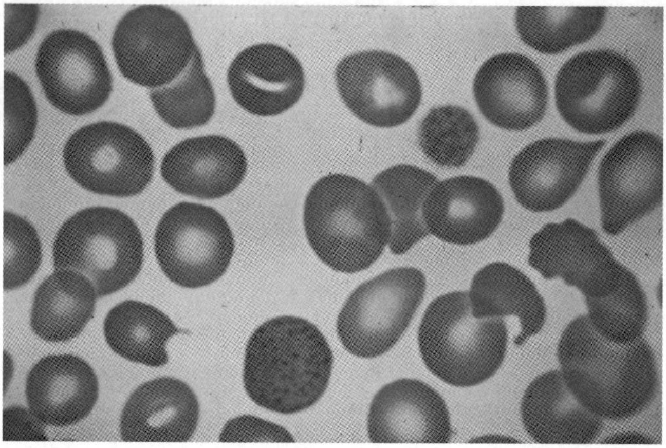

(Reproduced, with permission, from Lichtman MA, Shafer JA, Felgar RE, et al. Atlas of Hematology. *New York: McGraw-Hill; 2007: Fig. I.B.1. http://www.accessmedicine.com.)*

a. Porphyria
b. Kernicterus
c. Fragile X syndrome
d. Lead poisoning
e. Cretinism

467. A grammar school is going to start screening children for scoliosis and has asked for your recommendations regarding testing. Which of the following is the most appropriate screening test for this purpose?

a. Growth charts
b. Lateral radiograph of the thoracic spine
c. Forward bending test
d. MRI of the thoracic spine
e. Ortolani test

468. A 4-year-old boy is brought to the emergency room complaining of left ear pain that awakened him from sleep. The child has no past medical history and has been in good health. During the physical examination, the child is irritable and often tugs at his left ear. His temperature is 38.6°C (101.5°F), and he has no lymphadenopathy. The canals are normal but the left tympanic membrane is bulging and erythematous. Which of the following is the most likely diagnosis?

a. Otitis externa
b. Serous otitis media
c. Acute otitis media
d. Acute mastoiditis
e. Foreign body in the ear

469. The mother of an 11-month-old infant is concerned because her child is easily startled by slight noise and cannot sit alone without assistance. On physical examination, the child does not seem to respond to visual cues and is extremely hypotonic. Funduscopic examination reveals a macular cherry-red spot. Which of the following is the most likely diagnosis?

a. Pompe disease
b. Tay-Sachs disease
c. Adrenoleukodystrophy
d. Phenylketonuria
e. Cerebral palsy

470. A 2-year-old boy with 2 days of rhinorrhea is brought by his parents to the emergency room because of a barking cough and fever that started suddenly in the middle of the night. On physical examination, the patient's temperature is 38.6°C (101.5°F), and he appears frightened and anxious. He has a heart rate of 160 beats per minute and a respiratory rate of 36 breaths per minute. His breathing is labored, and he is using his accessory muscles of respiration. Marked inspiratory stridor is audible. His posterior pharynx is erythematous, but his lung examination is unremarkable. Which of the following is the most likely diagnosis?

a. Epiglottitis
b. Peritonsillar abscess
c. Acute laryngotracheobronchitis
d. Asthma
e. Bronchiolitis

471. A 2-year-old boy is having difficulty breathing. The mother states that he has had a cough since birth and that this visit to the emergency room is one of many for her sickly son. The neonatal history reveals that the boy did not defecate for some time after delivery. The growth chart reveals that the child is in the fifth percentile. Which of the following is the most helpful test to order in this patient?

a. HIV antibody test
b. Sweat chloride test
c. Urine toxicology screen
d. Lead level
e. MRI of the head

472. A 6-year-old girl is brought to your office by her parents, who believe that the child has been having brief episodes of unresponsiveness with fluttering of the eyelids and lip smacking. The child's schoolteacher has recently sent home a note stating that the girl is "daydreaming" in class and is often inattentive. She has no past medical history and is on no medications. Physical examination is normal, but at least twice during the examination, the child appears to look blank or be dazed for 20 to 30 seconds. Which of the following is the most likely diagnosis?

a. Atonic seizure
b. Absence seizure
c. Neonatal seizure
d. Focal seizure
e. Psychomotor seizure

473. A 6-week-old infant is constantly coughing. She is afebrile and began coughing about 10 days ago with increasing regularity. Vaginal delivery was uncomplicated, but when the girl was 10 days old a mild conjunctivitis developed, which responded well to topical antibiotics. On physical examination, her respiratory rate is 55 breaths per minute, and the infant is breathing by using accessory muscles of respiration. Lung auscultation reveals bilateral diffuse crackles. A chest radiograph reveals a bilateral diffuse interstitial infiltrate. Which of the following is the most likely diagnosis?

a. Chlamydial pneumonia
b. Pertussis
c. Respiratory syncytial viral (RSV) pneumonia
d. Foreign body aspiration
e. *Pneumocystis jiroveci* pneumonia (PCP)

474. A mother brings her infant son to your office for a well-baby checkup. On physical examination, you see that the boy's optic fundus is positive for a white reflex. Which of the following is the most likely cause of the white reflex?

a. Retinoblastoma
b. Retinocerebellar angioma
c. Choroidal angioma
d. Primary congenital glaucoma
e. Papilledema

475. A 9-month-old infant is brought to the emergency room by her parents. They report that the child has been irritable for the last several days and progressively lethargic. The infant vomited several times in the car on the way to the hospital. The parents state that the infant has not previously been ill. They deny any history of trauma or accidental ingestion of medication or poisons. On physical examination, the child is lethargic and difficult to arouse. Her vital signs are normal. There is no evidence of external trauma, but retinal hemorrhages are visible on funduscopic examination. Her anterior fontanel is bulging. Which of the following is the most likely diagnosis?

a. Bacterial meningitis
b. Oligodendroglioma
c. DiGeorge syndrome
d. Fetal alcohol syndrome
e. Shaken baby syndrome

476. A 4-hour-old full-term newborn had been doing well until the staff in the nursery attempted to feed her. The girl became cyanotic during the feeding challenge but improved with crying when the attempt to feed was discontinued. Which of the following is the most likely diagnosis?

a. Hyaline membrane disease
b. Choanal atresia
c. Meconium aspiration
d. Tracheoesophageal fistula
e. Tracheomalacia

477. A 10-year-old girl presents with several light brown maculae, each greater than 1 cm in diameter, on her trunk. Physical examination reveals axillary freckling and firm subcutaneous masses. Which of the following is the most likely diagnosis?

a. Von Hippel-Lindau syndrome
b. Tuberous sclerosis
c. Meningioma
d. Craniopharyngioma
e. Neurofibromatosis type 1

478. An 8-year-old girl presents with the acute onset of swelling of her hands, feet, legs, and face. Her past medical history is significant for a recent upper respiratory tract infection. Physical examination reveals normal vital signs. The patient has clear lungs but has pitting edema up to her sacrum. Heart examination is normal. Urinalysis reveals only 4+ proteinuria. Which of the following is the most likely diagnosis?

a. Rapidly progressive glomerulonephritis (RPGN)
b. Membranoproliferative glomerulonephritis (MPGN)
c. Minimal change disease
d. Focal segmental glomerulosclerosis
e. Membranous glomerulonephropathy

479. A 3-year-old boy with a 4-day history of upper respiratory tract infection presents to the emergency room for evaluation of pallor and fatigue. Physical examination reveals a pale child with normal vital signs. He has scattered petechiae on the chest and extremities and a palpable spleen tip. Laboratory data reveal a leukocytosis (white blood cell count of >30,000/μL). Hemoglobin is 7.4 g/dL, and platelet count is 50,000/μL. The peripheral blood smear reveals the presence of blasts. Which of the following is the most likely diagnosis?

a. Acute lymphoblastic leukemia
b. Acute nonlymphocytic leukemia
c. Chronic lymphocytic leukemia
d. Acute myelogenous leukemia
e. Chronic myelogenous leukemia

480. You are at a family friend's home when the friend starts screaming that her 18-month-old daughter is suddenly unable to breathe. The child's brother says that she was playing with his new Legos before this incident. Upon approaching the child, you note that she is in respiratory distress with stridor and is tiring but conscious. Attempts to ventilate do not result in a chest rise. What is the most appropriate next step?

a. Administer five back blows and five chest thrusts
b. Administer a series of five abdominal thrusts
c. Perform a finger sweep of the mouth
d. Perform chest compressions
e. Perform cricothyrotomy

481. A 7-year-old girl comes to the emergency room with fever, sore throat, and noisy breathing. She has no cough. On physical examination, she appears ill and speaks with a hoarse voice. She has obvious difficulty swallowing and is febrile, with a temperature of 39.9°C (103.8°F). Her pulse is 120 beats per minute and her respiratory rate is 18 breaths per minute. Her blood pressure is normal. She is drooling and prefers to remain in a sitting position, leaning forward with her mouth open. She has no palpable lymphadenopathy. Which of the following is the most likely diagnosis?

a. Group A *Streptococcus* pharyngitis
b. Epiglottitis
c. Croup
d. Diphtheria
e. Peritonsillar abscess

482. A 4-month-old infant is brought to the emergency room because of a swollen scrotum. On physical examination, the child is afebrile. The right side of the scrotum is distended but not taut. A mass is palpable that is firm, smooth, nontender, and transilluminates using a penlight. Which of the following is the most likely diagnosis?

a. Inguinal hernia
b. Spermatocele
c. Varicocele
d. Hydrocele
e. Cryptorchidism

483. A 5-week-old infant is brought to the pediatrician for a well-baby visit. The mother states that the child has been healthy. Physical examination reveals no cyanosis and no clubbing. Cardiac auscultation reveals a grade 4/6 holosystolic murmur heard best at the lower left sternal border. S_2 is loud but not split. Which of the following is the most likely diagnosis?

a. Atrial septal defect (ASD)
b. Patent ductus arteriosus (PDA)
c. Ventricular septal defect (VSD)
d. Eisenmenger syndrome
e. Endocarditis

484. A 13-year-old adolescent, who has recently recovered from an upper respiratory tract infection, presents to the emergency room with lethargy, vomiting, and delirium. While being transported to the emergency room, the boy has a seizure. On physical examination, the child is jaundiced and has hepatomegaly. He has no focal deficits on neurologic examination but is comatose. Which of the following is the most likely diagnosis?

a. Reye syndrome
b. Wilson disease
c. West Nile encephalitis
d. Viral hepatitis
e. Botulism

485. A 1-year-old boy is brought to the emergency room because of the passage of several maroon-colored stools per rectum. Abdominal examination reveals normal bowel sounds and no masses. Which of the following is the most likely diagnosis?

a. Biliary atresia
b. Intussusception
c. Meckel diverticulum
d. Zenker diverticulum
e. Pyloric stenosis

486. A 9-year-old girl is brought into your office by her mother, who states that the daughter has been losing weight and having difficulty at school. The mother discovered some yellow-colored discharge on the child's underwear. On physical examination, you notice erythema of all parts of the patient's vulva and the vagina. There is some yellow discharge visible. Which of the following is the most likely diagnosis?

a. Müllerian duct tumor
b. Wolffian duct tumor
c. Dermatitis
d. Sexual abuse
e. Straddle injury

487. A 10-year-old child presents with a confluence of pustular and vesicular lesions on the hands and face, some of which have ruptured and expressed a serous exudate with honey-colored crusts. A Tzanck smear is negative for multinucleated giant cells, but a Gram stain is significant for gram-positive cocci. Which of the following is the most likely diagnosis?

a. Folliculitis
b. Kawasaki disease
c. Staphylococcal scalded skin syndrome
d. Miliaria
e. Impetigo

488. A 2-year-old boy presents with progressive clumsiness and difficulty walking. Physical examination reveals that the child has large calves. He has difficulty walking on his toes and has a waddling gait. Gower maneuver is positive. Which of the following is the most likely diagnosis?

a. Becker muscular dystrophy
b. Myotonic dystrophy
c. Facioscapulohumeral dystrophy
d. Duchenne muscular dystrophy
e. Limb-girdle muscular dystrophy

489. A healthy 12-year-old boy is brought to your office by his parents because of a concern that he is much shorter than his peers. You note in the chart that he was in the 50th percentile for height and weight at birth and for the first year, and since then, has been in the 10th percentile. He is an A student at school and plays several sports well. Upon discussing this issue with his parents, who are of normal height, they reveal that each of them had a late growth spurt. What is the most likely cause of his growth problem?

a. Familial short stature
b. Constitutional growth delay
c. Failure to thrive
d. Hypothyroidism
e. Congenital pathologic short stature

490. A mother brings her 3-year-old child to the emergency room after finding an abdominal mass while bathing her. The mother states that the child has been losing weight and has been complaining of nausea and vomiting. Vital signs reveal a blood pressure of 135/85 mm Hg and a temperature of 38.9°C (102°F). Palpation of the abdomen reveals a mass that extends to the left flank. CT scan of the abdomen reveals a noncalcified tumor. Which of the following is the most likely diagnosis?

a. Neuroblastoma
b. Ewing sarcoma
c. Wilms tumor
d. Rhabdomyosarcoma
e. Hodgkin lymphoma

491. An 11-year-old girl with cystic fibrosis presents to her pediatrician with the chief complaint of weakness. Her mother states that the child has been lethargic and has lost 6 lb over a period of 2 weeks. Her bowel movements have increased and are foul smelling. Physical examination reveals a cachectic child. Abdominal examination is normal. Laboratory results reveal a prolonged prothrombin time (PT). Which of the following is the most likely cause of these findings?

a. Pseudocyst
b. Malabsorption
c. Iron-deficiency anemia
d. Underlying malignancy
e. *Pseudomonas* abscess

492. A newborn has an Apgar score of 0 at 1 minute and an Apgar score of 10 at 5 minutes. Which of the following statements is true regarding the Apgar score?

a. It has good predictive value regarding the newborn's long-term outcome.
b. It has no predictive value regarding the newborn's long-term outcome.
c. It has no predictive value regarding outcome in the neonatal period.
d. It tells you very little about the infant's respiratory efforts.
e. It should be repeated a third time at 10 minutes.

Questions 493 and 494

For each child with a rash, select the most likely diagnosis. Each lettered option may be used once, multiple times, or not at all.

a. Rubeola
b. Rubella
c. Varicella
d. Roseola
e. Erythema infectiosum

493. An 8-year-old child experiences a sudden onset of vesicles beginning first on the face and scalp and then spreading to the trunk and extremities. Some vesicles have evolved into pustules and crusts. The lesions are extremely pruritic. Two weeks ago, the child visited a nursing home on a school field trip.

494. A 1-year-old has had a high fever for 4 days. Today the child is afebrile but developed a blanchable, maculopapular rash over the trunk and neck. The child appears remarkably well.

Pediatrics and Neonatology

Answers

465. The answer is b. *(Kliegman, pp 1906-1912.)* The five congenital heart disorders listed in the answer **(the five T's)** cause right-to-left shunts and subsequent cyanosis. **Tetralogy of Fallot** is the most common type of cyanotic heart lesion and consists of **P**ulmonary stenosis, right ventricular hypertrophy (**R**VH), an **O**ver-riding aorta, and ventricular septal defect, or **V**SD **(PROV).** Children present with dyspnea, cyanosis after the neonatal period, irritability, easy fatigability, and retarded growth and development. Physical examination may reveal an RV lift, a murmur of VSD, and clubbing. The cyanosis of tetralogy is often relieved by increasing venous return to the heart by the knee-chest position **(squatting or tet spells).** Chest radiograph may reveal a **boot-shaped heart due to RVH.** Children with **transposition of the great vessels** (aorta connected to RV and pulmonary artery connected to LV), **tricuspid atresia** (no communication between RA and RV), **truncus arteriosus** (one great vessel arises from the heart to supply the arterial and pulmonary circulation), and **total anomalous pulmonary venous return** (blood drains into RA instead of LA) typically present with cyanosis during the neonatal period.

466. The answer is d. *(Kliegman, pp 2913-2917.)* **Lead poisoning** produces a motor neuropathy and is associated with anemia, a gingival lead line, colicky abdominal pain, and basophilic stippling of red blood cells (seen in the middle and bottom of the figure). The major source of childhood exposure is old lead-based paint. Patients with **acute intermittent porphyria (AIP)** present with recurrent bouts of abdominal pain, confusion, and peripheral and cranial neuropathies. **Kernicterus** is accumulation of bilirubin in the newborn that may cause neuronal death and scarring. Children with **fragile X syndrome** present with mental retardation, large ears, and a prominent jaw. The triad of macroglossia, abdominal distention, and constipation is consistent with **cretinism**.

467. The answer is c. *(Kliegman, pp 1843-1844.)* The presence of a hump or asymmetry when the child **bends forward** is the hallmark of a **scoliosis deformity. Radiographic evaluation** is used to determine the degree of scoliosis but would not be a cost-effective screening test because films of the entire spine are required. **Growth charts** plot a child's height and weight (the former of which may be affected by spinal curvature), but do not help diagnose scoliosis. The **Ortolani test** is used to identify congenital dislocation of the hip in an infant. While the patient is in the supine position, the examiner holds the legs with the thumbs against the inside of the knee and thigh and the fingers over the posterior aspect of the proximal femur. A click will be noted as the examiner applies anterior force to the femur and the hip is reduced into the acetabulum.

468. The answer is c. *(Kliegman, pp 2630-2643.)* The most likely diagnosis in this patient in whom the tympanic membrane is bulging and erythematous is **acute bacterial otitis media.** The organisms responsible for this infection are *Haemophilus influenzae, Streptococcus pneumoniae,* and *Moraxella catarrhalis*. Adenopathy is usually absent in simple otitis media. A mucopurulent discharge in acute otitis media occurs only if the drum perforates. Perforations of the eardrum may occur with infections, sudden changes in pressure, especially when diving, and trauma. **Serous otitis media** is a collection of fluid in the middle ear resulting from a blocked eustachian tube; if this remains chronically, it may cause the tympanic membrane to be retracted and scarred. **Otitis externa** is also known as **"swimmer's ear"** and manifests as acute ear pain with edema, erythema and discharge in the ear canal with periauricular lymphadenopathy. **Acute mastoiditis** is caused by the breakdown of the thin bony partitions between the mastoid cells and occurs when an otitis media continues, often with few symptoms, despite adequate treatment. Patients have a continuous discharge through a perforation in the eardrum and complain of swelling, tenderness, and erythema over the mastoid bone. A **foreign body** may be seen in the canal or if present for a longer period of time, it may cause an otitis externa.

469. The answer is b. *(Kliegman, pp 594-595.)* This child most likely has **Tay-Sachs disease,** a progressive autosomal recessive disorder resulting from a deficiency of the enzyme hexosaminidase A with the subsequent storage of ganglioside in the lysosomes of the neurons. Infants present with hyperacusis (startling to sound), hypotonia, and delayed motor development. Funduscopic examination will reveal a **macular cherry-red spot. Pompe disease** is acid maltase deficiency; infants present with weakness and floppiness. **Adrenoleukodystrophy** is an inherited demyelinating disease of males resulting in an enzymatic defect in peroxisomes. Children present with behavioral problems, spasticity, deafness, visual loss, dementia, and brown skin pigmentation. **Phenylketonuria (PKU)** is an autosomal recessive disease in which neonates present with growth failure, seizures, and mental retardation. Patients are diagnosed by obtaining elevated phenylalanine levels during required screening. **Cerebral palsy (CP)** is a group of disorders in which patients present with motor deficits (intelligence may be spared) acquired in the prenatal or perinatal period because of an episode of hypoxemia, ischemia, or infection.

470. The answer is c. *(Kliegman, pp 1762-1766.)* This child has a classical presentation of **croup (acute laryngotracheobronchitis)**, the most common form of acute upper respiratory obstruction, which usually occurs in the fall and winter months and is most often due to one of the **parainfluenzae viruses.** It occurs in boys more often than in girls, between the ages of 3 months and 5 years. The inflammation of croup is subglottic. Patients exhibit labored breathing, stridor, and use of the accessory muscles of respiration to assist breathing, sometimes needing immediate airway management. Temperature is typically less than 39.4°C (103°F). An anteroposterior radiograph of the larynx will show subglottic narrowing, known as the **hourglass sign** or the **steeple sign. Epiglottitis** is most often caused by ***H influenzae* type B.** It is seen in children between the ages of 2 and 7 and may cause life-threatening airway obstruction. Patients present with fever, dysphagia, muffled voice, inspiratory retractions, cyanosis, and drooling, with a cherry-red, enlarged epiglottis on examination. To keep the airway open, patients with epiglottitis often sit in the **sniffing dog position.** The **thumbprint sign** is seen in a soft tissue lateral radiograph of the neck, but these films are rarely done because children require immediate protection of the airway with intubation. A severe **asthma** exacerbation would cause expiratory wheezing along with the signs of respiratory distress, but not this characteristic barking cough seen in this patient. **Bronchiolitis** occurs in infants younger than 6 months and is most likely due to respiratory syncytial virus (RSV). There is characteristic hyperinflation of the lungs, and the infant appears anxious due to expiratory difficulty. A **peritonsillar abscess** could be accompanied by the vital signs seen in this patient, but there would be asymmetry of the tonsils and no barking cough.

471. The answer is b. *(Kliegman, pp 1803-1810.)* The child most likely has **cystic fibrosis (CF).** CF is a multisystemic autosomal recessive disorder that affects the sinuses, lower respiratory tract (bronchiectasis), exocrine function of the pancreas, intestinal function (deficiencies in fat-soluble **vitamins A, D, E,** and **K**), sweat glands, and urogenital tract (infertility). Patients have episodes of recurrent respiratory tract infections and a history of failure to thrive. In the proper clinical setting, an evaluation of the child's **sweat for its chloride content** is the standard diagnostic approach. A **meconium ileus** (obstruction from hardened meconium) as reported in this patient at birth occurs in only 15% of all patients with CF and may be the first manifestation of CF. **It is often pathognomonic for the disease.** Respiratory infections are most often due to *Pseudomonas aeruginosa* and *Staphylococcus aureus*. The recurrent infections produce large amounts of mucus that cause obstructive lesions in the bronchi and bronchioles. Diagnosis is made by combining the clinical presentation with an abnormal sweat chloride value (> 70 mmol/L).

472. The answer is b. *(Kliegman, pp 2462-2464.)* **Absence seizure** (petit mal) occurs in children between the ages of 3 and 10 years and is characterized by numerous daily episodes of unresponsiveness, often associated with lip smacking, eye rolling, eyelid fluttering, or lip movement. **Atonic (astatic) seizures** are called **drop attacks;** patients experience a sudden loss of tone in postural muscles. **Neonatal seizures** are various forms of seizures that may be seen in the newborn. **Focal seizures (partial complex)** involve one part of the body and are not associated with loss of consciousness. These seizures can spread to involve adjacent areas of the body **(Jacksonian march). Psychomotor seizures** (of the **temporal lobe**) are associated with automatisms (purposeless motor movements with altered consciousness).

473. The answer is a. *(Kliegman, pp 1283-1284.)* The clinical presentation is consistent with **chlamydial pneumonia,** which develops in 20% of infants born to women with *Chlamydia* infections. Newborns will present within 3 months of birth with a week of persistent symptoms. The majority will have bilateral crackles on lung auscultation. Inclusion conjunctivitis and pneumonia are often a consequence of the perinatal infection. The etiologic agent (***Chlamydia trachomatis***) is found in up to 25% of pregnant women. **Pertussis,** or **whooping cough**, is a highly contagious infection and is unlikely to be mild on presentation. The word *pertussis* means "violent cough," and the disease is often called the **cough of 100 days** because of its chronic nature. The cough of pertussis is described as being paroxysmal and staccato in character, ending with a high-pitched inspiratory whoop. Because of waning of immunity from childhood immunization, adults age 19 to 64 are recommended to receive a **Tdap** (which includes pertussis vaccine) once instead of their next tetanus and diphtheria booster (Td) in order to protect infant contacts. **Respiratory syncytial viral (RSV) pneumonia** presents like chlamydial pneumonia but with no history of conjunctivitis. Patients with RSV present with rhinorrhea and cough. **Aspiration of a foreign body** causes cyanosis, the abrupt onset of respiratory distress, stridor, intercostal retractions, wheezing, and asymmetric breath sounds. **PCP** may have a similar presentation to this case in immunocompromised patients (those with HIV or on chemotherapy) but is rarely found in infants.

474. The answer is a. *(Kliegman, pp 2151-2152.)* This infant likely has a **retinoblastoma,** which classically presents with a white corneal reflex **(leukocoria).** This is a life-threatening malignant tumor rarely seen in infants and children. Leukocoria may also be due to a cataract. **Retinocerebellar angiomatosis** is part of a rare autosomal dominant disease **(von Hippel-Lindau disease)**; patients present with nystagmus, retinal detachment, cerebellar hemangioblastoma, intra-abdominal cysts, and renal carcinoma. **Choroidal angioma** is found in **Sturge-Weber disease;** patients present with congenital glaucoma, cloudiness of the cornea, and marked enlargement of the eye at birth (buphthalmos). Infants with Sturge-Weber disease may also have facial angiomas. **Primary congenital glaucoma** is a condition of increased intraocular pressure caused by abnormal development of the aqueous drainage structures of the eye. In **papilledema,** the optic disc margins are bilaterally indistinct due to optic nerve swelling from increased intracranial pressure.

475. The answer is e. *(Kliegman, p 405.)* Retinal hemorrhages with no evidence of external trauma, along with a history of irritability, lethargy, vomiting, and a bulging fontanel, suggest increased intracranial pressure from a chronic subdural hematoma or **shaken baby syndrome.** Increased head circumference is also suggestive of increased intracranial pressure. **Bacterial meningitis** might cause irritability and lethargy but would be accompanied by fever and possibly a rash as well. **DiGeorge syndrome** is a congenital disorder that causes cardiac defects, tetany from hypocalcemia secondary to an underdeveloped parathyroid gland, facial abnormalities, and thymus gland maldevelopment causing an isolated T cell deficiency. **Oligodendroglioma** commonly involves the temporal lobe, and patients often present with seizures. **Fetal alcohol syndrome** is the number one cause of congenital malformations. Infants are born with developmental retardation and facial, heart, lung, and limb abnormalities.

476. The answer is b. *(Kliegman, p 1743.)* **Choanal atresia** is the most common congenital nasal anomaly (due to a septum between the nose and pharynx). Newborns are obligate nose breathers, and any nasal obstruction may cause respiratory distress. In choanal atresia, the baby appears to be fine when crying (breathing through the mouth) but becomes cyanotic when crying stops. The frequency of this disorder is 1 in 7000 live births. Treatment consists of maintaining the airway (which may be achieved with an oral airway or by making a large hole in a feeding nipple), which allows the infant to mouth-breathe. Fifty percent of infants with choanal atresia have other congenital anomalies **(CHARGE syndrome** = **C**oloboma, **H**eart disease, **A**tresia choanae, **R**etarded growth, hypo**G**onadism, and **E**ar abnormalities**)**. Newborns with **tracheoesophageal (T-E) fistula** may present within a few hours of birth with choking and respiratory distress or later in life with chronic respiratory problems like pneumonias. **Hyaline membrane disease,** the most common cause of respiratory distress in the premature newborn, is a deficiency of surfactant causing severe respiratory distress, usually in premature newborns. **Meconium aspiration syndrome** occurs immediately upon birth and is associated with significant pulmonary morbidity in the first few hours with tachypnea, grunting, and cyanosis. **Tracheomalacia** is a self-limited disorder that causes noisy breathing (wheezing or stridor) in infancy due to the lack of a rigid trachea.

477. The answer is e. *(Kliegman, pp 2483-2488.)* Neurofibromatosis is also called **von Recklinghausen syndrome.** Patients with **neurofibromatosis (NF) type 1** (classical or peripheral) typically present with multiple **café au lait spots**, axillary freckling, **cutaneous neurofibromas**, acoustic neuromas, neurilemomas, optic gliomas, **Lisch nodules** (hamartomas of the iris that appear as brown elevations), and skeletal abnormalities. Patients with **neurofibromatosis type 2** (central) present with bilateral acoustic neuromas and multiple meningiomas and rarely have café au lait spots or Lisch nodules. **Tuberous sclerosis (Bourneville disease)** is a multisystem disease; patients present with skin lesions, benign tumors of the central nervous system, seizures, and mental retardation. **Von Hippel-Lindau (VHL) syndrome** is characterized by cerebellar hemangioblastomas, renal and pancreatic cysts, renal cell carcinoma, and retinal angiomata. The neurocutaneous syndromes (NF, VHL, and tuberous sclerosis) are all autosomal dominant disorders. **Meningioma** is a slow-growing benign tumor that arises from the leptomeningeal arachnoidal cells and is rare in childhood. **Craniopharyngioma** is a slow-growing cystic tumor arising from the pituitary; patients present with visual field defects and endocrine abnormalities.

478. The answer is c. *(Kliegman, pp 2192-2194.)* **Nephrotic syndrome** is a clinical complex consisting of more than 3.0 g proteinuria in 24 hours, hypoalbuminemia, edema, hyperlipidemia, lipiduria, and hypercoagulability. **Minimal change disease (MCD)** accounts for 80% of nephrotic syndrome in children under the age of 16 and 20% of nephrotic syndrome in adults. Patients typically present with nephrosis and a benign urinary sediment. The etiology of MCD is unknown, but occasionally the syndrome develops after a respiratory tract infection or an immunization. Patients respond to steroids, and the prognosis is excellent. **RPGN** and **MPGN** are immunologically mediated diseases characterized by oliguria, subnephrotic proteinuria, edema, hematuria, red blood cell casts, and hypertension (acute nephritic syndrome). **Focal segmental glomerulosclerosis** can cause nephrotic syndrome but only 20% respond to steroid treatment. **Membranous nephropathy** is a rare cause of hematuria and nephrotic syndrome in children and is usually associated with autoimmune diseases, sarcoidosis and infections.

479. The answer is a. *(Kliegman, pp 2116-2120.)* **Acute lymphoblastic leukemia (ALL)** comprises 80% of all childhood leukemias (peak incidence is between 2 and 6 years of age). Most patients present with fatigue, mucosal bleeding, low-grade fever, and lower extremity bone pain. Patients may present with an infection due to the severe neutropenia. Physical examination is often remarkable for pallor, petechiae, purpura, mucous membrane bleeding, bone pain, generalized lymphadenopathy, and hepatosplenomegaly. The hallmark of ALL is **pancytopenia**—total leukocyte counts are less than 10,000/mcL, with circulating blast cells on peripheral smear, and a bone marrow that is replaced by at least 25% blasts—though half of patients with ALL have an elevated WBC. **Acute nonlymphocytic leukemia (ANLL)**, also called **acute myelogenous leukemia (AML)**, is primarily a disease of adults. The **Auer rod** is pathognomonic of AML. **CLL** is an indolent B cell malignancy of older patients. Patients present with lymphadenopathy and lymphocytosis, and half have splenomegaly. **CML** is a disease of middle age presenting with significant leukocytosis, fever, night sweats, fatigue, and splenomegaly. CML is characterized by an overproduction of myeloid cells, the Philadelphia chromosome and the bcr/abl gene.

480. The answer is b. *(Kliegman, pp 396-397.)* This child has likely **aspirated a foreign body**, obstructing her airway. **A conscious child should be left alone if he or she is able to cough**, but bystanders should **intervene once stridor or respiratory distress increase or the child becomes unconscious.** At this point, the airway should be opened with a head-tilt/chin-lift maneuver and ventilation should be attempted. If this fails, it should be attempted again. If there is no chest rise, attempts at removing the foreign body should begin. Since this child is **over the age of 1** and is still conscious, the **Heimlich maneuver (five abdominal thrusts)** should be used with the child standing or sitting (or lying down if unconscious). The airway should be examined thereafter and the foreign body removed with a **finger sweep** if seen. If not, ventilate and repeat the Heimlich maneuver. For a **baby** under the age of 1, a combination of **back blows and chest thrusts** should be given with the baby positioned on your forearm and lap with his or her head downward. **Chest compressions** are used when a patient's heart is not beating.

481. The answer is b. *(Kliegman, pp 1405-1407.)* **Epiglottitis** is a medical emergency and involves progressive cellulitis of the epiglottis and surrounding tissues due to *H. influenzae* type B in children (usual age is 2-7 years) or *S. pneumoniae* or *S. aureus* in adults. Patients like the one is this case with epiglottitis have a high fever and complain of sore throat, drooling (inability to swallow secretions), dysphagia, odynophagia, and a muffled voice. The mnemonic to remember the symptoms of epiglottitis is the **four D's** (**D**rooling, **D**ysphagia, **D**yspnea, and **D**ysphonia). Posture is usually upright, leaning forward, and in children is called the **sniffing dog position.** Stridor (a loud, high-pitched sound) may also be present. The diagnosis of a **cherry-red epiglottis** is confirmed by laryngoscopy. Patients with **exudative pharyngitis** due to **group A *Streptococcus*** present with fever and large, tender anterior cervical lymphadenopathy. **Croup** is caused by a viral illness and is characterized by fever, a barklike cough, inspiratory stridor, and often respiratory distress. **Peritonsillar abscess (quinsy)** occurs as a complication of bacterial tonsillitis and is the accumulation of pus between the tonsil and its bed. Patients complain of sore throat, unilateral otalgia, dysarthria, and trismus. On throat examination, an enlarged, medially displaced tonsil (abscess) is seen in the peritonsillar area and the uvula is displaced to the opposite side. A typical gray-white membranous exudate in the pharynx is consistent with **diphtheria**, but this infection is rare in North America where children are routinely immunized.

482. The answer is d. *(Kliegman, pp 1645-1646.)* **A hydrocele** is a fluid leak through the patent processus vaginalis (usually on the right side), causing swellings in the scrotum, along the spermatic cord or through the inguinal canal into the abdomen. Hydroceles are common in infancy; if the tunica vaginalis is not patent, the hydrocele will usually resolve in the first 6 months of life. A **spermatocele** does transilluminate, but it does not grow as large as a hydrocele and it remains localized as a cystic swelling on the epididymis. A **varicocele** is due to torsion of the pampiniform plexus that surrounds the spermatic cord. It usually occurs on the left side in boys or young men and is very painful. When palpated, a varicocele feels like a "bag of worms." An **inguinal hernia** is a protrusion of bowel into the scrotal sac; often bowel sounds can be auscultated and the hernia reduced on examination. **Cryptorchidism** is an undescended testis; the scrotum remains small, flat, and underdeveloped.

483. The answer is c. *(Kliegman, pp 1888-1891.)* The three congenital heart defects that cause left-to-right shunts are the **three D's** (VSD, ASD, and PDA). All three may progress to **Eisenmenger syndrome** (pulmonary hypertension that leads to right heart failure and shunt reversal) which is inoperable. This patient has the most common congenital heart abnormality, a **VSD.** Small shunts may be asymptomatic or close spontaneously, but large left-to-right shunts may cause dyspnea, exercise intolerance, and congestive heart failure. Typically, patients have a loud P_2, a palpable thrill, and a holosystolic murmur (a murmur with a thrill, by definition, is a grade 4/6). **PDA** murmurs are **continuous and "machinelike"** with a laterally displaced apical impulse, while **ASDs have a fixed-split S_2.**

484. The answer is a. *(Kliegman, p 1697.)* **Reye syndrome** is an often fatal sequela to certain viral illnesses. Patients present with encephalopathy and fatty infiltration and dysfunction of the liver. **Salicylates** are suspected of potentiating this syndrome in patients with a viral illness; however, the syndrome may occur in the absence of salicylate use. The mortality rate in Reye syndrome is 50%. **Botulism** bacillus is usually found in canned, smoked, or vacuum-packed foods. Patients present with dysphagia, dysphonia, visual disturbances, diplopia, ptosis, and fixed and dilated pupils. Infants may become flaccid after eating **honey** due to the inhibition of acetylcholine release (from ***Clostridium botulinum***). Patients with **Wilson disease** have **Kayser-Fleischer rings** (yellow-brown) in the Descemet membrane and neuropsychiatric involvement. **Viral hepatitis** causes fever, elevated liver enzymes, and jaundice and may be transmitted via the fecal-oral route (hepatitis A), from sexual activity, or blood transfusions (hepatitis B and C). Identified in 1999, the **West Nile virus** is an arbovirus (anthropod-borne agent) that causes malaise, lethargy, sore throat, stiff neck, nausea, and vomiting. It progresses to stupor, convulsions, cranial nerve palsies, paralysis of extremities, and exaggerated deep tendon reflexes (signs of upper motor neuron disease).

485. The answer is c. *(Kliegman, p 1563.)* A **Meckel diverticulum** rarely causes symptoms, but infants by age 2 may present with the painless passage of maroon-colored stools. The diverticulum is a remnant of the omphalomesenteric duct and **is the most common gastrointestinal tract congenital anomaly** (2% of the population). The mnemonic for Meckel diverticulum is called the "**rule of 2's.**" It is usually **2 cm long within 2 ft of the ileocecal valve**, and **males** (usually **< 2 years old**) are **affected two times more than females.** It is made of **two kinds of ectopic tissues** (stomach and pancreas) and has **two complications** (bleeding and inflammation). **Pyloric stenosis** is seen in newborns. Patients present with projectile vomiting, abdominal distention, and a palpable olive-sized mass in the right upper quadrant that appears after vomiting. Prominent peristaltic waves are often visible going from the left to the right side of the abdomen. **Intussusception** (one segment of the intestine prolapses into another) is the most common cause of obstruction in the first 2 years of life. Infants present with melena, abdominal pain, vomiting, and diarrhea mixed with mucus and blood, giving it a **red currant jelly** appearance. Often, a sausage-shaped mass is palpable in the upper midabdominal area. **Biliary atresia** is a congenital obstruction or absence of the bile duct system. Newborns (2-3 weeks old) present with light-colored stools, dark urine, hepatomegaly, pruritus, and jaundice. **Zenker diverticulum** is a disorder of adults in which the pharyngeal mucosa protrudes through an area of weakness in the musculature proximal to the upper pharyngeal sphincter. Patients present with halitosis from retention of food and saliva in the diverticulum.

486. The answer is d. *(Kliegman, pp 178-182.)* The majority of victims of **sexual abuse** have no physical examination findings. Swelling and erythema of the vulvar tissue (genital trauma) should be a red flag for child abuse, especially if associated with bruising or a foul-smelling discharge. In addition to the anorectal and genitourinary problems, there can be significant behavioral changes, such as sexually provocative mannerisms, excessive masturbation, inappropriate sexual knowledge, enuresis, depression, social withdrawal, anxiety, school problems, and weight changes. A **straddle injury,** often from a bicycle seat, occurs over the symphysis pubis, whereas signs of sexual abuse are more posterior around the perineum.

487. The answer is e. *(Kliegman, pp 2736-2737.)* **Impetigo,** which arises from minor superficial breaks in the skin, is caused by *S aureus* or β-hemolytic *Streptococcus* and usually occurs in children. It is a highly contagious epidermal rash characterized by vesicles, erosions, or ulcers that **crust and appear golden-yellow** and stuck on. **Folliculitis,** which is an infection of the upper portion of the hair follicle, may appear as an erythematous papule, pustule, erosion, or crust lesion and is usually due to *S aureus*. In folliculitis due to hot tub use, the etiology is *P aeruginosa*. **Kawasaki disease (KD)** or **mucocutaneous lymph node syndrome** is uncommon in children over the age of 8 years and is characterized by fever; a desquamating, edematous, blotchy-appearing mucocutaneous erythema; cervical lymphadenitis; and aneurysms of the coronary arteries. It is idiopathic. **Staphylococcal scalded skin syndrome (SSSS)** is most common in neonates during the first 3 months of life. It is a toxin-mediated epidermolytic disease characterized by tender erythema that wrinkles, resembling wet tissue paper. Bullous formation and desquamation may occur. Widespread detachment of the superficial layers of the epidermis resembles scalding. **Miliaria** or prickly heat is a burning and pruritic rash of infants localized to the upper extremities, the trunk, and the intertriginous areas. A **Tzanck smear** is most often used to diagnose **herpesvirus**.

488. The answer is d. *(Kliegman, pp 2540-2544.)* Children like this one with **Duchenne muscular dystrophy (DMD)** (the most common hereditary neuromuscular disorder) present between the ages of 2 and 6 years with fatigability, clumsiness, difficulty standing, difficulty walking on toes, pseudohypertrophy of the calf muscles, and a waddling gait. DMD results from a deficiency of dystrophin, while **Becker MD** is the result of abnormal dystrophin. Becker MD is less severe than DMD and boys are ambulatory until late adolescence. Both Becker and Duchenne MD are X-linked myopathies. The **Gower maneuver** (pushing off with the hands when rising from the floor because of proximal muscle weakness) is positive in muscular dystrophy.

The autosomal dominant myopathies are myotonic dystrophy and facioscapulohumeral dystrophy. **Myotonic dystrophy** causes characteristic slow relaxation after muscle contraction and **distal** muscle wasting (most other myopathies affect proximal muscles). It is also characterized by diminished facial movements, slurred speech, cataracts, and testicular atrophy. **Facioscapulohumeral dystrophy** occurs between the ages of 10 and 20 years and is characterized by facial and shoulder girdle weakness. Patients are often unable to close their eyes fully and lips protrude as if puckered. **Limb-girdle muscular dystrophy** affects muscles of the hip and shoulder girdles starting in late childhood, but does not affect intelligence or cardiac function.

489. The answer is b. *(Kliegman, p 2297.)* Children, like this patient, with **constitutional growth delay** have normal length and weight at birth and normal growth for the first year. Through childhood their height is sustained at a lower percentile, paralleling the norm, and their pubertal growth spurt is delayed. A careful family history often reveals that their parents or other relatives had short stature in childhood, with delayed puberty and eventually normal height. In **familial short stature**, both the child and parents are small. In **congenital pathologic short stature**, an infant is born small and growth tapers off through infancy. This child has no evidence of **failure to thrive** (associated malnutrition, reduced muscle mass, and often poor developmental or cognitive function) or other endocrine causes for his growth delay.

490. The answer is c. *(Kliegman, pp 2140-2143.)* The most common renal tumor in children (usually age 2-5) is **Wilms tumor** or **nephroblastoma** (an embryonal tumor of renal origin). Children present with an abdominal mass which may or may not be painful, hematuria, weight loss, nausea, and vomiting. Physical examination typically reveals fever, hypertension, and an abdominal or flank mass. **Neuroblastoma** is a tumor of neural crest cell origin and as such, may arise in many locations, most often in the abdomen. Patients present with fever, anorexia, malaise, a firm abdominal mass, diarrhea, neuromuscular symptoms, bluish subcutaneous nodules and periorbital bruises. Wilms tumor and neuroblastoma may be differentiated by seeing calcification of neuroblastomas on x-ray or CT scan, while **Wilms tumor does not calcify and originates in the kidney.** Patients with **Hodgkin lymphoma** usually present between the ages of 15 and 45 years or over the age of 60 years with the complaint of painless cervical lymphadenopathy. **Ewing sarcoma** is a tumor predominantly of white children that involves the diaphyses of long bones. **Rhabdomyosarcoma is the most common childhood soft tissue sarcoma.** It may occur anywhere in the body, but most often in the head and neck, GU tract, extremities; symptoms depend on the location of the progressively enlarging mass.

491. The answer is b. *(Kliegman, p 1807.)* Patients with **cystic fibrosis** are at risk for developing various nutritional deficiencies due to **malabsorption from exocrine pancreatic insufficiency.** These may include deficiencies of both the **fat-soluble** vitamins **(A, D, E, and K)** and the **water-soluble** vitamins **(B_6 and B_{12})**. B_{12} deficiency occurs because pancreatic enzymes are not available to cleave R-protein and assist in B_{12} absorption. Patients with cystic fibrosis have high caloric, protein, and fat requirements. Vitamin therapy and appropriate enzyme therapy are needed to prevent nutritional complications.

492. The answer is b. *(Kliegman, pp 679-680.)* The **Apgar score** has **no predictive value regarding long-term outcome** but tells you a great deal about the newborn's respiratory efforts and **does predict survival in the neonatal period.** It is repeated a third time at 10 minutes only if the score is poor at 5 minutes. The Apgar scoring system (a score of 0-10 is possible) is based on **APGAR** = **A**ppearance, **P**ulse, **G**rimace, **A**ctivity, and **R**espirations:

	0	1	2
Heart rate	Absent	< 100/min	> 100/min
Respiratory effort	Absent	Slow or irregular	Good
Muscle tone	Limp	Some flexion	Active motion
Response to catheter	None	Grimace	Cough/sneeze in nostril
Color	Blue/pale	Body pink/ extremities blue	All pink

493 and 494. The answers are 493-c, 494-d. *(Kliegman, pp 1366-1367, 1380-1382.)* **Chickenpox (varicella zoster virus)** is characterized by crops of pruritic vesicles that evolve into pustules, crusts, and even scars. Most cases occur in young children and may be complicated by pneumonia or encephalitis. The incubation period is approximately 14 days. Patients may remember an exposure to another child with chickenpox or to an older person with zoster. **Roseola** (exanthem subitum) is a childhood disease and is due to human herpesvirus type 6 and 7. It is characterized by high fever for several days before multiple blanchable macules and papules appear on the back as the fever resolves. **Rubella** (German measles or 3-day measles) is a common childhood infection manifested by a characteristic exanthem and lymphadenopathy. **Rubeola,** or measles, is highly infectious and is characterized by fever, **C**onjunctivitis, **C**oryza, **C**ough (the **three C's**), and **Koplik spots.** It has a significant morbidity and mortality. **Erythema infectiosum (fifth disease)** is caused by parvovirus B19 and is a benign childhood illness characterized by fever, upper respiratory symptoms and joint complaints accompanied by a **"slapped cheek" rash** that spreads as lacy macules to the trunk and proximal extremities.

Bonus Chapter: The Ten Toughest Physical Diagnosis Questions Ever Written

Questions

1. A 42-year-old man was diagnosed with AIDS (acquired immunodeficiency syndrome) 6 years ago. His viral load is 200/μL, and his CD4 count is 199/μL. He has been taking HAART (highly active antiretroviral treatment) since diagnosis and is compliant with his medications. For the last several months, he has been noticing muscle wasting in his buttocks and an increase in abdominal girth. He denies jaundice, fever, abdominal pain, nausea, vomiting, and diarrhea. He has no melena or hematochezia. On physical examination, the patient is afebrile; heart rate is 84 beats per minute and blood pressure is 110/70 mm Hg. There is no jaundice or jugular venous distention (JVD); heart and lung examinations are normal. Abdominal examination reveals central obesity, normal bowel sounds, and no tenderness. Liver size is 14 cm in the midclavicular line (MCL) and there is no splenomegaly. The patient has no caput medusa and no shifting dullness. There is no peripheral edema but there is muscle atrophy in his face and buttocks. The patient is alert and oriented to person, place, and time and has no asterixis. There are no motor or sensory deficits. Which of the following is the most appropriate next step in diagnosis?

a. Liver biopsy
b. Ultrasound of the abdomen
c. CT scan of the abdomen
d. Cholesterol and triglyceride levels
e. Paracentesis
f. Repeat viral load
g. Repeat CD4 count

2. A 23-year-old woman presents to the emergency room with a 4-day history of temperature spikes to 40.2°C (104.3°F), night sweats, and shaking chills. She has a sore throat and arthralgias but has no cough, shortness of breath, headache, neck stiffness, earache, abdominal pain, or genitourinary symptoms. She develops a nonpruritic rash that appears with a temperature spike. On physical examination, the patient is febrile (38.3°C [101°F]) and has an evanescent salmon-colored rash located primarily over the chest and abdomen. Head, ear, eye, nose, and throat (HEENT) examination is normal except for some bilateral shoddy posterior cervical lymphadenopathy. Lungs, heart, abdomen, and joint examinations are normal. Laboratory data reveal a mild anemia and a white blood cell count of 40,000/μL. Iron levels are normal, but her ferritin level is 600 ng/mL (normal female levels are 4-161 ng/mL). Chest radiograph, urine cultures, and blood cultures are normal. Which of the following is the most appropriate next step in management?

a. High-dose aspirin
b. Deferoxamine or chelating agent
c. Treatment for tuberculosis
d. Broad-spectrum antibiotics
e. Antimalarial treatment

3. A 16-year-old adolescent has recently emigrated from Mexico with her family. Through an interpreter, the mother states that the teenager suddenly developed a fever to 38.9°C (102°F), chills, sore throat, malaise, and "break-bone" aching of the head, back, and extremities the day prior to the office visit. The patient denies earache, cough, abdominal pain, nausea, vomiting, diarrhea, and genitourinary complaints. The adolescent has never been sexually active. She has no pets and denies animal bites and ill contacts. Temperature is 39.2°C (102.5°F). When the blood pressure is taken, petechiae develop at the cuff site. Additionally, she has conjunctival redness and a diffuse maculopapular blotching of the skin. The rest of the physical examination is normal. White blood cell (WBC) count is 2500/μL, and platelet count is $55 \times 10^3/\mu L$. The rest of the laboratory data are normal. Which of the following is the most likely diagnosis?

a. *Plasmodium falciparum* (Malaria)
b. Yellow fever
c. Influenza
d. Dengue fever
e. Hantavirus
f. Colorado tick fever

4. A 31-year-old high school teacher presents to your office with a 3-day history of cough productive of greenish-colored sputum. The patient has been feeling feverish but denies chills, night sweats, shortness of breath, and chest pain. Past medical history is remarkable for seven episodes of otitis media in childhood, three episodes of sinusitis, four episodes of pharyngitis, two episodes of bronchitis, and two previous episodes of pneumonia over the last 10 years. The patient denies tobacco use, alcohol abuse, and illicit drug use. She has no recent travel history and no ill contacts. On physical examination, she has a temperature of 38.9°C (102°F); pulse oximetry shows a saturation of 98% on room air. Respiratory rate is 18 breaths per minute, and the patient is in no distress. She has bronchophony and crackles at the right base; there is no clubbing. Laboratory data reveal a leukocytosis with bandemia; chest radiograph is positive for a right lower-lobe alveolar infiltrate. Her HIV test is negative. Which of the following is the most appropriate next step in diagnosis?

a. CD4 count
b. Serum immunoglobulin levels
c. Purified protein derivative (PPD) skin test
d. Bone marrow biopsy
e. Abdominal fat aspiration
f. Bronchoscopy with transbronchial biopsy

5. A 19-year-old man presents with muscle aches and fatigue for several weeks. He denies fever, chills, night sweats, and weight loss. He has no sore throat, cough, chest pain, shortness of breath, abdominal pain, nausea, vomiting, diarrhea, or genitourinary complaints. He has no rashes, weakness, incontinence, gait disturbance, or sensory deficits. He does not use tobacco, drink alcohol, or use illicit drugs. He has no past illnesses, no recent travel, and no ill contacts. He takes no medications or herbal medicines. His diet consists of milk shakes, hamburgers, and french fries with extra salt added; he works as a cashier in a fast-food restaurant. The patient is afebrile, with normal blood pressure and pulse and no orthostatic changes. HEENT, heart, lung, and abdominal examinations are normal. Musculoskeletal examination reveals no muscle tenderness or atrophy. There are no neurologic deficits. Chvostek sign is positive. Laboratory data show a normal WBC count and differential, normal platelets and no anemia. His basic metabolic profile reveals a sodium of 142 mEq/L, potassium of 2.1 mEq/L, chloride of 88 mEq/L, and bicarbonate of 29 mEq/L. His blood urea nitrogen (BUN) and creatinine are normal. Calcium and phosphorus levels are normal; magnesium level is 0.8 mg/dL. Urinalysis is unremarkable. Electrocardiogram shows a normal QT interval and diffuse *u* waves. The potassium and magnesium are replaced, and the patient becomes asymptomatic; *u* waves on ECG resolve. Which of the following is the most likely diagnosis?

a. Liddle syndrome
b. Dehydration
c. Rhabdomyolysis
d. Bartter syndrome
e. Gitelman syndrome

6. A 21-year-old man complains of fever, night sweats, weight loss, and fatigue. Nontender, freely moveable lymphadenopathy is present in the posterior cervical, submandibular, submental, and inguinal chains. Heart and lung examinations are normal. Abdominal examination shows hepatosplenomegaly. Laboratory data are normal except for anemia. Which of the following is the most likely diagnosis?

a. Castleman disease
b. Rosai-Dorfman disease
c. Mucocutaneous lymph node syndrome
d. POEMS syndrome
e. Acute disseminated encephalomyelitis (ADEM)

7. A 47-year-old woman is started on warfarin for paroxysmal atrial fibrillation. After 7 days of therapy, she develops sharply demarcated, erythematous lesions that are purpuric and indurated. Hemorrhagic bullae and eschar formation are evident over some of the lesions located over the breasts, thighs, and buttocks. Which of the following mechanisms best explains the etiology of the findings?

a. Protein S deficiency
b. Protein C deficiency
c. Antithrombin III deficiency
d. Lupus anticoagulant
e. Anticardiolipin antibody syndrome

8. A 32-year-old church pastor presents with the chief complaint of "first morning" reddish-brown urine for 3 weeks and a 3-day history of slowly progressive right-sided vision loss. He has no past medical history and takes no medications. He denies trauma, fever, chills, night sweats, and weight loss. He has no back pain, abdominal pain, dysuria, or frequency. He does not smoke cigarettes, drink alcohol, or use illicit drugs. Family history is unremarkable. On physical examination, vital signs are normal. Pupils are equal and reactive to light, and extraocular muscle movements are intact. Vision in the left eye is 20/20; vision in the right eye is limited to seeing fingers (patient reports that his vision 1 year ago was 20/20 bilaterally). Funduscopic examination is remarkable for a retina with a "blood and thunder" appearance. Lungs, heart, abdomen, and genitalia are normal. There is no costovertebral angle (CVA) tenderness. Rectal examination is fecal occult blood test (FOBT) negative, and the prostate gland is normal. Laboratory data are consistent with a normochromic normocytic anemia; there is leukopenia and thrombocytopenia. Peripheral smear shows schistocytes; leukocyte alkaline phosphatase level is decreased. BUN and creatinine are normal, but there is blood in the urine by dipstick but not microscopically. Bone marrow biopsy is consistent with erythroid hyperplasia. Which of the following is the most appropriate next step in diagnosis?

a. Ham test
b. Sucrose lysis test
c. Serum lysis test
d. LDH level
e. Flow cytometry
f. Serum iron level

9. A 5-month-old female infant is brought to your office by anxious parents for abnormal hand movements, which started several days ago. The parents at first thought that the movements were "cute" because they appeared as though their daughter was wringing her hands. There has been no loss of consciousness, fever, vomiting, or seizure activity. Although the child has never been ill and was a normal vaginal delivery, the parents sense that their daughter has poor language skills and is not as socially interactive compared to other children in her age group. They thought it might be secondary to shyness, which she would "grow out of." On physical examination, the child is afebrile and is breathing normally. Head circumference is reduced (20th percentile), but height and weight are normal. There is no cyanosis or neck stiffness. Heart, lung, and abdominal examinations are normal. The child has no neurological deficits. Which of the following is the most likely diagnosis?

a. Asperger syndrome
b. Oppositional defiant disorder
c. Autism
d. Attention deficit hyperactive disorder (ADHD)
e. Childhood schizophrenia
f. Rett disorder
g. Conduct disorder
h. Pervasive developmental disorder (NOS)

10. A 41-year-old woman presents with a 5-day history of a 4-cm linear lesion of her right breast. She complains that the breast is painful, tender, and swollen. She denies fever, chills, and weight loss. The patient is G2P2 (children are 11 and 9 years old), and her last menstrual period was 7 days ago. She does not think she can be pregnant, since she and her husband practice birth control. The patient had a mammogram 5 months ago, which was normal. There is no family history of breast cancer. She does not use tobacco, alcohol, or illicit drugs. She denies trauma. Physical examination is remarkable for a cordlike subcutaneous 4-cm lesion of the right breast that is fibrous and tender to palpation. The breast is swollen and tender; the nipple is normal. There is no erythema or lymphadenopathy. There are no other masses palpable. Which of the following is the most appropriate next step in management?

a. Anticoagulation with heparin
b. Nonsteroidal anti-inflammatory drugs
c. Oral antibiotics for 10 to 14 days
d. Schedule for repeat mammography
e. *BRCA1* and *BRCA2* genetic testing
f. Oral prednisone for 10 to 14 days
g. Schedule for fine needle aspiration

Bonus Chapter: The Ten Toughest Physical Diagnosis Questions Ever Written

Answers

1. The answer is d. *(McPhee, p 1229.)* Almost all protease inhibitor and nucleoside analogue use has been associated with a constellation of abnormalities referred to as **lipodystrophy.** This syndrome, which occurs in up to three-fourth of patients on these medications, causes changes in body fat composition (ie, abdominal obesity and often a "buffalo hump", with peripheral wasting most evident in the face and buttocks) as well as elevated cholesterol and triglyceride levels, insulin resistance, and diabetes mellitus. As a result, the correct answer is to order **cholesterol and triglyceride levels.** These changes do not indicate the need for imaging, liver biopsy, or closer observation of the patient's immune status and the patient does not have ascites, so paracentesis is unnecessary. If necessary, you should treat lipodystrophy with gemfibrozil and pravastatin or atorvastatin **(lovastatin and simvastatin should be avoided because of their interactions with protease inhibitors).** Similar changes in body habitus have been reported in patients with HIV who have never been treated with these medications.

2. The answer is a. *(McPhee, pp 751-752.)* The patient requires high-dose **aspirin** (1 g three times a day) or an NSAID for treatment of **adult Still disease.** Still disease is considered a **variant of rheumatoid arthritis** in which **high-spiking fevers are the predominant presenting symptom** rather than joint disease. Patients are usually between 20 and 30 years of age. Fevers can be as high as 40.5°C (105°F) and are accompanied by the **classic evanescent salmon-colored rash on the chest and abdomen,** shaking chills, and night sweats. **It is not uncommon for fevers to plunge**

to several degrees below normal intermittently. The fever pattern strongly suggests the diagnosis. Patients may have lymphadenopathy and pericardial effusions. Joint symptoms are mild in the beginning, but a destructive arthritis develops months later. Patients may have anemia, prominent leukocytosis, and **very high ferritin levels** (possibly as an acute phase reactant, though the cause is unclear). Half of patients require high-dose prednisone, but **aspirin is typically given first.** A third of patients have recurrent episodes.

3. The answer is d. *(McPhee, pp 1263-1264.)* This patient has **Dengue fever,** which is due to a flavivirus transmitted by the bite of an Aedes mosquito. Outbreaks have occurred on the border of the United States with Mexico and in Mexico. Worldwide there are approximately 100 million cases of dengue; several hundred thousand will go on to develop **dengue hemorrhagic fever.** The incubation period is usually 7 to 10 days. Dengue fever's presentation is nonspecific and may range from no symptoms (especially in children) to severe hemorrhagic shock. Patients will often complain of high fevers, chills, sore throat, a diffuse maculopapular rash sparing the palms and soles, and "**breakbone**" head, back, and extremity pain. Thrombocytopenia may cause a positive "**tourniquet sign**" in which petechiae develop when the blood pressure cuff is inflated. IgM and IgG ELISA tests usually confirm the diagnosis; treatment is supportive. **Yellow fever** is also a flavivirus more endemic in Africa and South America. Patients (who are usually adult male, due to work habits) may have retro-orbital pain, photophobia, leukopenia, proteinuria, and abnormal liver function tests. A positive **Faget sign (fever with bradycardia)** is often seen in patients with yellow fever. Patients with **Hantavirus** often present with a pulmonary syndrome that leads to acute respiratory distress syndrome (ARDS). **Colorado tick fever** is usually benign and is a self-limited syndrome of fever, myalgias, headache, and leukopenia and thrombocytopenia. Symptom resolution usually occurs within a week, but is closely followed in over half of patients by a relapse of fever and other symptoms for a few days more. **Influenza** is usually accompanied by fever, a nonproductive cough and coryza, without a rash or petechiae. Patients with **malaria** due to *P falciparum* will often have profuse sweating, abdominal cramps, vomiting, diarrhea, hemolytic anemia, dark urine **("blackwater fever")**, splenomegaly, and central nervous system involvement.

4. The answer is b. *(McPhee, pp 786-787.)* The patient most likely has **common variable immunodeficiency syndrome,** which is a defect in terminal differentiation of B cells with absent plasma cells and deficient synthesis of secreted antibody (decreased IgG levels). Patients present with **recurrent sinopulmonary infections** secondary to humoral immune deficiency **(panhypogammaglobulinemia).** Patients may also have diarrhea, malabsorption, hepatosplenomegaly, protein-losing enteropathy, and a spruelike syndrome. Interestingly, there may be an increase in autoimmune diseases (20%) as well as an increase in B cell neoplasms (lymphomas), gastric and skin cancers. Diagnosis is confirmed by the demonstration of **defects in antibody production.** Infections must be treated aggressively with antibiotics; monthly maintenance therapy with **intravenous immunoglobulin** should be considered in all patients (following serum IgG trough levels). As mentioned, this is a defect in B cells, so a **CD4 count** (T cells) is unnecessary. She does not require **bronchoscopy** at this time for what appears to be a community acquired pneumonia, and she does not need an **abdominal fat aspiration** which may be done to diagnose **amyloidosis** (sensitivity of 80%). She does not have risk factors for tuberculosis, so a **PPD** is unnecessary.

5. The answer is e. *(Kliegman, pp 2201-2202.)* The patient has **Gitelman syndrome** (a variant of Bartter syndrome) due to a gene defect in the distal convoluted tubule Na-Cl cotransporter (a distal tubule disorder). Patients present with **muscle aches, cramps, fatigue, and salt craving.** It is important to ask patients about adding extra salt or eating high-salt-content foods to determine salt craving. Patients with Gitelman syndrome will have a **hypokalemic metabolic alkalosis with hypomagnesemia, and hypocalciuria** (with normal serum calcium levels). In this case, the positive **Chvostek sign** is due to **hypomagnesemia** and not hypocalcemia. An electrocardiogram with ***u* waves** is consistent with hypokalemia; hypomagnesemia may cause **prolongation of the QT interval. Bartter syndrome** is a genetic defect affecting channels in the medullary thick ascending limb of Henle's loop. Patients have a metabolic alkalosis, hypokalemia, hypomagnesemia, and hypocalcemia (positive Chvostek sign). **Patients with Bartter syndrome present in childhood** (there is evidence of growth failure), while **patients with Gitelman syndrome present in early adulthood. Liddle syndrome** is a rare inherited tubular disorder causing distal nephron hyperfunction and is characterized by alkalosis, hypokalemia, and hypertension. The patient has no blood (false-positive dipstick) in the urine to suggest **rhabdomyolysis** and no orthostatic changes to suggest **dehydration**.

6. The answer is a. *(Kliegman, pp 2094-2095.)* Patients with **Castleman disease** (angiofollicular lymph node hyperplasia) present with anemia, fever, night sweats, malaise, and weight loss. Patients with localized disease present with an isolated enlarged node in the mediastinum or abdomen, while those with disseminated disease have lymphadenopathy, hepatosplenomegaly, and polyclonal hypergammaglobulinemia. The condition has been associated with an overproduction of interleukin 6 most likely caused by human herpesvirus type 8. Patients with disseminated disease are treated with steroids, monoclonal antibodies to IL-6, antiviral agents, and interferon alpha. **Rosai-Dorfman disease** is a nonprogressive self-limited disease found in children and young adults; patients present with bulky lymphadenopathy. **Kawasaki disease, formerly known as mucocutaneous lymph node syndrome**, causes severe vasculitis of all blood vessels including the coronary arteries with myocarditis. Symptoms include fever, conjunctivitis, pharyngeal erythema with strawberry tongue, erythema of the hands and feet, rash, and cervical lymphadenopathy. The features of **POEMS syndrome** (osteosclerotic myeloma or Crow-Fukase syndrome) are Polyneuropathy, Organomegaly, Endocrinopathy, M-protein, and Skin changes. Besides the progressive sensorimotor neuropathy, patients present with lymphadenopathy and organomegaly. Skin changes consist of hypertrichosis, hyperpigmentation, skin thickening, and digital clubbing. Endocrine manifestations may include type 2 diabetes, amenorrhea, erectile dysfunction, adrenal insufficiency, hypothyroidism, and hyperprolactinemia. The pathogenesis of POEMS syndrome is unknown but is probably related to high-circulating cytokine levels. Treatment of the multiple myeloma may result in improvement of manifestations. **Acute disseminated encephalomyelitis (ADEM)** is associated with antecedent smallpox, measles, chicken pox, or rabies immunization; patients present with sensory loss, hemiplegia, quadriplegia, and brainstem involvement.

7. The answer is b. *(Fauci, p 345.)* The rare reaction of **warfarin-induced skin necrosis** occurs in patients with **protein C deficiency** between the third and tenth days of therapy with warfarin derivatives. Protein C is a vitamin K–dependent protein that has a shorter half-life than the other coagulation proteins. **Warfarin creates a vitamin K–independent state and will transiently deplete protein C before it leads to anticoagulation.** Without protein C, there is a transient **hypercoagulable state**, and thrombosis of the skin vessels leads to what is known as warfarin-induced necrosis. The development of the syndrome is unrelated to drug dose or underlying condition. The most common areas for the skin necrosis are **thighs, buttocks, and breasts** (the reaction is more common in **women**). Using heparin for 5 to 7 days until warfarin induces anticoagulation can prevent the syndrome. Warfarin-induced necrosis is treated with heparin and vitamin K. Protein C concentrates may be helpful in patients with known protein C deficiency. The course is not altered by discontinuation of warfarin after onset of the eruption.

8. The answer is e. *(Kliegman, pp 2024-2025.)* The most common manifestations of **paroxysmal nocturnal hemoglobinuria (PNH)** are hemolytic anemia, venous thrombosis, and defective hematopoiesis acquired at the stem cell level. Patients have evidence of intravascular hemolysis, that is, **hemoglobinuria and hemosiderinuria;** they often have **leukopenia** and **thrombocytopenia** (further reflection of impaired hematopoiesis). The activation of complement indirectly stimulates platelet aggregation and hypercoagulability, which leads to thrombosis (in this case, retinal vein thrombosis). Bone marrow may appear normocellular. For many years, the diagnosis of PNH depended upon demonstrating red blood cell (RBC) lysis after complement activation by either acid **(Ham test)** or by reduction in ionic strength **(sucrose lysis test)**, but the Ham and sucrose lysis tests are no longer reliable. They have been replaced by **flow cytometry** analysis of complement defense proteins (either **CD59** or DAF). These proteins block complement activation on the cell surface, and if absent, RBCs will be sensitive to complement lysis and have a tendency for platelets to abnormally initiate clotting. Hemoglobinuria (as well as myoglobinuria) should not be confused with hematuria. A urine microscopy that reveals more than 3 RBCs/HPF would support the diagnosis of hematuria.

9. The answer is f. *(Kliegman, pp 2504-2505.)* Females are more likely than males to present with **Rett syndrome,** an X-linked dominant disorder of early brain development with a prevalence of 1/20,000 (males usually die at birth). Clinical features include **reduced head circumference (microcephaly), loss of social relatedness, and classic "hand wringing" movements.** They also have impaired language function, scoliosis, and impaired mental functioning. Children are approximately 5 months of age at the time of diagnosis and death usually occurs in adolescence. Children with **autism** have severe deficits in social responsiveness and interpersonal relationships. Speech and language development are abnormal; children often demonstrate peculiarities, such as ritualized behaviors, rigidity, and lack of interest in age-typical activities. Children may lack attention to the primary caregiver's face and fail to respond to voices. Most autistic children function at the mentally retarded level. Onset is usually in early childhood, and more boys than girls are affected. Children with **Asperger syndrome** (also more common in males) are of normal intelligence but have a limited ability to appreciate social nuances, display motor clumsiness, and they have eccentric interests. Children with **childhood schizophrenia** have hallucinations and delusions. Thought content is bizarre and morbid; speech is rambling and illogical. **Attention deficit hyperactive disorder (ADHD)** is characterized by distractibility, short attention span, and impulsiveness. Children may engage in aimless activity and display hyperactive behavior at home and on the playground, in the classroom (this is usually where it is first recognized), and even in the doctor's office. The disorder is more common in boys than in girls. **Oppositional defiant disorder** is characterized by persistent disobedience and opposition to authority figures, especially in the home. However, children still respect the basic rights of others, and age-appropriate societal rules and behavior are not violated. Before puberty, the disorder is more frequently found in males than in females; after puberty, the ratio evens out. The typical child with **conduct disorder** is a boy with academic difficulties who is constantly fighting, running away, throwing tantrums, and in general is defiant of authority. With increasing age, truancy, vandalism, fire setting, theft, sexual promiscuity, substance abuse, and other criminal behaviors may occur. **Pervasive developmental disorder (PDD)** denotes a group of disorders with the common findings of impairment of socialization skills and characteristic behavioral abnormalities. Patients may also have speech and language deficits. PDD may be autistic, nonautistic (ie, Rett disorder), or NOS (not otherwise specified).

10. The answer is b. *(Fauci, pp 563-570.)* The patient with the sudden appearance of a subcutaneous cord of the breast, which is initially red and tender and subsequently becomes a painless, tough, fibrous band, has **Mondor disease**, or thrombophlebitis of the subcutaneous veins of the anterolateral chest wall. It is a self-limited benign disease that responds to **nonsteroidal anti-inflammatory drugs (NSAIDs)**. Mondor disease is more common in women but may be seen in men. It is **associated with breast cancer**, so yearly mammograms are recommended.

High-Yield Facts
Helpful Hints and Mnemonics by Organ System

GENERAL INSPECTION

Body Mass Index

- Normal BMI is defined as 18.5 to 24.9 kg/m^2.
- Overweight is a BMI of 25 to 29.9 kg/m^2.
- Obesity is a BMI of 30 to 39.9 kg/m^2.
- Morbid obesity is a BMI of more than 40 kg/m^2.
- Mild malnutrition is defined as a BMI of 17 to 18.4 kg/m^2.
- Moderate malnutrition is a BMI of 16 to 16.9 kg/m^2.
- Severe malnutrition is a BMI of less than 16.0 kg/m^2.

CAGE QUESTIONNAIRE to evaluate for ALCOHOL ABUSE

1. Have you felt the need to Cut down on your drinking?
2. Have you ever felt Annoyed by criticisms of your drinking?
3. Have you ever felt Guilty about your drinking?
4. Have you ever needed an Eye-opener in the morning?

SAFE QUESTIONNAIRE to evaluate for DOMESTIC ABUSE

S = Do you feel Safe or Stressed in a relationship?

A = Have you ever been Abused or Afraid in a relationship?

F = Are your Friends and Family aware of your relationship problem?

E = Do you have an Emergency plan if needed?

DEPRESSION mnemonic "**SIG E CAPS**" (at least one of the symptoms must be depressed mood or loss of interest)

Sleep (too much or too little)

Interest (anhedonia—lack of interest)

Guilt (excessive/inappropriate)

Energy (loss/fatigue)

Concentration (diminished)

Appetite (increased or decreased)

Psychomotor retardation

Suicidal thoughts or attempt + depressed mood

PANIC DISORDER mnemonic is **PANIC** (4 out of 5 required)

Palpitations

Abdominal pain

Nausea

Increased perspiration

Chest pain, **C**hills, or **C**hoking

HYPERSENSITIVITY REACTIONS

Type I (Immediate) are IgE mediated and cause urticaria and anaphylaxis (eg, atopic dermatitis).

Type II are antibody-mediated. They are due to transfusions (ABO mismatch) or use of medications and typically cause hemolysis, thrombocytopenia, and nephritis (eg, Rh hemolytic disease of the newborn).

Type III are immune complex-mediated (eg, serum sickness).

Type IV are delayed hypersensitivity cause a contact dermatitis, pulmonary fibrosis, photosensitivity, and toxic epidermal necrolysis.

DERMATOLOGY

Morphologic warning signs of **MELANOMA** (mnemonic **ABCD)**

Asymmetry

Border

Color variation

Diameter increase

Possible causes of **ACANTHOSIS NIGRICANS** (mnemonic **PAID COb**)

Polycystic ovarian disease

Acromegaly

Insulin resistance

Diabetes mellitus

Cancer (colon, stomach)

Obesity

Possible cause of migratory necrolytic erythema: **GLUCAGONOMA**

Possible cause of acrodermatitis enteropathica: **ZINC DEFICIENCY**

Precursor lesion of **SQUAMOUS CELL CARCINOMA** of the skin: **ACTINIC KERATOSIS**

Precursor lesion of **MELANOMA**: **DYSPLASTIC NEVUS**

Erythemas

ERYTHEMA NODOSUM associated conditions (mnemonic **BUMP SIS**)

Behçet syndrome, **B**irth control pills (BCPs)

Ulcerative colitis

***M**ycobacterium tuberculosis* (MTB)

Parasites

Sarcoidosis, **S**ulfonamides

Inflammatory bowel disease (IBD)

Streptococcal and fungal infections

ERYTHEMA CHRONICUM MIGRANS (ECM): Lyme disease

ERYTHEMA MIGRANS LINGUALIS: geographic tongue (erythema migrans of the tongue)

ERYTHEMA MARGINATUM: rheumatic fever

ERYTHEMA MULTIFORME: Stevens-Johnson syndrome, sulfonamides, NSAIDs, Dilantin

PITYRIASIS ROSEA: initial lesion "**herald patch**"; other lesions follow a "**Christmas tree**" pattern, resolves spontaneously in weeks

PSORIASIS: associated with **pitting** of the nails

NAIL CLUBBING is associated with the following:

- Lung diseases: lung cancer, chronic bronchitis (not emphysema), TB, bronchiectasis, hypoxemia due to pulmonary shunts
- GI diseases: IBD (Crohn disease/ulcerative colitis), cirrhosis
- Cardiac diseases: infective endocarditis, cardiogenic shunts, hypertrophic pulmonary osteoarthropathy
- Pregnancy
- Amyloidosis

HEENT

A CENTRAL CRANIAL NERVE VII PALSY spares the forehead, while a **PERIPHERAL one (BELL PALSY)** does not

ARGYLL ROBERTSON PUPILS: "prostitute pupils"—"they accommodate but won't react (to light)." Mnemonic for causes: **SAD**

Syphilis (tertiary)—**classic association**

Alcoholism (Wernicke encephalopathy)

Diabetes

(LR_6 SO_4)$_3$ = **L**ateral **R**ectus is innervated by cranial nerve **VI**, **S**uperior **O**blique by CN **IV** and all the rest by CN III

MARCUS GUNN PUPIL: afferent pupillary defect on swinging flashlight test, dilates on direct light seen in **OPTIC NEURITIS, CENTRAL RETINAL ARTERY OCCLUSION**

BLUE SCLERAS: hallmark of **OSTEOGENESIS IMPERFECTA**

PAPILLEDEMA: most common causes (associated with increased intracranial pressure) mnemonic is **HAM TIP**

Hematoma

Abscesses

Meningitis

Tumors

Intracranial hemorrhages

Pseudotumor cerebri

BULLOUS MYRINGITIS

- Pathognomonic for *Mycoplasma pneumoniae* infection
- May occur in Ramsay Hunt syndrome
- Viral and bacterial infections

WEBER TEST: base of vibrating fork over the midline of the SKULL

In CONDUCTIVE hearing loss:	Weber sign lateralizes to the **bad** ear
In SENSORINEURAL loss:	Weber sign lateralizes to the **good** ear

RINNE TEST: base of vibrating tuning fork over the MASTOID

In CONDUCTIVE defect:	bone conduction lasts longer than air conduction (bone > air)
In SENSORINEURAL loss:	air and bone conduction are equally affected so air conduction lasts longer than bone conduction (air > bone)

Example, left cerumen impaction: Weber lateralizes to left ear while Rinne bone > air on left

RESPIRATORY DISEASES

Respirations

KUSSMAUL **respirations: fast and deep** respirations seen in patients with **diabetic ketoacidosis (DKA)**

BIOT **respirations:** irregular, unpredictable periods of **apnea alternating with periods of noisy hyperventilation** seen in patients with **increased intracranial pressure**

CHEYNE-STOKES **respirations: a rhythmic, gradually changing pattern of apnea and hyperpnea** that is **cardiac or neurologic** in origin

APNEUSTIC **breathing:** characterized by a **long period of inspiration or gasping** with almost no expiratory phase

HOARSENESS: a helpful mnemonic for causes is **VINDICATE**

- **V**ascular (thoracic aneurysm)
- **I**nflammation
- **N**eoplasm
- **D**egenerative (ie, amyotrophic lateral sclerosis)
- **I**ntoxication (smoking, alcohol)
- **C**ongenital (laryngeal web)
- **A**llergies
- **T**rauma
- **E**ndocrine (thyroiditis)

SADDLE NOSE DEFORMITY: mnemonic is **CRoWS**

- **C**ocaine abuse
- **R**elapsing polychondritis
- **W**egener granulomatosis
- **S**yphilis

Criteria for **ALLERGIC BRONCHOPULMONARY ASPERGILLOSIS (ABPA):** mnemonic is **ESCAPE A** (escape ABPA)

- **E**osinophilia
- **S**kin reactivity to *Aspergillus* antigen
- **C**entral bronchiectasis
- **A**sthma
- **P**ulmonary infiltrates
- **E**levated serum IgE levels
- **A**ntibodies to *Aspergillus* antigen

The most sensitive physical sign and most common ECG finding of **PULMONARY EMBOLISM: sinus tachycardia**

Livedo reticularis + shortness of breath following **fracture** of femur: **FAT EMBOLI**

Blue **b**loater: **CHRONIC BRONCHITIS**

Pink puffer: **EMPHYSEMA**

CHEST EXAMINATION PHYSICAL FINDINGS				
Disease	**Trachea**	**Fremitus**	**Percussion**	**Breath Sounds**
Pleural effusion (large)	Shifted to opposite side	Decreased	Dull	Decreased
Consolidation (pneumonia)	Midline	Increased	Dull	Bronchial
Tension Pneumothorax	Shifted to opposite side	Decreased	Hyperresonant	Decreased
Atelectasis	Shifted to same side	Decreased	Dull	Decreased
Emphysema	Midline	Decreased	Hyperresonant	Decreased

CARDIOLOGY

Mnemonic for the **four auscultatory sites**: **A**ll **P**hysicians **T**ake **M**oney (or Meds)

All = **A**ortic (second right intercostal space [RICS])

Physicians = **P**ulmonic (second left intercostal space [LICS])

Take = **T**ricuspid (along left lower sternal border)

Money = **M**itral (fifth LICS, midclavicular line)

MURMURS are caused by turbulent blood flow and **GRADED 1 to 6:**

Grade 1 murmurs are barely audible.

Grade 2 murmurs are quiet but audible with a stethoscope.

Grade 3 murmurs are easily heard and should not be missed.

Grade 4 murmurs are loud with a palpable **thrill**.

Grade 5 murmurs are very loud and can be heard with the diaphragm barely on the chest.

Grade 6 murmurs can be heard with the stethoscope off the chest.

- **RIght** = **R**ight sided murmurs get louder with **I**nspiration
- **LEft** = **L**eft sided murmurs get louder with **E**xpiration

SYSTOLIC MURMURS	DIASTOLIC MURMURS
Tricuspid regurgitation (TR)	Tricuspid stenosis (TS)
Mitral regurgitation (MR)	Mitral stenosis (MS)
Pulmonic stenosis (PS)	Pulmonic insufficiency (PI)
Aortic stenosis (AS)	Aortic insufficiency (AI)

Characteristic Cardiac Findings

AORTIC REGURGITATION/AORTIC INSUFFICIENCY:

- Wide arterial pulse pressure
- High-pitched decrescendo diastolic murmur
- Diastolic rumble (from the aortic regurgitant flow displacing the mitral valve, often called the **Austin Flint murmur**)
- **Musset sign** (head bobbing with the heartbeat)
- **Water-hammer pulse or Corrigan pulse** (rapidly rising and collapsing pulse)
- **Hill sign** (an increase of > 40 mm Hg in femoral artery systolic BP compared to brachial artery BP)
- **Quincke pulse** (nail-bed capillary pulsations)
- **Pistol-shot pulse** (booming sound heard over the femoral arteries)
- **Duroziez sign** (bruit auscultated over the femoral artery when compressed)

PATENT DUCTUS ARTERIOSUS: **"continuous machinery murmur"**

PULMONIC STENOSIS: **systolic ejection murmur** with a **thrill at the UPPER LEFT sternal border**

VENTRICULAR SEPTAL DEFECT (VSD): **holosystolic** murmur with a **thrill at the LOWER LEFT sternal border**

MITRAL REGURGITATION: **holosystolic** murmur best heard at the **APEX, radiating to the AXILLA**

AORTIC STENOSIS: **crescendo-decrescendo midsystolic ejection** murmur along **LEFT STERNAL BORDER radiating to the CAROTIDS** with **palpable S4**

MITRAL VALVE PROLAPSE: **midsystolic click** with **late systolic murmur**

MITRAL STENOSIS: **opening snap** soon after P_2, loud S_1, **diastolic rumble**

CONSTRICTIVE PERICARDITIS: **pericardial knock**

ATRIAL FLUTTER: "sawtooth" pattern on ECG

ATRIAL FIBRILLATION:

- **Physical examination:** "irregularly irregular" rhythm, pulse deficit, **NEVER associated with an S_4**
- **ECG:** absent P waves, and irregular baseline
- A useful mnemonic for causes of atrial fibrillation is **PIRATES**:

  P—pericarditis, pulmonary disease, pulmonary embolism

  I—ischemia, infarction, infection, and inflammation

  R—rheumatic heart disease

  A—atrial septal defect

  T—thyrotoxicosis

  E—elevated blood pressure, ETOH excess and withdrawal

  S—sleep apnea, surgery (cardiothoracic)

BACTERIAL ENDOCARDITIS:

- **Splinter hemorrhages** under the nails
- **Roth spots** (oval retinal hemorrhages with a pale center)
- **Osler nodes (tender** nodes on finger or toe pads)
- **Janeway lesions** (small **nontender** hemorrhages on the palms and soles)

ATRIAL MYXOMA: associated with a "**tumor plop**"

IMPORTANT PULSE PATTERNS

Pulse Finding	Conditions
Pulsus alternans	Cardiac tamponade
Pulsus bisferiens	Aortic regurgitation and HCM/IHSS
Pulsus paradoxus	Cardiac tamponade, asthma, constrictive pericarditis
Pulsus tardus	Aortic stenosis

EXTRA HEART SOUNDS

Extra Sound	Conditions
Midsystolic click	MVP
Opening snap	Mitral/tricuspid stenosis
Pericardial knock	Constrictive pericarditis
Pericardial friction rub	Pericarditis

FIRST HEART SOUND	
Loud	**Soft**
Mitral stenosis	Mitral regurgitation
Short PR interval (WPW)	Long PR interval
Left atrial myxoma	LBBB
MVP with regurgitation	AR, TR

SECOND HEART SOUND			
Wide Split	**Narrow or Paradoxical**	**Fixed Split**	**Summary**
RBBB	**L**BBB	ASD	**Fixed split = ASD** (the only 1)
MR, VSD	**H**TN		Narrow/paradoxical mnemonic = **LHAIM**
RV volume overload (l-r shunt)	**A**ortic stenosis		All others have a wide split
RV pressure overload (PS, PAH)	**I**HSS		
	Acute **MI**		

Jones criteria for **RHEUMATIC FEVER**: mnemonic is **FEAR CASES**

Minor Criteria*	Major Criteria*
Fever	**C**arditis
ECG changes (PR prolonged)	Migratory **A**rthritis
Arthralgias	**S**ydenham chorea
Reactant, acute phase	**E**rythema marginatum
	Subcutaneous nodules

*To fulfill the Jones criteria, either two major criteria or one major and two minor criteria plus evidence of an antecedent streptococcal infection is required.

GASTROENTEROLOGY

Abdominal distension is caused by the **six Fs:**

Fat, Fluid, Food, Fetus, Feces, and Flatus

CHARCOT TRIAD: indicates **acute cholangitis** in 70% of cases

1. Biliary pain
2. Jaundice
3. Fever (with chills and rigor)

REYNOLD PENTAD: positive in only 10% of patients with cholangitis
Charcot triad (1, 2, and 3 above) plus:
4. Mental confusion
5. Refractory sepsis manifested by hypotension

MANEUVERS/SIGNS and their associations:
Signs of retroperitoneal bleeding:

- **Cullen sign**—periumbilical discoloration ("C" fits around the umbilicus)
- **Grey Turner sign**-flank discoloration ("Turn" on your side)

Murphy sign: inspiratory halt with palpation of RUQ, indicating acute cholecystitis

Caput medusae: vascular engorgement around the umbilicus, indicating liver cirrhosis

Courvoisier gallbladder: nontender RUQ mass, indicative of cancer of the biliary tract or pancreatic head

Kehr sign: Acute pain in tip of the shoulder, may indicate splenic rupture

Obturator test, reverse psoas maneuver: diagnoses retrocecal appendicitis

Markle sign: pain with jarring movement (eg, hit bottom of foot), specific for peritonitis

Succussion splash: indicates intestinal obstruction or gastric dilatation

Bedside maneuvers to detect **ASCITES:**

- Inspection for bulging flanks
- Percussion for flank dullness
- Shifting dullness maneuver
- Fluid wave maneuver

Causes of **CIRRHOSIS**: mnemonic is **ABCDEF**

Alpha-1-antitrypsin deficiency

Budd-Chiari syndrome, hepatitis **B**

Hepatitis **C**, **C**opper overload

Drugs

Ethanol

Fe overload

Physical findings seen in **HEMOCHROMATOSIS:**

- Bronzed skin pigmentation (sun-exposed areas)
- Hepatomegaly with or without cirrhosis
- Degenerative arthritis of the hands and fingers (proximal PIPs)
- Testicular atrophy

Irreversible complications of **HEMOCHROMATOSIS** (despite therapy):

- Arthropathy
- Hypogonadism
- Cirrhosis

NEPHROLOGY

Causes of **HIGH ANION GAP ACIDOSIS**: mnemonic is **C MUDPILES**

Cyanide

Methanol

Uremia

Diabetic ketoacidosis

Paraldehyde

Isoniazid, **I**ron

Lactic acidosis

Ethylene glycol, **E**thanol

Salicylates, **S**tarvation

Causes of **NON–ANION GAP ACIDOSIS** (hyperchloremia): mnemonic is **USED CARP**

Ureteroenterostomy

Spironolactone

Expansion acidosis (saline)

Diarrhea

Carbonic anhydrase inhibitors, **C**yclosporine

Amiloride: **A**ddison disease

Renal tubular acidosis

Pancreatic fistula, **P**entamidine

Indications for **EMERGENT HEMODIALYSIS**: mnemonic is **AEIOU**

Acidosis unresolved with bicarbonate treatment

Electrolyte abnormality (refractory hyperkalemia despite kayexalate)

Ingestion (barbiturates, bromide, chloral hydrate, ethanol, ethylene glycol, isopropyl alcohol, lithium, methanol, procainamide, theophylline, salicylates, and heavy metals)

Overload (fluid) unresponsive to diuretics

Uremia (pericarditis, encephalopathy or coagulopathy)

Causes of **HEMATURIA:** mnemonic is **SWITCH GPS**

Stones, **S**ickle cell disease, **S**cleroderma, **S**LE, **S**ulfonamides

Wegener granulomatosis

Infections, **I**nstrumentation, **I**atrogenic, **I**nterstitial nephritis

Trauma, **T**B, **T**umor, **T**TP, **T**ubulointerstitial disease

Cryoglobulinemia, **C**yclophosphamide

Hemolytic uremic syndrome, **H**enoch-Schönlein purpura, **H**emophilia

Goodpasture disease

Papillary necrosis, **P**olycystic kidney disease, **P**olyarteritis nodosa

Schistosomiasis, **S**ponge disease (medullary)

URINARY TRACT INFECTIONS (UTIs) (most common organisms responsible) mnemonic is **SEEK PP**

Serratia marcescens

Escherichia coli

Enterobacter cloacae

Klebsiella

Proteus mirabilis

Pseudomonas aeruginosa

ENDOCRINOLOGY

Complications of **ACROMEGALY:**

- Sleep apnea syndrome
- Carpal tunnel syndrome
- CH (LVH)
- Increased risk of colon cancer
- Increased risk of osteoarthritis
- Hypertension

BITEMPORAL HEMIANOPSIA	vs.	**HOMONYMOUS HEMIANOPSIA**
(on optic chiasm)		(behind the chiasm)
Etiologies:		
Craniopharyngioma Aneurysm Pituitary tumor		Occipital lesions secondary to AIDS, herpes, tumor

SYNDROME OF INAPPROPRIATE ADH SECRETION (SIADH)	vs.	**DIABETES INSIPIDUS (DI)**
Decreased serum sodium		Increased serum sodium
Increased urine osmolality		Decreased urine osmolality
Increased urine sodium		

TSH: single best test of thyroid function

Lid lag and stare: most important physical findings to suggest **GRAVES DISEASE**

Delayed deep tendon reflexes (DTRs): most important physical finding in **HYPOTHYROIDISM**

CHVOSTEK and **TROUSSEAU SIGNS**: suggest **hypocalcemia**

HYPERCALCEMIA

- "**Stones**"—renal calculi
- "**Bones**"—fractures, osteitis fibrosa
- "**Groans**"—constipation, vomiting, peptic ulcers, pancreatitis
- "**Psychic overtones**"—anxiety, depression, insomnia, psychosis

Causes of **HYPERCALCEMIA**: mnemonic is **CHIMPANZEES**

Calcium supplements

Hyperparathyroidism

Iatrogenic (thiazides), **I**mmobility

Milk-alkali syndrome

Paget disease

Addison disease/Acromegaly

Neoplasm

Zollinger-Ellison syndrome (MEN-1)

Excess vitamin A

Excess vitamin D

Sarcoidosis

POLYCYSTIC OVARIAN DISEASE (Stein-Leventhal syndrome, PCOD): amenorrhea, obesity, hirsutism, elevated LH:FSH ratio (>3)

MEN-I (Wermer Syndrome)	MEN-2A (Sipple Syndrome)	MEN-2B
PPP **P**ituitary adenoma **P**ancreatic islet cell tumor **P**arathyroid hyperplasia	PPT **P**arathyroid hyperplasia **P**heochromocytoma Medullary **T**hyroid cancer	PNT **P**heochromocytoma **N**euromas Medullary **T**hyroid cancer

A man with gynecomastia + small testes + tall stature + female hair distribution: think **KLINEFELTER SYNDROME**

A patient with pigmented mucosa of the gums + hypokalemia + pigmentation of skin creases: think **ADDISON DISEASE**

Hypogonadism + anosmia: **KALLMANN SYNDROME**

PHEOCHROMOCYTOMA: "rule of 10": bilateral, malignant, extraadrenal, familial, children

HEMATOLOGY AND ONCOLOGY

HENOCH-SCHÖNLEIN PURPURA (HSP): purpuric rash + abdominal pain + glomerulonephritis in a child/young patient mnemonic is **AGAR**

Abdominal pain

Glomerulonephritis

Arthralgia

Rash

Purpura (livedo reticularis) after a coronary angiogram: think **CHOLESTEROL ATHEROEMBOLIC DISEASE**

Purpura (livedo reticularis) + hepatitis B + abdominal pain after meals + footdrop + HTN: think **POLYARTERITIS NODOSA**

THROMBOTIC THROMBOCYTOPENIC PURPURA (TTP): mnemonic is **FAT RN** Pentad:

1. **F**ever
2. Microangiopathic hemolytic **A**nemia (+ schistocytes)
3. **T**hrombocytopenia
4. **R**enal abnormalities
5. **N**eurologic abnormalities (confusion, aphasia, headache, coma, seizures)

HEMOLYTIC UREMIC SYNDROME (HUS): mnemonic is **RAT**

Renal failure

Microangiopathic hemolytic **A**nemia

Thrombocytopenia

"The FAT RN has TTP and her HUS has a RAT"

TTP and HUS both have the following:

1. Normal coagulation tests (normal PT/PTT)
2. Elevated LDH

HUS is similar to TTP, except that it only affects the RENAL system

For patients with chronic low-grade lymphoproliferative disorders for years who develop **new lymphadenopathy**, consider transformation to a **high-grade lymphoma**.

Patients with **ACUTE LEUKEMIAS** usually present with low to normal WBC, whereas patients with **CHRONIC LEUKEMIAS** may present with splenomegaly and high WBC

Eosinophilia causes: mnemonic is **NAACP**

Neoplasia

Addison disease

Allergy/Asthma

Connective tissue disorders

Parasites

More Common Peripheral Smears and Genetic Markers

- **Smudge cells** (mature lymphocytes): chronic lymphocytic leukemia
- **Auer rods**: acute myelogenous leukemia/promyelocytic leukemia
- **Reed-Sternberg cells**: Hodgkin disease
- **Burr cells**: uremia, DIC
- **Spur cells**: liver disease, DIC
- **Reactive lymphocytes**: infectious mononucleosis
- **"Fried egg" appearance of cells** that are TRAP (+): hairy cell leukemia
- **Target cells**: liver disease, iron deficiency, thalassemia
- **Helmet cells**: traumatic hemolysis, DIC
- **Polychromasia and spherocytosis**: implies autoimmune hemolytic anemia
- **Young patients with unexplained pancytopenia**: consider paroxysmal nocturnal hemoglobinuria
- **Philadelphia chromosome** t(9;22)/bcr-abl gene: chronic myelogenous leukemia
- **Bite cells/Heinz bodies**: think glucose-6-phosphate dehydrogenase (G6PD) deficiency

	IRON-DEFICIENCY ANEMIA	VS.	ANEMIA OF CHRONIC DISEASE
IRON	Decreased		Decreased
FERRITIN	Decreased		Increased
TIBC	Increased		Decreased

LEAD POISONING signs: mnemonic is **LEAD**

Lead lines in gingiva

Erythrocyte stippling

Abdominal pain

Drop (foot, wrist)

RHEUMATOLOGY

CHURG-STRAUSS SYNDROME: mnemonic is **RAVE**

Rhinitis

Asthma

Vasculitis

Eosinophilia

BEHÇET SYNDROME: mnemonic is **GOES**

Genital ulcers (recurrent)

Oral ulcers (recurrent aphthous ulcers)

Eye lesions (uveitis)

Skin lesions (erythema nodosum, vasculitis)

DRUGS THAT MAY INDUCE LUPUS (SLE): mnemonic is **Be HIPP DAQ**

Beta blockers

Hydralazine

Isoniazid

Procainamide

Phenothiazine

Dilantin

Aldomet

Quinidine

REITER SYNDROME: mnemonic is **CUBA**

Conjunctivitis ("can't see")

Urethritis ("can't pee")

Balanitis

Arthritis ("can't bend my knees" or "can't climb a tree")

SAUSAGE-SHAPED DIGITS: mnemonic is **RAP** (rap those digits)

Reiter syndrome

Ankylosing spondylitis

Psoriatic arthritis

"Ice pick"–like pitting of the nails: specific for **PSORIASIS**

STILL DISEASE (adult onset)	vs.	**FELTY SYNDROME**
Rheumatoid arthritis		Rheumatoid arthritis
Splenomegaly		Splenomegaly
Leukocytosis		Neutropenia
Rash (salmon colored)		
Fever		

NEUROLOGY

- Cranial nerves involved in Ramsay Hunt syndrome: CN VII and VIII
- Facial palsy + herpes zoster of the face: think Ramsay Hunt syndrome
- CN III palsy + pupil sparing: think diabetes or hypertension
- CN III palsy + dilated pupil: think compression by a tumor or aneurysm
- CN III palsy + CN V palsy: think tumor/aneurysm/ thrombosis in the cavernous sinus

Triad of **NORMAL PRESSURE HYDROCEPHALUS: "wet, wobbly, and weird"**

1. Urinary incontinence ("wet")
2. Ataxic gait ("wobbly")
3. Altered mentation/dementia ("weird")

WERNICKE ENCEPHALOPATHY: mnemonic is **COAt**

Confusion

Ophthalmoplegia

Ataxia

KORSAKOFF PSYCHOSIS: confusion, confabulation, antegrade, and retrograde amnesia

Triad of **NIACIN DEFICIENCY/PELLAGRA**: **D**ementia, **D**ermatitis, **D**iarrhea **(triple D)**

CLASSIC MIGRAINE: mnemonic is **A POUND**

Aura

Pulsatile

One-day duration

Unilateral

Nausea

Interferes with **D**aily activities

Eye examination: all the eye muscles are supplied by CN III (cranial nerve III) except **LR_6 SO_4**

LR_6: lateral rectus/CN VI

SO_4: superior oblique/CN IV

CLAWHAND DEFORMITY: ulnar nerve paralysis

WRISTDROP: radial nerve palsy

CARPAL TUNNEL SYNDROME: median nerve compression

BRAIN TUMORS	
Adults	**Children**
Supratentorial 1. Astrocytoma 2. Meningioma 3. Pituitary	Infratentorial 1. Medulloblastoma 2. Astrocytoma 3. Ependymoma

METASTASIS TO THE BRAIN: mnemonic is **L**ots of **B**ad **S**tuff **K**ills **G**lia (**LBSKG**)

Lung

Breast

Skin

Kidney

GI

GERIATRICS

ACTIVITIES OF DAILY LIVING (ADLs): mnemonic is **DEATH**

Dressing

Eating

Ambulating

Toileting

Hygiene

INSTRUMENTAL ACTIVITIES OF DAILY LIVING (IADLs): mnemonic is **SHAFT**

Shopping

Housekeeping

Accounting

Food preparation

Transportation

COMMON CAUSES OF ACUTE URINARY INCONTINENCE: mnemonic is **DRIP**

Delirium

Restricted mobility

Impaction

Polyuria

COMMON CAUSES OF CHRONIC URINARY INCONTINENCE: mnemonic is **DIAPPERS**

Delirium

Infection

Atrophy (postmenopausal)

Pharmacologic

Psychogenic

Endocrine

Restricted mobility

Stool impaction

Causes for **DELIRIUM** mnemonic is **I WATCH DEATH**):

Infections (UTI, pneumonia, meningitis, etc.)

Withdrawal (alcohol, sedatives)

Acute metabolic causes (acidosis, electrolyte disturbances, liver or kidney failure)

Trauma (heat stroke, burns, postoperative)

CNS pathology (abscess, tumor, hemorrhage, stroke, etc.)

Hypoxia (from hypotension, PE, CHF)

Deficiencies (vitamin B_{12}, niacin, thiamine)

Endocrine abnormalities (hyper- or hypoglycemia, hyper- or hypothyroidism, etc.)

Acute vascular problems (hypertensive encephalopathy)

Toxins/drugs (drugs of abuse, medications, ingestions)

Heavy metals (lead, mercury)

COMMON SYMPTOMS OF DEPRESSION IN THE ELDERLY: mnemonic is **PAGE SICS** or **SIG E CAPS**

Psychomotor retardation/agitation

Appetite loss

Guilt feelings

Lowered **E**nergy level

Sleep problems

Decreased **I**nterest in life

Decreased **C**oncentration

Suicidal ideation

COMMON CAUSES OF VISUAL LOSS IN THE ELDERLY:

1. Macular degeneration
2. Cataracts
3. Glaucoma
4. Diabetes mellitus

OBSTETRICS AND GYNECOLOGY

PREECLAMPSIA: mnemonic is **HEP**

Triad:

1. **H**ypertension (> 140/90 mm Hg)
2. **E**dema
3. **P**roteinuria (> 0.5 g in 24 h)

ECLAMPSIA: preeclampsia (HEP) + seizures

HELLP SYNDROME:

Hemolysis

ELevated liver enzymes

Low **P**latelets

PLACENTA PREVIA: sudden, painless vaginal bleeding in the third trimester

ABRUPTIO PLACENTA: premature separation of the placenta with unremitting abdominal (uterine) and low back pain; visible or concealed bleeding in the third trimester

CONDYLOMA LATA: flat warts that are lesions of secondary syphilis

CONDYLOMA ACUMINATA: genital warts caused by human papillomavirus (HPV)

Purulent-appearing cervical discharge: harbinger of **PURULENT CERVICITIS**

CHANDELIER SIGN or cervical motion tenderness: indicator of **PELVIC INFLAMMATORY DISEASE**

CHADWICK SIGN: bluish-violet appearance of the cervix or vagina

Sign of PREGNANCY that appears after the seventh week of pregnancy

May also be associated with a PELVIC TUMOR

GOODELL SIGN: softening of the **cervix** associated with pregnancy; occurs at about the eighth week of gestation

HEGAR SIGN: softening of the **uterus** at the junction between the cervix and the fundus; occurs in the first trimester of pregnancy

Differential diagnosis of **ADNEXAL TENDERNESS:**

Ectopic pregnancy

Tubo-ovarian abscess

Ovarian cysts

Endometriomas

Appendicitis

PEDIATRICS

TETRALOGY OF FALLOT: mnemonic is **PROVe**

Pulmonic stenosis (PS)

Right ventricular hypertrophy (RVH)

Overriding aorta

Ventricular septal defect (VSD)

CONGENITAL RIGHT-TO-LEFT SHUNTS: mnemonic is **five Ts**

Tetralogy of Fallot

Transportation of great vessels

Tricuspid atresia

Total anomalous pulmonary venous return

Truncus arteriosus

CONGENITAL LEFT-TO-RIGHT SHUNTS: mnemonic is **three Ds**

Ventricular septal **D**efect

Atrial septal **D**efect

Patent **D**uctus arteriosus

The four **CARDINAL SIGNS OF CONGESTIVE HEART FAILURE** in small children

1. Tachycardia
2. Tachypnea with shallow respirations and retractions
3. Cardiomegaly
4. Hepatomegaly

VENTRICULAR SEPTAL DEFECT (VSD): most common congenital heart disease

Forced pharyngeal examination may precipitate acute airway obstruction in kids with **EPIGLOTTITIS** and should not be attempted in those who have stridor

INTUSSUSCEPTION: sausage-shaped mass on abdominal examination and passage of "currant jelly" stools

INTRAUTERINE ACQUIRED INFECTIONS: mnemonic is **TORCHES**

Toxoplasmosis

Rubella

Cytomegalovirus

HErpes, **H**IV

Syphilis

Bibliography

Fauci AF, Braunwald E, Kasper DL, et al. *Harrison's Principals of Internal Medicine*. 17th ed. New York, NY: McGraw-Hill; 2008.

Kliegman RM, Behrman RE, Jenson HB, et al. *Nelson's Book of Pediatrics*. 18th ed. Philadelphia, PA: Saunders; 2007.

LeBlond RF, Brown DD, DeGowin RL. *DeGowin's Diagnostic Examination*. 9th ed. New York, NY: McGraw-Hill; 2009.

McPhee SJ, Papadakis MA. *Current Medical Diagnosis & Treatment 2010*. 49th ed. New York, NY: McGraw-Hill; 2010.

Seidel HM, Ball JW, Dains JE, et al. *Mosby's Guide to Physical Examination*. 6th ed. St. Louis, MO: Mosby; 2006.

Simel DL, Rennie D. *The Rational Clinical Examination: Evidence-Based Clinical Diagnosis*. New York, NY: McGraw-Hill; 2009.

Wolff K, Johnson RA. *Fitzpatrick's Color Atlas & Synopsis of Clinical Dermatology*. 6th ed. New York, NY: McGraw-Hill; 2009.

Index

NOTE: Page numbers followed by *f* and *t* denote figures and tables, respectively.

I